The Toronto
General Hospital,
1819-1965:
A Chronicle

The Toronto General Hospital, 1819-1965:

A Chronicle

W.G. COSBIE, MD

Macmillan of Canada
Toronto

Library of Congress Catalogue Card No. 74-10299
ISBN 0-7705-1184-8

The support of the Medical Staff Association of the Toronto General Hospital, without whose financial assistance this chronicle could not have been published, is gratefully acknowledged. The assistance provided by the Toronto General Hospital during the period of its preparation is also acknowledged with thanks. Permission to reproduce the illustrations has been granted by the Toronto General Hospital.

Printed in Canada for
The Macmillan Company of Canada Limited

Contents

Preface

THE STORY OF THE TORONTO GENERAL HOSPITAL REFLECTS THE growth and development of the community in which it has flourished, the generous service of the good citizens who have supported and guided its destiny and particularly the long line of physicians and surgeons who, in an ever-changing atmosphere, have spent time within its walls.

As a centre for the training of the medical and paramedical professions, the hospital has shared its development with that of the University of Toronto and its medical schools: their stories are inseparable.

Professor Robert Janes was the inspiration of the author. It was his idea that this story should be told, and his research provided a foundation for the studies that made it possible. Tribute must be paid to Mrs. Catharine Windeyer and Mrs. Sheila Swanson and her staff at the William Bond Library of the Toronto Academy of Medicine for their constant help. The author is greatly indebted to Dr. Henry Doyle, for many years Assistant Superintendent Medical, as he has provided information otherwise unobtainable. Dr. Arthur Kelly's advice influenced the material of the narrative, and the candid recollections of many others who have contributed to the fame of this old institution have been received with thanks by the author, though by their own wishes they must remain anonymous.

The measurement of time by the calendar and anniversary dates is artificial; for the epochs of history are the work of original minds. This story ends where it does, for the present, because the judgment of time is necessary to resolve the effects of radical change and controversy.

W.G.C.

The Toronto
General Hospital,
1819-1965:
A Chronicle

I

York and Its Hospitals

IT WAS THE GOOD HARBOUR BEHIND THE LONG, LOW PENINSULA that decided John Graves Simcoe to choose the site at Toronto for the new capital of Upper Canada.

Lord Dorchester, the Governor at Quebec, had already negotiated the "Toronto Purchase" in 1787, acquiring an ill-defined area of 250,000 acres stretching eastwards for fourteen miles from the Etobicoke Creek. The price had been £1,700, some bales of cloth, some axes and various trinkets "dear to the heart of the simple savage." But the Mississauga Indians apparently were satisfied, and Dorchester felt he had secured the fur trading route from the Georgian Bay, which reached Lake Ontario by way of the Holland River, the old Toronto Portage and the Humber. Next year Captain Gother Mann of the Royal Engineers surveyed and made a map of the harbour and a possible town site at "TORENTO."

It was Simcoe, however, who in 1794 came by boat around the head of the lake from the first capital of the province at Newark (Niagara) and began to build the fort to protect the harbour, and who organized the small civilian community which soon began to develop to the west of the swampy mouth of the Don River.

Under the old French régime, apart from those manning military and trading posts, Jesuit missionaries and fur traders had been practically the only white inhabitants of this western country. But now people from all walks of life began to settle in little villages and on the pioneer farmlands cleared from the primeval forest along the St. Lawrence and on the shores of Lake Ontario and Lake Erie. Most of them were

United Empire Loyalists who, following the American Revolutionary War, preferred to live under the British Crown rather than remain in the new republic. Later their numbers were to be augmented by a steady flow of veterans from the Napoleonic War and the North American struggle that coincided with it. From the beginning their settlements were British, and it was as a result of the demands of the Loyalists that the Constitutional Act of 1791 was passed at Westminster to establish a Province of Upper Canada, separate from Lower Canada, where British law and culture would form the basis for the government under which they desired to live.

With the establishment of the new capital at York, the undeveloped hamlet began to grow rapidly. While Simcoe's decisions were governed by military expediency, his successor, the Hon. Peter Russell, directed the further development of the town on a more permanent and civilian basis. During his time land was reserved for a church, a school, a court house, a jail, a hospital and a market, but only the jail was built. However, this did provide, at a later date, accommodation for the mentally ill, for when a better prison was built the old jail became a lunatic asylum.

In 1806 Joseph Cawthra announced the opening of the first apothecary shop which, according to the advertisement, differed little from a modern drug store:

> J. Cawthra wishes to inform the Inhabitants of York and the adjacent Country, that he has opened an Apothecary's Store in the House of A. Cameron, opposite Stoyle's Tavern in York, where the public can be supplied with most articles in that line. He has on hand also, a quantity of Men's, Women's and Children's Shoes, Men's hats; also for a few days will be sold the following articles, Table Knives and Forks, Siscars, Silver Watches, Maps and Prints, Profiles, some Linen, and a few Bed Ticks, Teas, Tobacco, a few casks of fourth Proof Cognac Brandy and a small quantity of Lime Juice, about twenty thousand Whitechapel Needles.
>
> York, June 14, 1806[1]

It was a time when home remedies took care of most minor illness. Few, if any, physicians had accompanied the original settlers, and as a rule only the military surgeons attached to the regiments on garrison duty were available to take care of any seriously ill civilians.

[1]Edith G. Firth, ed., *The Town of York, 1793–1815* (Toronto: Champlain Society, 1962), D32, p. 130.

In low-lying areas throughout the province "fever and ague" were endemic and in York the civilian population, exposed to the "miasma" from the very extensive swamps at the mouth of the Don, suffered to a much greater extent than did the soldiers living in the fort on the high ground to the west. Since screens were unknown and most houses lacked even window glass there was little protection against the snow in wintertime and the hordes of mosquitoes in summer, though no one at this time associated the insects with the ever-prevalent malaria.[2]

Vaccination against smallpox was just beginning to be used, when a doctor was available. But yearly variations in the juvenile population figures are mute evidence of the toll taken by recurring epidemics of infectious fevers.

The first civilian doctor to practise in York was Dr. William Warren Baldwin, a graduate of Edinburgh University, who had come to Canada with his family in 1789, moving to York in 1802. Oddly enough, he apparently did not find enough work to keep him busy in the practice of medicine, and so he undertook to establish a boys' school. This was announced in an advertisement in the *Upper Canada Gazette*:

> Understanding that some of the Gentlemen of this Town have expressed much anxiety for the establishment of a Classical School, Dr. Baldwin begs leave to inform them and the Public, that he intends to open a School, in which he will instruct twelve Boys in Writing, Readings, the Classics and Arithmetic—the Terms are, for each Boy eight Guineas per annum, to be paid quarterly, one Guinea entrance and one cord of Wood to be supplied by each Boy on opening the School.
>
> York, Dec. 17, 1802[3]

A few years later he took up the practice of law, which became his major interest in spite of his continued but rather infrequent medical practice. He was in York when the Americans took the fort and the town in 1813 and he attended many of the wounded soldiers. The story is also told that while he was engaged in arguing a case in court he was called away to attend a childbirth and returned an hour or so later to inform the judge that child and mother were doing very well.[4]

[2]W. R. Riddell, "The Mosquito in Upper Canada," *Transactions, Ontario Historical Society*, II (1960).

[3]Firth, *Town of York, 1793–1815*, G10, p. 196.

[4]William Canniff, *The Medical Profession in Upper Canada, 1783–1850* (Toronto: William Briggs, 1894), p. 232.

He was followed by James Glennon, who announced his arrival in a glowing advertisement:

> Dr. Glennon, (Late from Europe) Respectfully begs leave to inform the public and the inhabitants of York in particular, that he has commenced practice at the house of Mr. Paul Marion. He flatters himself that the opportunity he has had in acquiring knowledge of his profession at one of the first colleges in Europe will enable him to permit the approbation of those who may be pleased to favour him with their commands.
>
> N.B.
> He has on hand an assorted stock of genuine medicines carefully chosen under his immediate inspection.
> July 1807[5]

Competing with Dr. Glennon were three practitioners of less reputable status, namely two tavern keepers and one who had a general store.

The first Act to control the practice of medicine in Canada had been passed in 1788, and a further Act was brought into force for the Province of Upper Canada in 1795. But this was later repealed and it was not until the Medical Board was authorized in 1818 that authoritative control came into force. Prior to this the province was overrun with self-made physicians who had no pretensions to knowledge of any kind. The Rev. John Strachan, who was later to become such a powerful influence in the church and in education, gave in an early letter to the press his opinion of the situation.

> It is indeed preposterous to expect judgment and skill, a nice discrimination of diseases or a proper method sure from men who have never been regularly taught, who cannot pronounce, much less explain the terms of the art they profess and who are unable to read the books written upon the subject. . . . They treat all disease with two specifics, opium and mercury.[6]

Britain was still engaged in a life-and-death struggle with Napoleon when war broke out with the United States in 1812. As there were fewer than 5,000 regular British soldiers in North America, volunteers from Upper Canada played a major part in many battles fought in the Niagara Peninsula, which determined the future existence of their country. York, which was almost isolated by land, was open to attack by water. As a result of a combined operation, a large American force

[5] *Ibid.*, p. 389.
[6] *Ibid.*, p. 27.

was landed, took Fort York and held the town for a number of days in April 1813.

In the early years of the war the only hospital was the Garrison Hospital located north of the fort in the ravine through which ran the Garrison Creek. It was a small building about seventy feet long by twenty feet wide, and when heavier fighting developed in 1814 it was quite inadequate to accommodate the casualties which were sent to York by boat to be farther away from the battle areas. The Rev. John Strachan rose to the occasion, however, and cleared the interior of his Church of St. James: both the sick and the wounded benefited from the greatly improved accommodation which this building provided.

A military surgeon of that time has left us his observations regarding the conditions that existed in York:

> York, the seat of government and capital of the Province is built on a level plain, along the northern bank of an extensive bay, which communicates on its west side with the lake. This bay is long and narrow, and fed by many streams from the contiguous soil, which in summer supply its waste of evaporation. It is navigable to vessels of considerable burden; and its shores in many parts are overgrown with rushes. Those winds which at times agitate the surface of the lake, seldom or never disturb its stagnant waters.
>
> The site which the town occupies appears to have once been a deep meadow, interspersed with pools of water. Some spots of ground which border upon the town are as yet in a state of nature. Even those fields which have been cultivated, are not sufficiently intersected with drains to carry off the collection of water, which, in the rainy season of the year, often inundate the soil. The inhabitants of the town do not exceed 600, a number extremely small when contrasted with the whole population of the Province. The town on its west side is defended by a fort, which was erected on a dry and level spot of ground. Here was established the general hospital, in rear of the army, to which the sick and wounded were conducted as necessity or contingency required. In sickly seasons the inhabitants of York are liable to be attacked by intermittent fever.[7]

The war had a great and unifying influence throughout British North America, and nowhere was this feeling more apparent than in York, where the new patriotism led, indirectly, to the first serious provision for civilian hospital facilities. In those early years the administrative

[7]John Douglas, "Account of the Wounded at York," *Douglas Medical Topography of Upper Canada*, pp. 15–17, 82–85, 104–105. (John Douglas was the Assistant Surgeon to the 8th Regiment of Foot, the King's Liverpool Regiment, with which the Royal Regiment of Canada is allied.)

power and leadership of the Lieutenant-Governor were much greater than they became with the full development of responsible government. But in this instance it was a group of prominent civilians who organized a "Flannel Fund" and, a month later, formed the Loyal and Patriotic Society of Upper Canada. This society had two purposes: to alleviate war-time distress, especially as it might affect the volunteer soldiers or their widows and orphans, and to provide recognition of distinguished service and bravery.

Response to the demands of the society was generous and from many different sources. Naturally, the townspeople of York rose to the occasion, and many pledged an annual subscription of a tenth of their income. Their example was followed by other donors throughout the province, in Quebec and Montreal, and by supporters in London, England, under the patronage of the Duke of Kent, the father of Queen Victoria. Nova Scotia and Jamaica also gave generous support. By October 17, 1817, receipts had brought in a total of £13,000. The contributions from Jamaica included fifty puncheons of rum, much tobacco and many doubloons.

In 1813, the society gave £253 43s. 9d. for the support of the hospital in the town of York, which had become a civilian responsibility when it was left without a surgeon, a commissary or any medical stores, following the capture of the town and evacuation by the commander of the forces and units of the regular army. At the conclusion of hostilities in 1815, the society had £8,000 on hand, but within the next three years most of this had been expended in efforts to relieve the wounded veterans and assist those whom the war had reduced to a state of indigence.

The society was faced with the need to implement its second obligation, namely to "commemorate the glorious exploits by bestowing medals . . . for extraordinary incidence of personal courage and fidelity in the defence of the Province." For this purpose the society arranged to have medals struck in England. The first design was unsuitable, and only after prolonged discussion did a heraldicly appropriate medal finally become available. This medal was 2½ inches in diameter. On the obverse there was a laurel wreath surrounded by the legend "Presented by a grateful country" and enclosing the words "for Merit." The reverse was more symbolic: "A Streight between two lakes, on the North side a Beaver (Emblem of peaceful industry), the ancient armorial bearing of Canada. In the background an English Lion slumbering. On the South side the American Eagle, planing in the air, as if checked from seizing the Beaver by the presence of the Lion." The legend read "Upper Canada Preserved."

When the medals arrived in 1817 at a cost of £750, bitter arguments arose as to who was entitled to receive them. The society found itself with 62 gold medals intended for generals and senior officers and 550 silver medals of two varieties for junior officers and for non-commissioned officers and private soldiers. When no solution to this bitter problem was found, the medals were placed for safe-keeping in the Bank of Upper Canada.

While the controversy continued, an unexpected contribution of £4,000 came to the society from England. This was most opportune, because with the end of the war a steadily increasing flow of immigrants was coming from the British Isles, a large percentage of them poor and often sick and destitute after the long sea voyage. To meet this serious situation a Society for the Relief of Strangers in Distress was formed to take care of the new arrivals, but it was soon in great need of financial help as it faced an ever-increasing demand on its services. The Loyal and Patriotic Society, having in mind the source of its recent contribution, felt that it could not do better than make a liberal donation to help this good cause.

By this time the people of York had become seriously aware of the need for a proper hospital to accommodate those who did not have the resources to look after themselves, and the question of building a hospital appealed strongly to the members of the Loyal and Patriotic Society. Consequently, it decided, with the approval of its London and Montreal committees, to assign £4,000 for building a hospital. At first it was thought that this would be a provincial hospital for the reception of wounded and disabled veterans, but the increasing demands of the civilian population changed all this. The society's contribution was qualified by the condition that the government should provide land grants for the building and that an endowment must be set up to maintain it. As a matter of fact, the government had already set aside land for this purpose and had appointed as trustee the Hon. Chief Justice Powell, the Hon. James Baby and the Hon. and Rev. Dr. John Strachan. The total area held under the trustees was 399 acres, comprising: six acres on the west side of Church Street and north side of Newgate Street (Adelaide Street); six acres, Lots 12 and 13 on the north side of King Street, 11 and 12 on the south side of Newgate Street, and 14, 15, and 16 on the west side of John Street; one acre on the corner of King and York streets; the tract of land known as "Park

Reserve" bounded south and east by the Don River, west by Parliament Street and north by Elm Street, containing about 380 acres; and a lot purchased by the trustees on the Garrison or Military Reserve containing six acres.

While plans were being developed for the hospital, a meeting of the Loyal and Patriotic Society was held in February 1820 where it was "resolved, that it is the opinion of this meeting that as the gold and silver medals cannot now be distributed in any manner to answer the original purpose for which they were designed, it is expedient that the same be sold as bullion and the net proceeds to be put to interest, for the purpose above stated. . . ."

Despite this resolution, the medals remained in the bank, and in the legislature "the delay in the distribution of the medals was taken up as a public grievance."[8] Several further meetings were held that year, and finally in June it was decided that the £4,000 held in trust and the money coming from the sale of the bullion made from the medals should be given for the establishment of the York General Hospital and that it should be called a "provincial hospital."

However, this was not the end of the matter so far as the medals were concerned for it was twenty-three years later, after another parliamentary investigation, that the surviving members of the society empowered Messrs. Allan and Wood "at once and without delay to engage the services of a well known blacksmith and his two apprentices, in order to deface the medals."[9] This sentence was duly carried out upon an anvil in Mr. Wood's garden with a large hammer, the face of which had been roughened for the purpose, the rings and chipped edges flying off among the vegetables. The mangled medals were sold to two watchmakers of the city, "and realized, after deducting expenses which included £1 to P. Bishop and his 2 assistants, £393 12s. 1d."[10] Thus the activities of the Loyal and Patriotic Society came to an end, and its financial responsibilities were closed by the following receipt:

> Bank of Upper Canada,
> Toronto, 11th November, 1840
>
> Received from the Honourable William Allan and Alexander Wood, Esquire, the Sum of Three Hundred and Ninety-Three Pounds,

[8]C. K. Clarke, *A History of the Toronto General Hospital* (Toronto: William Briggs, 1913), p. 22.
[9]*Ibid.*, pp. 24, 30.
[10]Toronto Medical Historical Club, "R. I. Harris, Christopher Widmer and the Toronto General Hospital," February 1965.

Twelve Shillings and One Pence, Currency, for Account of the Trustees of the Provincial Hospital.

THOMAS G. RIDOUT
Cashier[11]

In addition to the grant of lands to the trustees, the Chief Justice, William Dummer Powell, the Hon. James Baby, the Hon. and Rev. Dr. John Strachan and the Lieutenant-Governor Sir Peregrine Maitland organized a plan by which subscribers could support the hospital on an annual basis. It was proposed that a subscription of ten pounds would entitle the person to be enrolled as one of the governors of the hospital, and that a president, two vice-presidents and a secretary would be elected from their number. Each subscriber of five pounds would be entitled to admit a patient to the hospital but would also be obliged to pay one shilling per day for his support. The right to sponsor more patients would be dependent on the size of the subscription. The Lieutenant-Governor and the Chief Justice headed the list of primary donations with gifts of twenty pounds, and the total amount received was £385. Twenty-two subscribers qualified as governors of the new institution.

The Hon. James Baby, George Cruikshank and Dr. Grant Powell were empowered to proceed with the erection of the hospital, Mr. William Allan acting as treasurer. Even as early as this, however, the trustees undertook to sell some portions of the original land grants and at a meeting on June 25, 1821, the disposal of lots in the Park Reserve and on Richmond Street and King Street was reported.

In 1819 a Medical Board was appointed by the authority of the Parliament of Upper Canada. Its primary function was to control the practice of medicine in the province and to examine candidates desirous of having a licence to practise physic, midwifery and surgery. The members of this board were James MacAulay, Christopher Widmer, William Lyons and Grant Powell. The influence of the members of the board obviously extended beyond their judicial services and on November 25, 1819, the *Upper Canada Gazette* reported:

> That the Profession led by the Medical Board was alive to the interest of the public as well as to their own is shown by the following announcement: "Proposals for building by contract a brick hospital in the Town of York will be received at the Post Office by William Allan, Esquire, where a plan, elevation and particular description of the intended building may be seen and any information

[11]Clarke, *A History of the T.G.H.*, p. 24.

respecting it obtained. The proposals would be given within one month from this date."

York,
November 24th, 1819.

The tender submitted by John Ewart was the lowest of those who bid for this work and the contract was awarded to him. He was a builder of good reputation and was responsible for the construction of many structures in York, including the Parliament Buildings, Osgoode Hall, the Court House and two historic churches, St. Andrew's at King and York streets and St. Paul's Roman Catholic Church. His youngest daughter married Sir Oliver Mowat, later Prime Minister and subsequently Lieutenant-Governor of the Province of Ontario.

The hospital was erected on a six-acre lot which is bounded today by King, John, Adelaide and Peter streets. It was a spacious, plain, two-storey structure of red brick, 107 feet long by 50 feet wide, with a flattish hipped roof and conveniently designed interior with recessed galleries on the north and south sides. It stood with its four sides facing north and south and east and west, without regard to the direction of the streets that bounded the area.

The peculiar location of the building was the responsibility of Dr. Grant Powell, at that time a prominent member of the medical profession. The son of Chief Justice William Dummer Powell, he was born in Norwich, England, in 1779 and received his medical education in England prior to his arrival in America in 1804. He first settled in New York State and practised medicine there until 1807 when, because of the possibility of war with the United States, he moved to Montreal. He arrived in York in 1812. With the outbreak of war, General Brock appointed him surgeon in charge of all military arrangements along the Niagara frontier. He was in York on both occasions when the Americans took it, in April and July 1813. At the end of the war he resumed his practice, but he was never enamoured of the practice of medicine. To use his own expression, "the theory was beautiful but the practice was damnable."[12]

Powell welcomed the arrival of Dr. Christopher Widmer, to whom he handed over what practice he had. He was, however, a member of the first Medical Board of Upper Canada, and while he practically retired from practice in 1817, he remained an examiner on the Board until his death in 1838. He was also a very conscientious member of

[12]Canniff, *The Medical Profession in Upper Canada*, p. 560.

the Board of Health when it was established to meet the critical situation that developed in 1832, but his paramount interests were political and led to his appointment as Clerk of the Assembly of Upper Canada and later as judge of the Home District Court. His dual career in medicine and the law closely resembled that of two of his contemporaries, Dr. William Warren Baldwin and Dr. John Rolph.

The building of the hospital proceeded very slowly and by the end of 1824 the only occupant of the building was a female housekeeper. Then on Christmas Eve a fire destroyed the Parliament Buildings that had been erected five years before on the site of the original buildings, which had themselves been destroyed during the invasion in 1813. At a meeting of the trustees of the hospital a letter was received from Major Hillier, Secretary to the Lieutenant-Governor, informing the chairman, "that on the recent accident by fire, which destroyed the public buildings appropriated to the use of the Legislature, His Excellency, the Lieutenant-Governor in consideration of the near approach of the Sessions, has not hesitated to direct the hospital to be prepared for the reception of the two Houses." It is recorded that the Board of Trustees unanimously and cheerfully concurred in this arrangement.

The General Hospital was, therefore, hastily adapted to accommodate the legislature, and it continued to be occupied for this purpose until 1829. The trustees, however, insisted that it should be recognized as very temporary accommodation. At a meeting in November 1825, they addressed a letter to the Lieutenant-Governor, stating that they were now prepared to make the hospital useful for the purpose for which it was erected and that they felt it proper to make this known to His Excellency.

As there was no response, a petition was sent by the trustees early in 1828 to the Lieutenant-Governor and recorded as follows in the *Upper Canada Gazette*:

> The trustees of the Hospital beg leave respectfully to represent to your Excellency, that during the whole period in which the building has been unavoidably occupied by the Legislature, the most urgent occasion has existed for its being applied to the purpose for which it was designed.
>
> It was well known to your Excellency, how great a number of poor immigrants resort hither every summer and how many cases of extreme distress from sickness arise every year, for which no relief exists, but in the charitable exertions of the humane inhabitants of this Town.
>
> As patron of the society for their relief, your Excellency, in com-

mon with most of the Trustees who are members of that society, is well aware of the truth of the representations made by the medical gentlemen, of the misery to which the sick are exposed in this town, for want of a proper place for their reception, and of the great inconvenience and expense which, from that circumstance, attends the benevolent efforts to relieve them.

The Trustees are, from the circumstances, induced to beg that Your Excellency will represent to the Legislature the necessity of making such provision for their future accommodation, as may enable the Trustees speedily to apply the hospital for its proper purpose, and that Your Excellency will express to them the hope of the Trustees, that in consideration of the time for which the building has been hitherto occupied, a sum may be granted to the Trustees to be applied for furtherance of the objects of their charitable institution.

Dated at York (Signed) WILLIAM CAMPBELL
This 20th March, 1828 Chairman of the Board of Trustees.[13]

The reply of the new Lieutenant-Governor, Sir John Colborne, endorsed this request, as reported in the *Loyalist*, York, June 24, 1828. He said that he was fully aware of the great need for immediate hospital services and as a result the hospital finally opened its doors to patients on June 3, 1829. In January 1830, Dr. Christopher Widmer submitted the first report of the York Hospital to the House of Assembly:

> The Hospital was first opened for the reception of patients on the third of last June and a plentiful supply of medicine having been procured, the Dispensary was commenced on the same day—Fifty-two cases have been admitted into Hospital—Thirty-five have been discharged cured—Two incurable—one for irregularity of conduct—Seven have died, Etc.—Seven remain under treatment—Ninety-five persons have received advice and medicine at the Dispensary.
>
> The occurrence of Fever was frequent amongst the indigent poor during the summer months, and it is believed that a great proportion of these cases would have proved fatal but for their early removal into the Hospital, where the benefits of free ventilation and a cooler atmosphere soon manifested their influence upon the disease, indeed it was obvious that the saving of human life in this class of complaints at the period mentioned was considerable.
>
> Many serious cases of surgery have been admitted from various parts of the Province, and several persons afflicted with severe ulcers of the limbs which totally incapacitated them from labour have been cured and restored to their occupations.

[13]Edith G. Firth, ed., *The Town of York, 1815–1834* (Toronto: Champlain Society, 1966), F10, p. 230.

> Of diseases of the Eyes, so common amongst the poor, and so liable to become serious from neglect, there have been several instances that would have probably terminated in blindness had they not been received into the hospital.
>
> It is much to be regretted that so commodious a structure as this Hospital should be so limited in its usefulness by want of funds: the inhabitants of the Province could not fail to regard with satisfaction any extension of the means by which the full advantage of the Institution might become available.
>
> York Hospital, (Signed) C. WIDMER[14]
> 27th January, 1830

At the time that this report was submitted the hospital provided accommodation for approximately fifty patients.

During the inactive years of the hospital its function was becoming more clearly defined. In the first place, the rapidly increasing civilian population was creating a major demand for service, while with the passage of time the obligation to disabled veterans had ceased to be anything more than an occasional occurrence. Moreover, the trustees had apparently settled on a more realistic scope of operation: whereas at their first meeting they were designated as the Trustees of the General Hospital of Upper Canada, the next meeting in January 1825 saw the hospital described as the General Hospital of the Town of York, and so it continued until July 1834.

The early and rather infrequent meetings of the board had largely to do with the financial problems which seem to be inherent in the existence of all hospitals. Originally the building was erected at a cost of £3,051 12s. 8d. and Mr. Allan had purchased 320 shares of the stock of the Bank of Upper Canada with the residue of £800. The shares were held in the names of the Rev. Dr. Strachan and Mr. Allan himself, as trustees of the General Hospital. There were other and smaller financial transactions, but it is clearly evident that the sale of land never produced the amount of money that might have been expected. The financial security that ought to have resulted for the institution was delayed and the records fail to answer many obvious questions.

The next annual report showed that the work at both the hospital and the dispensary increased very markedly in the second year:

> During the past year from the first of January to the thirty-first of December 136 patients have been admitted into the Hospital, of

[14]*Ibid.*, F14, p. 234.

these 124 were discharged as cured, 6 incurable, and 10 have died. Fifty-one cases of fever of various descriptions and 23 of small-pox were the principal acute diseases; the remainder, excluding of a few cases of internal inflammation, consisted of chronic diseases in surgical patients—442 persons have been prescribed for at the Dispensary.

One of the most important benefits derived from this Institution in the course of the past year has been the prevention of Small-Pox—23 cases of this disease were landed upon our wharves, many in a highly aggravated form of it; these being speedily removed to our airy and cool wards had their suffering mitigated and were rescued from impending destruction; out of these 23 cases of Small-Pox only 2 deaths occurred. If no asylum had been open for their reception not only the mortality amongst these poor people would have been great, but from the carelessness of the lower class of the population in neglecting the benefits of vaccination, which is here constantly offered to them gratuitously, the rapid extension of the disease would have been inevitable.

A number of instances of insanity exist amongst the indigent poor in this District; and the mode of securing persons labouring under this infirmity in the District Jail is so objectionable that some other means of providing for their safekeeping and treatment becomes a duty of the community. The internal construction of our Hospital will not admit of their reception into it, but the erection of a suitable lunatic ward would be effected at small expense. The medical treatment, cleanliness and security of these, our fellow beings, and the consequent recovery of many of them, would, by the adoption of such a measure be ensured.

York Hospital, (Signed) C. WIDMER[15]
17th Jan'y, 1831

There was growing concern with regard to the problem of proper accommodation of severely ill mental patients. In January 1830, the Grand Jury for the Home District appealed to the legislature to provide a proper asylum for insane persons rather than continue to confine them to the District Prison where they "were greatly annoying to the Debtors and Criminals confined to the said Prison, to the discomfort of the Gaoler and his family and the Surrounding Inhabitants by their cries and impious language."[16]

In February 1830, a special committee reported to the legislature on an inspection of the Gaol of York, which was made after a petition had been received from the prisoners regarding conditions in that institution. This report stated that

[15]*Colonial Advocate*, February 23, 1831.
[16]Firth, *Town of York, 1815–1834*, F13, p. 233.

in the cells below ground your committee found 3 female lunatics confined, one of them from England, and who is understood to be the mother of a family, who became deranged on her husband leaving her; another from Ireland, a young woman, and the third a native of Canada. It was stated by the Jailor that they have as wholesome and nutritious food as himself and family, and there is a stove in the dungeon, but they are lodged in locked up cribs, on straw, 2 in one crib and the other by herself; one of them contrived to set fire to the Jail some time ago, but it was providentially discovered in time to save the building by cutting down a door that was in flames. A gentleman confined for debt, complained that the smell from the dungeon in which these poor lunatics are confined, which is below his room is almost unsupportable, and their constant howlings and groans were annoying in the extreme. The smell is certainly most disagreeable and confinement in such a noisome place will be likely to aggravate the disorder; who, were they taken to a particular ward in the hospital, and the usual restraints put on their persons, (strait-waistcoats) and gently treated, might either wholly recover their reason, or at least become convalescent. Their confinement is severe beyond that of the most hardened criminal, although their situation entitles them to a double portion of the favourable regard of all in whom the blessing of reason has been bestowed.[17]

The Lieutenant-Governor himself had by this time become greatly concerned with the problem of accommodation for mental patients, and at a meeting of the Board of Trustees on May 4, 1831, he submitted to them the question of a contract that had been entered into by him for the erection of an addition on the west end of the hospital that would cost £215. This was disapproved by the Board of Trustees because in their opinion it would cut off the light to the staircase.

The matter was concluded at a meeting on May 21, 1831, when the board read a communication from the Secretary to the Lieutenant-Governor:

Sir:
I am directed by the Lieutenant Governor to acquaint you that he has ordered the contract of the building entered into for the reception of the insane persons to be cancelled, and that he thinks it is better that the magistrates should make their own arrangements for them.

The indifference of the board to the responsibility for the restraint, accommodation and care of mental patients was not unusual, but quite in keeping with conditions at that time. The early history of the mentally ill in Canada was characterized by the same neglect and

[17]*Ibid.*, p. 281.

cruelty shown to this unfortunate class by all other countries at the same period. Even down to the first half of the nineteenth century, those persons suffering from mental afflictions were allowed to roam at will, or cared for at home by their "friends" under deplorable conditions (in cages, closets, sheds and barns); while those requiring more rigid supervision were placed in jails and dungeons, like ordinary criminals. They were brutally ill-treated, neglected and starved, and no provision whatever was made for their medical care or treatment. It was some time before their condition would improve.

II

Cholera

WHAT WAR COULD NOT ACCOMPLISH PESTILENCE ALMOST DID. For over twenty years, recurring epidemics of cholera and typhus drove the fearful from the town, while literally thousands died during the hot summer months when disease was rampant. Throughout these years of tribulation the little hospital expanded temporarily with each new onslaught and grew more and more to be an integral part of the life of the growing community.

Asiatic cholera was pandemic in India and by 1818 it had spread by way of the trade routes to Indo-China and Japan. In 1821 it reached the Near East, and by the summer of 1831 it arrived in Moscow. Ships sailing from the Baltic brought it to England, the first case occurring in the Yorkshire port of Sunderland in October 1831. From there it spread inexorably to all the towns and cities of the British Isles. Even before this, however, the British government had warned Canadian authorities of the threat of this rapidly spreading disease and the danger of its being carried by the ever-increasing emigration. As a result, an act was passed on February 25, 1832, which empowered the Governor to name a Board of Health, a Health Commissioner and a Resident Physician, and to establish a Quarantine Station at Grosse Ile, twenty miles below Quebec. Here a military post was organized to enforce obedience from passing vessels, and a few wooden sheds were hurriedly erected to serve as a very indifferent quarantine hospital for the sick immigrants.

In spite of the best intentions, however, the health control of emigrants was confined to their examination before sailing, and to the separation on arrival of the obviously sick from the probably healthy.

No thought was given to isolating convalescents, carriers, or contacts, but this is understandable considering contemporary ignorance regarding the nature and cause of the disease. The tremendous flood of immigrants in 1832 was far too great for the primitive quarantine control, for nearly 40,000 persons arrived during the month of June, and from the end of April the reports of the Atlantic crossings of the emigrant-laden ships were most alarming. The *Constantia* from Limerick, Ireland, reported that 20 of her 170 passengers had died at sea; the *Elizabeth* from Dublin had 22 deaths among 200 passengers; and the *Carrick,* from the same port, docking on June 3, reported that 45 of her 145 passengers had been buried at sea.

It should be realized that these people had endured a voyage of anywhere from 36 to 80 days in cramped discomfort and lacking all sanitary arrangements. To reach their destination in York, they were still faced with a further journey by ship to Montreal, by stage coach over rough corduroy roads, and then another voyage from the upper St. Lawrence along the north shore of Lake Ontario. As a result their condition on arrival, often penniless, always weary and discouraged, and not infrequently ill, presented a challenge both to the health officials and to the benevolence of those whose fellow citizens they were to become.

When all the warning signals were flying, the Lieutenant-Governor of Upper Canada, Sir John Colborne, proclaimed May 16 as a day of "public fasting, humiliation and prayer . . . for beseeching God to turn from our people that great calamity with which parts of our Dominion are at this time afflicted. . . ."[1]

A few weeks passed, and then the steamship *Great Britain* dropped anchor in the harbour on the evening of June 21, 1832, bringing with her the beginning of the cholera epidemic that would almost decimate the little community of York. Dr. John King, the Health Officer of York, visited the ship and a "medical gentleman on board," he reported, "informed me that a passenger named Mrs. Lucas had been attacked with cholera and had been landed at Kingston; another woman passenger had been landed at Cobourg in a dying state and two children had died on board from diarrhoea, but could not be proven cholera."[2] Dr. King found two cases of cholera and ordered them to hospital, and

[1]M. E. Patterson, "The Cholera Epidemic of 1832 in York, Upper Canada," *Bulletin of the Medical Library Association*, XLVI (April 1958): 170.
[2]*Ibid.*, pp. 170–173.

so the fears of the townspeople, which had been mounting steadily, were realized.

Asiatic cholera in its most malignant form ran an appallingly short course. Victims first suffered nausea and diarrhoea, then passed rapidly into a state of shock and circulatory collapse. Hospital records showed, and the public soon came to realize, that death often occurred within hours of the onset of the disease. It was not unnatural, therefore, when skilled physicians were unable to alter the course of the disease, that many turned to quack remedies and home-made nostrums. One of these, with a typically Canadian basis, was credited with good effect on thirty cases occurring in Montreal:

> 2 Tablespoonsfull of Ground Maple Char Coal
> 2 of Hogs Lard and
> 2 of Maple Sugar.
> To be mixed and given at 3 doses every half hour.[3]

At this time there was no organized health control in York or in Upper Canada. The Quarter Sessions of the Peace, composed of magistrates, included in their responsibilities the alleviation of disaster, besides the administration and the building of roads and bridges. In response to the new crisis, the magistrates now adopted regulations to combat the unsanitary conditions in the town by appointing inspectors, and also drafted regulations governing the inspection of all ships prior to entering the harbour.

Some idea of the conditions in York can be gathered from an article in the *Canadian Freeman*, April 5, 1832:

> It is really astounding how the magistrates can allow the horrible nuisance which now appears on the face of this Bay. All the filth of the town—dead horses, dogs, cats, manure, etc., heaped up together on the ice, to drop down, in a few days, into the water which is used by almost all the inhabitants on the Bay Shore. If they had no regard for the health of their fellow beings, are they not afraid to poison the fish that supply their own tables? We hope that His Excellency will take cognizance of the state of the Bay from the Garrison down and see the carrion-broth to which the worshipful magistrates are about to treat the inhabitants when the ice dissolves. There is not a drop of good well-water about the Market-square and the people are obliged to use the Bay water, however rotten.—Instead, therefore, of corrupting the present bad supply, we think the authorities ought rather

[3]Firth, *Town of York, 1815–1834*, F23, p. 242. (Extracts from the diary of James Leslie.)

adopt measures to supply the town from the pure fountain that springs from the Spadina and the Davenport Hill, which could be done at a trifling expense. There is nothing more conducive to health than good water—nothing more destructive than bad—and what ought the authorities to watch over and protect before the health of the community?[4]

On May 17 this same paper described the sanitary conditions of the town:

We understand that the Medical Board has appointed a Health Officer (Dr. John King) for this Port. We do not know the exact duties of this officer, or whether his services will be confined altogether to the Port—but we think that the Town is more in need of a Health Officer than the Port, as much sickness prevails at present and the approach of the warm weather is likely to increase the evil.—Therefore, the cleanliness of the Town, or rather its filthiness, ought to engage the first attention of this Officer. Stagnant pools of water, green as a leek, and emitting deadly exhalations, are to be met with in every corner of the Town—yards and cellars send forth a stench already from rotten vegetables sufficient almost of itself to produce a plague —and the state of the Bay from which a large portion of the inhabitants are supplied with water is horrible.[5]

Filthy privies, open drains and the haphazard collection of offal and night waste completed a situation almost beyond hope of control.

A Board of Health was established on June 21. It consisted of seven laymen and the fourteen medical practitioners of the town. Dr. William Warren Baldwin was appointed chairman. The board commenced its duties without delay, but almost from the beginning it was handicapped by insufficient financial support and a lack of recognized authority.

Help was soon forthcoming from the Medical Board of the York Hospital, who had met on June 18 to consider the need for hospital accommodation for cholera patients. They offered to convert the hospital for this purpose, and proposed the erection of a temporary building on the hospital grounds for ordinary patients. As the President of the Board, Christopher Widmer, stated:

The many advantages of the above arrangement are so obvious that they cannot escape the most superficial consideration of the subject, amongst them are the nature of the building, built with brick, its lofty and commodious rooms, its easy and quick access for cholera patients to whom a rapid removal to a hospital is of first importance, and the

[4]*Ibid.*, F18, p. 236.
[5]*Ibid.*, F21, p. 238.

great inconvenience for Medical men to neglect their various professional duties to attend at a remote spot.[6]

The Board of Health took advantage of this offer, and stationed a proper carriage close to the Court House to transport the sick immigrants to the hospital as quickly as possible. Regulations were drawn up requiring medical practitioners to make daily reports of cases, and the Health Wardens, whose primary duty was to inspect and report on the sanitary conditions in various parts of the town, were to report any sickness to the nearest physician and advise householders of the necessity of calling a regular medical practitioner when sickness occurred.

In 1832 the population of York was only 5,550, and slightly over 40,000 people were living in the surrounding countryside. The arrival of 11,000 immigrants that summer completely over-taxed all available accommodation. In order to meet the immediate situation, immigrant sheds were built on the shore near the Commissariat and Reeves' Wharf and within a few weeks it was necessary to build an immigrant hospital and cholera sheds on the grounds of the York Hospital.

The value of isolation was evident, for cholera did not affect the garrison in the early months of the epidemic nor were there any cases among the masters and boys of Upper Canada College, who lived so close to the hospital that they were constantly exposed to the sight of the coming and going of the victims of the disease. John Ross Robertson has left an account of this in Dr. George Dixon's history of that famous school:

> Directly west of the College on Russell Square was the large and squarish building of the General Hospital. . . . Back of the hospital proper was a long row of wooden buildings known as the "cholera sheds" and these were the dread of the boys, especially the resident pupils. The first cholera epidemic came in 1832 and then every boy in the College had his tiny bag of camphor hung around his neck, an amulet, so the youngsters claimed, that was proof against that dreamless sleep into which so many sank to rest in that dread year. . . . The boys could see the Hospital grounds from the windows in the rear and they gazed with sympathetic eyes on the covered wagons that hourly gathered up the dead for burial and brought the sick to the meagre comforts of the Hospital sheds. Fortunately the boys escaped infection; indeed a bag of gold could not have tempted them to go near the dismal sheds where the sick and the dying held grim communion, while the dead lay on their "lone couch of everlasting rest."[7]

[6]*Ibid.*, F22, p. 240.

[7]George Dixon and G. Mercer Adam, eds., *History of Upper Canada College* (Toronto: Rowswell and Hutchison, 1893), p. 83.

As the epidemic continued, people developed an increasing fear of being sent into hospital, many feeling that this was a fate worse than death, and tales of misdemeanours by the hospital staff circulated about the town. To put an end to one such rumour, the Grand Jury undertook to investigate the story that a woman had been placed in a coffin while still alive and had been rescued by her husband from the death house. After a full investigation the jury reported that the "report in question is utterly without foundation. . . . The Medical Gentlemen and servants of the hospital have discharged their very labourious and dangerous duties in a manner alike creditable to themselves and satisfactory to all who have witnessed their labour."

Public prejudice continued, however, and the Board of Health appointed a committee of George Ridout, James Smith and George Munroe "to wait on the medical gentlemen and ascertain their opinion relative to the providing of one or more Receiving Houses for that part of the cholera sick in York who cannot be prevailed upon to go to the Hospital." To this Dr. John Rolph wrote a reply:

York:
August 3rd, 1832.

> . . . The most cruel injustice is done to the Institution and to the physicians at the head of it from the hopeless state of the disease in which its victims are carried there for relief. . . . But without considering the correctness—if the treatment of patients should be conducted as hitherto had been done there will be formed a lasting source for the propagation of this disease to an extent that cannot fail to prove as disastrous a scourge to the higher circles as it has already proven to the humbler ones. It would be expedient to establish a receiving hospital. . . .

After some controversy the Board of Health asked the Lieutenant-Governor for the old District Grammar School so that it might be converted into a receiving hospital. This building, known as the Old Blue School, had become vacant when Upper Canada College moved to its new buildings, but the site at the corner of March (Lombard) and New (Jarvis) streets, although convenient, was considered "insalubrious" as it was adjacent to Stuart's Half Acre, a low-lying piece of land where even in the healthiest season "the effluvia is sufficient to produce pestilence and where from the tainted atmosphere of which neighbourhood the prevailing disease has appeared in its worst form."[8]

The Lieutenant-Governor informed the board in a letter of August

[8]Patterson, "The Cholera Epidemic of 1832," pp. 170–180.

10 that Dr. W. Turner, the resident physician of the permanent hospital, had reported that of 88 patients admitted to the hospital, 40 were in the blue stage (terminal stage), and many of them had been attended by private physicians. Thirty-five patients had recovered and been discharged from hospital, while 52 deaths had occurred and, of 109 persons who had been buried in the Western Burying Ground, 57 had died out of hospital.[9] He also felt that the board should prompt the inhabitants of York to maintain "habitual cleanliness in York, where almost every yard is favourable to the continuance of the prevailing disease from the putrefactive process going on in the want of drains. The immigrant shed should also be attended to as the positive filth which has been allowed to accumulate near it should be removed daily."

One can only imagine the task that confronted Dr. Turner, Mr. Sullivan (an apprentice of Dr. King who was the hospital apothecary), the matron, a few practical nurses and an "active servant" in their efforts to care for the desperately ill patients admitted to the hospital. On August 11 Dr. Turner complained that "he must not be troubled at all hours of the day and night by demands on the part of the carter for assistance in removing the dead bodies from the cart or to provide coffins for those who died on their way to the hospital."[10]

The epidemic continued through the hot weeks of summer and the board faced its continuing problems with an increasing sense of frustration. Finally, on August 8, a letter was sent to the Lieutenant-Governor to make him aware of

> its total inefficiency in carrying into effect any salutary regulations for the public good, not from any want of unanimity amongst its numbers—nor of concord on the part of the Magistracy of the District—but from the absence of any legal means to which it might resort, to compel the observance of its ordinances and regulations. The sum placed by Your Excellency at the Disposal of the Magistrates, the Board is given to understand is nearly exhausted and no further aid can be furnished by Your Excellency. Thus without power and without funds the Board is reluctantly compelled to address Your Excellency, praying Your Excellency (in the emergency in which this District and other parts of the Province are placed) will at as early a period as the law will allow summon the Legislature for the especial purpose of providing for the appointment of an efficient Board with sufficient funds, to act summarily and with promptness and decision during the continuance of the dreadful malady which is now raging in this Province.

[9]R. I. Harris, "Cholera—1832" (unpublished MS).
[10]Patterson, "The Cholera Epidemic of 1832," p. 181.

His Excellency's answer did not provide the help which was sought and the Board passed its final resolution on August 11.

> Resolved that the Board of Health being at length fully convinced from their want of legal enactment as well as from the want of funds . . . of their total inability to be of any further service to their fellow Townsmen have this day dissolved themselves as a public body.[11]

Another board was appointed in a few days, but without the strong guiding hand of Dr. William Baldwin. It served throughout the declining period of the epidemic, which ended in the latter part of September. This board finally reported that to its knowledge there had been 535 cases of cholera, with 205 deaths. It is difficult, however, to say how many people died in York from cholera in 1832. Bishop Strachan described his personal experience: "Often I have been in the malignant ward with 6 or 8 expiring around me, the foulness of the air, too, was at times overpowering. The cholera epidemic is probably the most melancholy chapter in our history." He estimated that one in every four adults was attacked and that one-twelfth of the whole population had died within the space of three months. In later years, during subsequent epidemics, the health authorities in Toronto admitted their inability to determine the number of deaths occurring and as a last resort acquired their statistics from the persons in charge of burial grounds. A re-examination of the records of the burial grounds at that time indicates that even this source was not dependable, as death certificates usually indicated major symptoms rather than a diagnosis of the cause of death.

In the practice of medicine there is no substitute for experience, and in 1832 there was no rationale for treatment. Vigorous purgation or heavy sedation were two accepted extremes. It is interesting, however, that some physicians, while not appreciating the full significance of the situation, undertook to combat dehydration and severe electrolyte imbalance by intravenous therapy and sedation; and in one of the later epidemics Bovell and Hodder claimed with some satisfaction the first use of intravenous fresh cow's milk, reporting the recovery of two extremely ill patients after this procedure.

The importance of isolation and the great need for improved sanitation were reflected in later experience of subsequent epidemics. An act passed by the legislature in February 1833 authorized the establishment of local boards of health and resulted in the mayor and his chosen

[11]Harris, "Cholera—1832."

colleagues on the city council assuming this responsibility in the newly incorporated City of Toronto in 1834.

On June 9, 1834, an Act to Establish a Board of Health ordered that the board

> during the existence of any epidemical disease, or upon a probable approach shall have power at the public expense to open lazarettos or such other place or places as they shall deem proper for the accommodation of the sick and to make such rules and regulations for their admission, reception and treatment as they may think proper, hereby authorizing such Board to employ such and so many Physicians and Nurses and to procure such nourishment, food and necessaries for the use of the sick so admitted as well as for the use of the sick of the City as they may deem just.

Other sections of this act gave the board "power to remove or order the removal of all persons and things within the said City infected by, or tainted with pestilential matter to such place or places as may in their opinion best conduce to the preservation of the health of the City." And after describing practical sanitary regulations, the act ordered that "no Tub shall be removed from any privy or necessary house within the City, except between the hours of eleven at night, and three in the morning, from the first day of May to the first day of October."[12] It also empowered some suitable person "to enter in the daytime and examine in any building of any kind, a cellar, lot of ground, alley, vault or privy which they may have reason to believe are foul, damp, sunken or ill-constructed, directing the cleaning, altering and amending of the same and the removal of all nuisances in and about the said premises." Finally, it directed that "no person shall inter any corpse in any cemetery unless in vaults or graves at least six feet deep and without removing, disturbing or disposing any other dead body or coffin."

Ten days later another act dealt with the cleaning and repairing of streets and the construction of common sewers. It forbade anyone to drain a sewer or privy into the common sewer without special permission. It also defined the duty of the street survey to "cause a cart to pass once in every day except Sunday through all the streets in the city and the drivers of such cart shall give notice of their approach by ringing a hand bell and shall receive all vegetables and ashes, offalls or garbage which shall be delivered at such carts." Both these acts were signed by the strong-minded little mayor, William Lyon Mackenzie, whose administration embarked on an ambitious program of public

[12]*An Act to Establish a Board of Health*, Toronto, June 9, 1834.

works and health measures following the incorporation of the city.

In 1834 cholera did not reach epidemic proportions until late in July. Even early in August the *Patriot* wrote optimistically:

> The general health of our City is good, perhaps never better with the exception of a few cases of cholera which terminate fatally, perhaps more from previous neglect than from anything else. It is greatly on the decrease, and from the time that it has now been with us we may expect it to quit altogether; its sojourn in a place is generally understood to be about 40 days; it has now been with us upwards of 30 days. It has not interrupted business for a single hour, nor called forth the slightest manifestation of panic, while the triumph of good sense has saved many lives. We verily think that in 1832 the Press killed more on this continent than the cholera.[13]

The situation, however, worsened rapidly and on August 14 the *Toronto Freeman* reported:

> The health of the City, we lament to say has never been so bad as it has been for the last fortnight. The cholera continued its ravages with unexampled mortality and most of those who escaped its vengeance have been borne down by stress of weather, accompanied by some sickness or another. We never experienced such weather as last week, so sultry, so oppressive, so suffiocating, that had it continued or increased we think it would have threatened destruction to the whole human family. The atmosphere heavy and lowering, the sky mostly obscured by motionless clouds, the lightning's flash was weak but the thunder rolled alternately with gentle growl and terrible peal, the rain fell mostly in light showers, but sometimes in torrents, yet all this never produced a breeze and only served to increase suffocation. Add to this the awful spectacle of cholera victims, some on carts, in white deal coffins, attended by only two or three poor friends, others in hearses, followed by a large train of respectable mourners and the scene was gloomy in the extreme.[14]

The *Christian Guardian* also echoed the reaction of the public to the growing crisis:

> We believe that no public evil has fallen upon us which will bear any comparison with the cholera, either in its destruction of human life or its effect upon the commercial and general interest of the Province. We doubt whether as many human lives were sacrificed during the late war with the United States as have fallen victims to this destructive pestilence.
>
> As the present visitation is more destructive to human life than the former [referring to the epidemic of 1832] the loss of life, depression

[13]Clarke, *A History of the T.G.H.*, pp. 44–45.
[14]*Ibid.*, p. 45.

> of business, value of property, agriculture and the settlement of the country, who can estimate the consequences of this direful disease to this Province? . . . The total number of cases of deaths in this City since the commencement of the cholera mounts to, we believe, upwards of 400. Many actively engaged in business and in health one day have been buried the next and the hand that now writes may, before the sun sets, be cold in death. The lesson it is constantly teaching is "be thou always ready."[15]

In Upper Canada nearly every town and village was affected. Several thousand people left Toronto in dread of the disease, and the severity of the epidemic was evident in the death of 342 patients in a period of nineteen days. A special cholera hospital was opened in the east wing of the new Parliament Buildings, but this, as well as the accommodation in the Toronto General Hospital and the cholera sheds, was greatly overtaxed.

The public was by now becoming aware of the efforts that were being made to take care of the sick. The *Patriot* reported:

> We have had occasion to visit the cholera hospital, which is under the able management of Dr. Charles Sheward, who most obligingly showed us through all the wards and explained to us the nature of every case. We were particularly struck with the cleanliness and order of the place and felt, on behalf of this City, much gratitude to His Excellency for his humane thoughtfulness and care in assigning the east wing of the public building for this charitable use. The situation is as healthy as any that could have been chosen, the rooms are spacious and airy and the internal arrangements are highly creditable to Dr. Sheward whose assiduity and skill render him an acquisition of incalculable importance at so distressing a time. The eleven who have died within an hour after arrival at the hospital speaks volumes as to the state in which the patients are introduced to the institution and at once accounts for the number of deaths which have occurred in the hospital. Will it be believed that no one of the Board of Health visits the hospital except Dr. Morrison, who goes there daily, but our braggadocio mayor and his squad of aldermen and common councilmen shun the place as they would a pest house. We have been charmed by the account given to us by the worthy Dr. Sheward of the Christian-like conduct of the Venerable Archdeacon Strachan whose attendance at the hospital is regular and constant.[16]

Two physicians, Dr. James Cathcart and Dr. Muttlebury, died of cholera in 1832, and the young resident physician at the Toronto General Hospital, Dr. Isaac Stephenson, died during the 1834 epidemic.

[15]*Christian Guardian*, August 20, 1834.
[16]*Patriot*, August 19, 1834.

The latter was held in high regard. A year before, he had been appointed secretary of Upper Canada's first medical society—the Medico Chirurgical Society of Upper Canada—and he had prepared a paper on cholera shortly before his death.[17]

The epidemic of 1834 came to an end early in September, but by this time it was estimated that of the 10,000 inhabitants of Toronto one-quarter had suffered from the disease. Once again with sickness came poverty and the citizens responded generously at a meeting organized by the Rev. Dr. Strachan in providing relief for the widows, orphans and others left almost destitute in their midst.

Thirteen years later Toronto faced the worst immigrant-generated epidemic to occur in its history. By 1847 the population of the city had increased to 21,000, but the facilities for handling the impending deluge were terribly inadequate and the accommodation in the General Hospital had suffered greatly from the wear and tear of time. Following the failure of the potato crop in Ireland a tremendous number of starving immigrants arrived in Canada, bringing with them a typhus epidemic of terrifying severity. Of nearly 90,000 persons embarking in British ports, six-sevenths of them from Ireland, over 5,000 died on the voyage and another 8,000 on arrival in the Quarantine and Emigrant hospitals at Grosse Isle, Quebec and Montreal. And before the epidemic was over, nearly 2,000 deaths were reported by the boards of health in Kingston and Toronto.

The appalling condition of the new arrivals has been described by a Dr. Douglas who was in charge of the quarantine station at Grosse Isle:

> All the Cork and Liverpool passengers were half dead from starvation and want before embarking and the least bowel complaint . . . finished them without a struggle. I never saw people so indifferent to life. They would continue in the same berth with a dead person until the seamen or captain dragged out the corpse with boat hooks. . . . The fever sheds were miserable affairs; most of the patients were attacked with dysentery and the smell was dreadful: It was impossible to separate the sick from the well or to disinfect or clean the bedding. The very straw upon which they had lain was often allowed to become a bed for their successors.[18]

[17]This society remained in existence until 1862, and maintained the largest medical library in the province, which it had inherited from the College of Physicians and Surgeons of Upper Canada when the college lost its charter in 1841.

[18]John J. Heagerty, *Four Centuries of Medical History in Canada* (Toronto: Macmillan, 1928), p. 121.

From this human maelstrom more than 38,000 utterly destitute immigrants arrived in Upper Canada, the great majority coming to Toronto. Once again the resources of the community were completely overtaxed. Records show that 3,876 patients were admitted to the hospitals and before the epidemic subsided 863 deaths had occurred in Toronto.

As a result of an addition that had been built at the rear of the General Hospital, the bed capacity had been increased to about a hundred beds, but the medical officers objected to the admission of sick immigrants into the General Hospital in the fear that they might spread contagious diseases. They urged the Board of Health of the city to provide a fever hospital for their reception beyond the limits of the city. As an alternative, the trustees of the hospital reported that they were considering renting apartments on King Street in the Temple Chambers with a view to occupying this area as a general hospital so that the present General Hospital might be surrendered to the Board of Health as an immigrant fever hospital. As a matter of fact the trustees proceeded to rent the new accommodation while the Board of Health erected five immigrant fever hospital sheds on the grounds of the hospital, for which the Toronto General Hospital provided bedsteads and bedding and equipment.

Sanitary regulations were also drawn up directing that all immigrants should be landed at Reeves' Wharf at the foot of Simcoe Street and that those who were arriving but not staying on in the town were to leave immediately. All tavern keepers with whom immigrants stayed were to report new arrivals immediately and the medical officer in charge of the immigrant hospital was required to visit them once daily. The severity of the epidemic is evident in the weekly report of July 5–11, which showed that there had been 149 patients admitted, 23 discharged, 28 dead and 345 remaining in hospital. Dr. George Grasett, the Superintendent of the hospital, reported to the Board of Health that the work entailed was too much for the attending physicians, and the following day Dr. Edward Henwood was appointed as his assistant. The next week the report showed 175 patients admitted to hospital, 41 dead, 44 discharged and 463 remaining in hospital. On July 22 a request was made to the Board of Health that a sufficient number of covered tin slop-pails should be obtained to supply each ward of the old hospital building and each of the hospital sheds, into which all the slops should be emptied for removal. The nurses and servants were strictly forbidden to throw any kind of slops, garbage or other unwholesome matter upon the ground near the hospital sheds; the order also went out to obtain sufficient gauze to make veils "to cover and protect from the flies the faces of the immigrant patients who may be too feeble and helpless to protect themselves from such annoyance and irritation." By August 1 there were 643 patients in hospital. About this time a house was rented from the Hon. Henry Dunn at the corner of Simcoe and Front streets to be used as a convalescent hospital, and the report on July 31 showed that while there were 655 patients in the fever hospital there were now 176 in the convalescent hospital.

The epidemic continued, however, without abating and in the worst week of August the number of patients in the fever hospitals increased from 747 to 798, while 278 patients were still in the convalescent hospital. At the same time, some patients had to be refused admission to the General Hospital because of lack of accommodation and the Board of Health reluctantly rented another building.

Even with the advent of cooler weather, the epidemic continued and early in October the weekly report showed 536 people in the fever hospitals, with 29 deaths and 45 transferred to the convalescent hospital, to make a total of 169 patients in that institution.

The toll of those who through their service succumbed to the fever included the Superintendent of the Emigrant Hospital, Dr. George Robert Grasett, and Dr. Joseph Hamilton. But it was particularly the death of Michael Power, the first Roman Catholic Bishop of Toronto, on October 1 that had a profound effect on everyone in Toronto, for it was said he had laid down his life for the stricken members of his flock; a sacrifice commemorated by a monument near the entrance to his old church, St. Paul's on Queen Street, where in those days so many of his people were buried. The *Globe* reported editorially on October 9:

> We regret to mention the death of Dr. Michael Power, Roman Catholic Bishop of Toronto. He fell a victim to the malignant disease which has been raging amongst the immigrants, having caught the infection while visiting the hospital. Deceased was in the vigour of life, only 44 years of age and from his appearance it might have been expected that many days were yet before him, but, as in the case of the lamented Dr. Grasett, a few days of this destructive pestilence was sufficient to bring this strong man down and number him with the dead.

Even in those days government remuneration for medical services was a cause for considerable difference of opinion, to quote from the *Globe* of November 6:

> The order from Government which obliges surgeons attending the hospitals to attend 200 patients each and restricting their remuneration to $5.00 per day is a disgrace to the country and the Government. It is certainly possible for the doctor to around the ground twice a day where 200 patients are laid down and to feel the pulse of each. If he is within the atmosphere of the hospital 10 hours a day he can thus give a minute and a half to each patient. Such a description of the superveillance may satisfy a government conscience but what family would be satisfied with such attendance on one of their number? How can the various stages of the disease be watched and proper remedies applied suitable to the condition or the age of the patient?
>
> Except in some remarkable cases the practitioner will not be able to recollect the particular cases he has attended and will lose the connecting link to aid him in the treatment and prescriptions. If the 200 were reduced to 50 patients for each doctor there would only be six minutes for each, but the patients might be oftener visited and each case kept in distinct recollection.

The final conclusion was that the remuneration was too small and "will lower the standard of the medical attendance."

It was late in 1847 before the strain on hospital accommodation eased. The Board of Trustees of the Toronto General Hospital were by this time considering plans for the enlargement of the hospital, and negotiations were carried on with the Chief Immigrant Agent regarding the transfer of patients from the immigrant and convalescent hospitals to the General Hospital. The trustees requested that if this occurred the government should pay one shilling ninepence per day for the patients so transferred and a sum of thirty shillings per day for the additional medical attendants who would be required. As a matter of fact, however, it was not until May 1, 1848, that the transfer took place.

The strenuous days of 1847 had made great demands on the staff of the General Hospital and had been accompanied by repeated replacements of stewards and matrons. It was also difficult to keep a full complement of nurses engaged in the hospital, and the trustees ordered that the nurses in the hospital should be paid, until otherwise ordered at the rate of two pounds per month for night nurses and one pound fifteen shillings for day nurses. The secretary was also asked to advertise for day and night nurses, for a man and his wife to fulfil the duties of steward and matron, and for a resident medical officer.

During the epidemic the Toronto General Dispensary, which had been re-established in the latter part of 1845, provided very valuable service. The object of this institution was to afford medical and surgical relief and medicines to the distressed poor, either at the dispensary or, if they were unable to attend, at their own homes:

> This institution will not in any way interfere with the General Hospital, as by far the greater number of cases that are likely to apply to the dispensary will be such as are unfit to be in-patients in a hospital or who cannot, without risk, attend as out-patients. On the contrary, where cases occur in the practice of a dispensary of such a nature as to require long and careful nursing as an essential auxiliary to the medical treatment they will be recommended to apply to the hospital. This institution is desirous of co-operating with its kindred charity the Indigent Sick Society, whereby a greater amount of good will be bestowed at a much smaller cost than can be effected by each remaining distinct and separate.[19]

It can be realized how active the dispensary must have been during the summer of 1847, and the Senior Physician to the Dispensary, Dr. John Edward Rankin, was prompted to protest to the Board of Health that it had made no provision "for the bathing of the newly landed immigrants for both the sick and the well before they leave the docks and that the accumulation of dirt on steerage patients must carry infection as well as on their clothes."

Fortunately 1848 was a year free of any major outbreak of contagious disease. But cholera made its appearance again in 1849. An editorial in the *Mirror* on June 8, 1849, stated that "from east to west and south the tidings of the onward march of the destroyer reach us. It prevails in Chicago and in Boston, in New York and New Orleans and every intermediate town and village lying between these four points. . . ." It was also noted that a vessel named the *Mary* had arrived at Grosse Isle from Limerick with only 9 persons remaining alive out of 111, the rest having died at sea of cholera. Another *Mirror* editorial of July 6 stated:

> Up to the present no extra hospital accommodation has been provided for the poor who may be affected with cholera in the event of the disease reaching us. . . . We believe that the Board of Health have used every possible exertion to meet the threatened emergency but we regret to learn that their efforts have been completely paralyzed by a few selfish and terror-stricken individuals. We would dare say it would hardly be believed that the "cholera shed" erected last week by permission of the Hospital Trustees on the Hospital Reserve west of Brock Street, was in the night after its completion torn to pieces and the broken fragments were scattered along the contiguous streets.

[19]*British Colonist*, August 5, 1845.

The hospital trustees also received protests asking for reduction in rent for the houses that had been built on the west side of the hospital grounds because of the cholera sheds being erected too close to them.

A report appearing in the *Globe* on July 19, 1849, stated that there had been 79 cases to date with 46 deaths. By the middle of August this increased to 414 cases with 254 deaths, and by September 1 to 656 cases with 449 deaths. The various burial grounds in the city reported that in the month of July there were 326 interments, and of 230 interments in the first two weeks in August, 168 were reported as due to cholera. This epidemic apparently was under control by the middle of September, but the striking feature that year was the high death rate. Possibly this was due to more accurate diagnosis, as in previous years it seems very likely that severe dysentery was often mistaken for cholera. From August 9 to 15, when the epidemic apparently was at its height, there had been 425 cases of cholera admitted to hospital with 260 deaths.

Once again in 1854 the citizens were warned by their newspapers of the danger of another epidemic year. The *Leader* on February 10 stated:

> If the truth must be told, and it would be criminal to conceal it, we were never at any previous time so badly prepared as at this moment. The water which is chiefly used for culinary purposes and is swallowed in an alarming extent by the citizens, has been described by the owner and vendor of it as "poison." We took credit unto ourselves for having described in pretty strong terms the abominable filth served out by the water company, but our description was mildness itself compared to that given by Mr. Furness, the proprietor of the Water Works. The sewage of the city is very greatly increasing in amount and is all discharged into the Bay at one point or another and from the Bay the water company draws its supplies; even now when no epidemic prevails the physicians forbid a drop of this vile compound to enter the lips of the families under their care. It is impossible that this water can form a beverage of any considered proportion of the population of the city without immensely aggravating the effects of Asiatic Cholera. But that terrible scourge, in accordance with every present probability, will visit us next summer.

By July the same paper wrote further:

> With no desire to create unnecessary alarm, we cannot disguise from ourselves that the city may soon be the scene of an epidemic against which it is the duty of the Corporation to take all possible preventive measures. Some cases of sickness having an epidemic form have, within the last few days terminated fatally. . . . The city has not been

> half cleansed; it is in a worse state than Kingston or Montreal or Quebec. On the back lanes of some of the central portions of King Street, filth lies several feet thick. The time when this could have been without any fear of danger is past. . . . The pigs have it all their own way, both in the streets and in the yards. All the prohibitions and restrictions of the Corporation being a dead letter. The drains in the city in some places emit offensive gases through the gratings. . . . Perhaps the greatest source of pestilence in a city like this is the practice of crowding together great numbers of cows in inadequate space, where they are fed on swill, and allowing large accumulations of filth to lie reeking in the sun infecting the whole neighbourhood. Where are the city Inspectors, that they do not see to the worst and most notorious of these? Then our back streets, in what condition are they? A great deal of filth has been removed in several places but the work is by no means complete.

The sanitary arrangements that were presented in the by-laws in 1834 did not seem to have had very much effect on the condition of the city, as the *Leader* points out:

> It may be a question of whether a city of 40,000 inhabitants does not require the official appointment of public scavengers, but, at least in a time like this of dread and danger from these influences something should be done to meet the exigency. . . . We may advert to another point in connection with this—the presence of hogs about the streets is a subject of public disgust and is not without its annoyances in a great commercial city. So is that of the hyena in Abyssinian cities, yet both the one and the other have their uses. While things are as they are we scruple the wisdom of the authorities in forcibly checking as of late the wandering of the porcine tribe, at least at night which, while they pick up a slight addition to their substance by the vegetables thrown into the street, act as the only scavengers in the city.

The epidemic this year, however, did not reach the proportions of the previous epidemics, and on July 22 the Board of Health reported that the number of cholera patients had remained stable at nineteen, with six deaths and two discharges. During this epidemic the accommodation at the Toronto General Hospital seems to have been sufficient to take care of all the patients, and on September 4 the *Daily Leader* announced the cessation of cholera in the city.

In the twenty years of the great epidemics it was only natural when a specific routine was lacking that active treatment was not very effective. The control of some cases of "choleraic diarrhoea" before they progressed to "cholera" may have depended upon faulty diagnosis rather than treatment influencing the course of the disease. Thoughtful physicians, however, came to realize the advantage of the "astringent principle" of chalk and opium over methods of forcing "elimination" with calomel, castor oil, turpentine, enemata and emetics. At the same time the routine of hospital care improved very greatly and must have been a factor in the recovery of many patients. The greatest benefit probably came from the persistent, if often inefficient, efforts of the Board of Health to improve sanitary conditions. However, while serious thought was given to improving the water supply of the city nothing of real consequence was accomplished and Dr. James Bovell, in concluding an account of his treatment of cholera, expressed the hope in January 1855 that as "the proper authorities have this matter under consideration, . . . the detestable liquid quaffed last year and even at this time will not be much longer supplied to us."[20]

[20] *Canadian Journal*, 1855, p. 192.

III

The Tory and the Radical

In the hospital's early days on King Street, two men dominated the medical profession in Toronto. Both were imbued with the high ideals of their calling, to the great benefit of their patients and the inspiration of their students. But here the similarity ended. One, with the disciplined mind of an old regimental surgeon, supported the establishment—seeking change by exerting the kind of leadership of which the establishment would approve. The other, with a restless and questioning mind, attacked entrenchment with the zeal of an impatient iconoclast and sought the changes which he judged necessary in things affecting church and state, as well as the medical profession, by overthrow and bloodless revolution.

Christopher Widmer and John Rolph were contemporaries, but Widmer became a permanent resident in York, later Toronto, whereas Rolph came and went at the dictates of his ambitions and interests. Widmer, through his long association with the Toronto General Hospital, left his imprint as the Father of Surgery in Upper Canada. Rolph, with his interest in the basic sciences, such as they were, pursued an equally active career as the Father of Medical Education, though the hospital actually profited more by the service of his students and disciples than from his personal association with the institution.

Christopher Widmer was born in 1780 in the historic little town of High Wycombe, a few miles northwest of London. His medical education, like that of many others at this time, began with a military association. After training in the Conjoint School of Guy's and St. Thomas's hospitals, he obtained his M.R.C.S. in March 1803. Shortly afterwards he was appointed as a Hospital Mate and in August 1805 he was gazetted as Assistant Surgeon to the 14th Light Dragoons.

The regiment was sent to Portugal in December 1808 and became one of the crack cavalry regiments serving under Wellington in his great Peninsular army. In later life Widmer wore with pride a medal with five clasps in recognition of his service at Talavera, Busaco, Fuentes D'Onoro, Salamanca and Vittoria. When peace came to Europe, Britain was still involved with the war in America, and Widmer was sent out to Upper Canada on military duty. At the end of the War of 1812, he took his discharge from the army and decided to settle in York, where he began his practice in 1815.

From the beginning, he established his position as the leading medical practitioner in the town of York. At this time the government of Upper Canada, alarmed by the appalling hold that irregulars and quacks were developing in the province, established a Medical Board to "hear and examine all persons desirous to apply for a licence to Practise Physick, Surgery and Midwifery." Widmer was appointed to the board and, constant in its service, he became its president in 1823. This board also served as a pension tribunal for the veterans of the War of 1812–1814 and was recognized as the representative body for the profession in the province for the next twenty years.

John Rolph was born in Gravesend, England, in 1792, the son of a surgeon, Thomas Rolph. His family came out to Upper Canada and settled in Norfolk County in 1807, but John Rolph remained in England to complete his education. Both Widmer and he were pupils of Astley Cooper in the Conjoint School of Guy's and St. Thomas's hospitals. But Rolph had a unique career, as he studied both law and medicine concurrently: he was enrolled as a member of the Royal College of Surgeons the same year that he qualified as Master of Law in the Inner Temple.

When he rejoined his family in Canada he chose to live in St. Thomas in what was then known as the Talbot Settlement, situated along the north shore of Lake Erie. Here he practised both law and medicine, and in 1824 he organized the first medical school in Upper Canada, announcing his plans to his patron, Col. Thomas Talbot, with remarkable optimism and a full measure of regional pride:

> Everything that is great and useful should begin in Talbot Settlement under our auspices. It was proposed by Dr. Duncombe more than a year ago to form an institution at the City of St. Thomas for the instruction of candidates in Medicine and Surgery. No school of that

> description has yet been formed in any part of the Province nor is the hospital at York ever likely under its sleepy patrons to become a source of public usefulness. . . . Dr. Duncombe and myself will join our libraries for the institution which I am satisfied will exceed very far any in this or the sister Province. To it we will add other valuable works and periodical publications. To these I will the anatomical preparations which were the work of my labour when a pupil of Sir Astley Cooper. . . . There will be about 12 pupils to begin with.

The school only survived two years, and then Rolph added politics to his two primary interests. In 1828, dissatisfied with an adverse judgment, he threw off his gown and left the court to confine his interests to the practice of medicine. Three years later he moved to the Town of York, and in 1831 resumed the teaching of medical students in his home on Lot Street (later Queen Street).

Rolph was soon appointed to the Medical Board and joined with Widmer in making an appeal to the public for a properly developed educational system as a means of providing students to be trained for the practice of medicine:

> The Medical Board are deeply impressed with the conviction that the success of the medical candidate must especially depend upon the proper direction of his early studies and the systematic pursuit of the various branches of science belonging to his profession.
>
> Under this conviction they wish earnestly to impress on the minds of parents and others how very important it is to the interest of the public and to the future credit and respectability of the practitioner, that all who desire to become candidates for the profession should avail themselves of the increasing advantages afforded by the Province for a liberal education.
>
> The public, it is hoped, will fairly appreciate their anxiety to improve the education and qualifications of those who are hereafter to have the care of the health of the community committed into their hands, while the student who is actuated by honourable and conscientious motives, must feel that the due observance of the regulations and advice urged upon him is necessary to enable him to enter upon the duties of his profession with credit to himself and justice to the public.
>
> They are inclined to hope that medical practitioners in every part of the Province will be disposed to second their endeavours by encouraging the young men who are placed under their care, or who may apply to them for advice, in the study of the languages and general sciences, the high character which the profession has acquired in the world and the arduous duties imposed upon its members, justify the expectation of the Board and of the public that the future qualifications of candidates will be commensurate to the means of education within their reach.

The Board, therefore, must hereafter require that each candidate at the commencement of his examination shall translate into English some portion of a Latin author that they may be satisfied he has acquired a competent knowledge of a language in which the formula of medical authors and extemporaneous prescriptions of practitioners are written and from which are derived so many terms used in all the sciences with which he must be conversant.

That for the attainment of a Science to Practise Medicine the candidate will be required to understand Anatomy, Physiology, the Practise of Physick, Chymistry, Materia Medica and Pharmacy, Medical Botany and Medical Jurisprudence.

The candidate for Surgery will be required to understand Relative and Surgical Anatomy, Physiology, the Principles and Practice of Surgery, Materia Medica and Pharmacy and Jurisprudence.

The candidate for Midwifery will be required to understand the Anatomy of the Pelvis, its contents and their appendages, Physiology as far as it is connected with the same, a knowledge of the diseases of parturient women and of children and the necessary acquaintance with Materia Medica and Pharmacy.

The York Hospital is now in successful operation and affords to students daily opportunities of observing diseases and their treatment and they feel it a duty to point out to students that it is at such institutions they can best acquire, at the bedside of the patient, under experienced practitioners, the practical information most essentially befitting them to render professional services to their fellow-creatures.

(Signed) C. WIDMER,
President[1]

With the meagre non-clinical instruction that was available, the most important part of the medical student's education was received within the wards of the hospital, chiefly under the guidance of Christopher Widmer, John King and John Rolph. The final reward the student received was a licence to practise after passing the examination by the Medical Board. The students working on the wards of the hospital felt that they could profit by recognition of a common bond, and they organized themselves into the York Students' Medical Society at a meeting held in the hospital on December 7, 1832.

The sole object of the society, as stated in a resolution adopted unanimously by those present, was "to impart reciprocally for the purpose of general improvement the knowledge of the various branches of the medical science. . . ."[2] It was this organization, however, that presented to the Lieutenant-Governor its opinion of the teaching the

[1]Canniff, *The Medical Profession in Upper Canada*, p. 61.
[2]*Ibid.*

students received in the hospital, and having in mind the age-old tendency of students to criticize their teachers and to advise their governors, it is worth noting their high regard for Christopher Widmer and the influence he exerted in the hospital:

> The petition of the Members of the Students' Medical Society humbly sheweth; That it is with feelings of unfeigned regret that we are obliged to present your Excellency with this humble petition regarding the General Hospital, and are induced to do so, being fully aware of the great interest your Excellency has always hitherto shewn towards promoting any object, which may contribute towards the support of so valuable and necessary an Institution; being a means not only of restoring the sick and destitute to health and comfort, but the only source by which your petitioners may obtain that knowledge by which they may render themselves useful members of society.
>
> Your Excellency is perfectly aware of the necessity for those studying the Medical Profession, to be constant in their attendance at the bedside of the sick, under the direction and instructions of an experienced and skilful practitioner, under one who will not only take a pleasure in communicating that knowledge which a long intimacy with disease has taught him, but will take an interest in pointing out the treatment to be adopted, and directing the course of study by which the student may attain the honour of being numbered amongst the Members of a profession so useful to suffering mankind.
>
> That no one is better calculated for this office, your petitioners have had ample experience, whilst attending Dr. Widmer in his professional capacity at the Hospital, and we have too good reason to fear that any successor whom the Trustees may appoint would fall far short of the kindness and attention with which he has always regarded us, we humbly hope that your Excellency will be pleased, by your gracious interference, to prevent an occurrence so highly detrimental to the present prospects of your petitioners.
>
> The harmony and good feeling which have hitherto subsisted between the medical gentlemen attending the Hospital, have long been felt by those who have had the honour of being instructed by them, and for ought we can determine, the introduction of strangers amongst them, would induce their resignation also, and deprive the public of the advantage of their tried and valued services.
>
> Not only would it be injured by so unexpected and uncalled for a circumstance, but the poor who have always placed the most implicit confidence in their advice, and who have come from various parts of the Province, for the benefit of being attended by the most eminent men which Upper Canada affords in the Medical Profession, would be thus debarred the privilege which is now afforded them, and would be left to perish by disease and want out of the reach perhaps of any assistance. If Doctor Widmer were no longer able to sustain the

arduous duties which he has to perform for their and our benefit, then we would not be justified in making this humble appeal to your Excellency, to endeavour by your influence to prevent his resignation, but as we are fully aware of his perfect ability to perform those duties for which time and disposition has so well adapted him, we beg your Excellency will take into consideration our humble petition and your petitioners as in duty bound will ever pray.[3]

Society's Room	(Signed)	JOSEPH ORR
York Hospital,	Select Committee	GEO. H. PARK
Jan'y 13th, 1834	appointed by the Society	DANL. STEERS
		F. CAMERON
		H. B. BOSTWICK
		JOHN O'HARE

The Medical Board, consisting as it did of physicians and surgeons closely associated with the hospital, was not popular with the other members of the profession in the town. After a meeting held in the Court House in January 1836, a note of protest was submitted to the Lieutenant-Governor which maintained, however obliquely, that the hospital was failing in its function by operating in an ivory tower:

It is the opinion of this meeting that no institution has been devised better calculated to lighten the afflictions of the poorer portion of society labouring under disease, or suffering from accident, than an hospital constituted on wise and liberal principles and conducted by an adequate number of skillful practitioners.

Resolved—it being a subject of general notoriety that there exists in the minds of the poorer classes in all countries a prejudice against all such institutions that it is the opinion of this meeting that this prejudice, partly natural, arises principally from an ill-grounded apprehension that medical men requite themselves for unpaid services by the extensive field of experimental practice thus open to them, remote from the observation of the public and of the friends and relations of the patient.

Resolved—that it is of the utmost importance to remove this prejudice as far as may be and that it appears to this meeting that nothing is better adapted to this end than the precautions of such institutions at home, viz. appointing particular days in the week for important operations that admit of delay when medical men and their pupils and all persons interested are at liberty to attend—publishing periodically full statements of persons admitted, their ailments, recovery or death, etc.,—and generally by affording to visitors such easy access to the wards as is consistent with the comfort and accommodation of the patients.

Resolved—that it is the opinion of this meeting that over the hospital in this city a veil of obscurity impends which it is highly

[3]Firth, *Town of York, 1815–1834*, D41, p. 176.

> advantageous to have removed. No appointed days invite the attendance of medical men in connection with the institution; no published reports to inform the public of the number of those who have been restored to their friends, cured of their diseases or healed of their infirmities; the passing bier alone affords the melancholy proof that the institution still exists in active operation.
>
> Resolved—that it is contrary to the practice in other countries and manifestly inexpedient that *two* or *three* medical practitioners holding their inquisition in utter darkness should have from year to year the power of pronouncing *without appeal* on the professional merit of *their own* pupils or those of others with whom they may possibly be at variance.
>
> Resolved—that a respectful petition be presented to the Lt. Governor praying him to introduce such changes in the Constitution of the Medical Board of Canada as may seem to His Excellency best calculated to restore to it the confidence of the medical men of this country and of those who are to submit to their decision their future prospects in life.[4]

As a result of this protest a number of physicians were added to the board, the most prominent being W. C. Gwynne, an Irish graduate and at that time one of the most highly regarded practitioners in the town. In addition, the board submitted a detailed report to the Lieutenant-Governor. The introductory letters of Christopher Widmer and John Strachan drew attention to the financial problems endemic in any charitable institution:

> Toronto Hospital,
> January 12, 1837
>
> The medical officers of this institution in transmitting the annual report feel it incumbent upon them to represent the necessity of appropriation of funds for the purpose of hospital bedding, the present stock being worn out and nearly useless. The bedsteads which are of wood are also much in want of repair but the medical officers recommend the substitution of cast iron bedsteads, which are now universally adopted in all hospitals. It is impossibleto keep the present wooden beds free from vermin. The subject is respectfully pressed upon the early attention of the Trustees.
>
> (Signed) CHRISTOPHER WIDMER[5]
>
> Toronto,
> March 19th, 1839
>
> I have the honour to enclose for the information of His Excellency the Lieutenant Governor, the report of the General Hospital for year

[4]Canniff, *The Medical Profession in Upper Canada*, p. 86.

[5]Archives of the Province of Ontario, Legislative Assembly of Upper Canada, 1836–1837.

> ending the 31st of December last. . . . I regret to say that from these documents it appears that notwithstanding the greatest economy, the expenses of supporting the hospital and the great number of patients, has, for the last 3 years, averaged nearly £1300 per annum—a sum more than double its income during that same period. The statement of the Treasurer proves that the funds are almost entirely exhausted; that the capital rising from the sale of lands given for its endowment has been of necessity used in meeting current expenses, and that matters are so nearly at a stand that if assistance be not promptly obtained from some quarter, the doors of the hospital must soon be closed. To prevent such a calamity (for the benefit of the institution may be considered rather provincial than national) I see no recourse but that of applying to the Legislature for relief.
>
> (Signed) JOHN STRACHAN[6]

This report, and those that followed, showed that most admissions to the hospital were for malaria, typhus, pneumonia and gastro-intestinal infections. Ophthalmalia was common and typhus, consumption and pneumonia caused the most deaths. An 1836 misprint referring to eight "obstinate women" became "obstetric women" in 1838. More amputations were performed in the latter year for a variety of reasons and with only an occasional death. Significantly, the out-patients outnumbered those who were admitted to the hospital during these years by over two to one—an active out-patient service, considering the size of Toronto at this time.

The explosive year of 1837 proved too much for the volatile nature of John Rolph. His legal background had made him a reformist and prompted him to criticize the thoroughly inbred government of the Family Compact. Never loath to voice his opinions, whether in the city council or as a member of the legislature for Norfolk County, he joined with William Lyon Mackenzie in fomenting the agitation which culminated in armed rebellion.

The arrest of Dr. T. D. Morrison, another prominent Toronto physician, was witnessed by one of Rolph's devoted students, who hurriedly informed him of his danger. Rolph lost no time. While his young friend rode his horse out to the crossroads of Lot Street (Queen Street) and the Dundas Road, he walked along quietly to meet him. Then, with changes of horses, he hurried through the night to cross the Niagara River and seek sanctuary. Twice on his way he was apprehended and only freed through the good offices of former students who

[6]"Report from the Trustees of the Toronto General Hospital," *Journal of the Legislative Assembly of Upper Canada*, II (1839), 298.

testified that it would be impossible for such a good citizen to have been involved in the action that had taken place. There is no doubt that his escape was timely, as within a few days a reward was offered for his capture.

£500 REWARD
PROCLAMATION

By His Excellency, Sir Francis Bond Head, Baronet, Lieutenant-Governor of Upper Canada, Etc., Etc.

Whereas it appears that Dr. John Rolph of Toronto absconded hastily from his residence on the breaking out of the insurrection.

And whereas, from facts which have come to the knowledge of His Excellency the Lieutenant-Governor . . . it appears that he has been concerned in the traitorous attempt, which has happily been defeated, to subverse the Government of his Province, the above reward of 500 Pounds is hereby offered to anyone who will apprehend the said John Rolph and deliver him up to justice, in the City of Toronto.

December 11, 1837[7]

Rolph lived for five years in Rochester, New York, where he taught as well as practised. Two of his students who were to figure prominently in the medical history of Toronto were H. H. Wright and J. H. Richardson. After the amnesty of 1843, he returned to Toronto and reorganized his school. Later, Dr. Joseph Workman was associated with him in the years when the Rolph School was progressing towards incorporation as the Toronto School of Medicine.

The Medical Board continued an unrelenting campaign to have a medical school established in connection with King's College (later the University of Toronto). In the autumn of 1837 almost continuous correspondence was maintained between the Medical Board and the secretary to the Lieutenant-Governor, who was Chancellor of King's College. His Excellency repeatedly maintained that the demands for a medical faculty had his personal approval, and explained that the council of the university was delaying its establishment until other faculties at the university were firmly established. The best efforts of the board were, therefore, unproductive and in 1839 its duties and responsibilities were taken over by a newly incorporated College of Physicians and Surgeons of Upper Canada, which acted under the same council with Widmer as president.

With the establishment of this college, the status of the Licentiates

[7]Canniff, *The Medical Profession in Upper Canada*, p. 597.

was elevated, as they now became Fellows of the college after examination. It was not long, however, before the licensing jurisdiction of the college was questioned by the Royal College of Surgeons of London, some of whose members had been refused the right to practise medicine and midwifery in Upper Canada without satisfying the provincial board examiners. As a result of this dispute the college lost its incorporation, and early in 1841 the Medical Board was re-established, with Widmer continuing as its president until his death in 1858.

The struggle to establish a medical faculty in King's College finally came to a successful conclusion in 1843 after the board had found it necessary to state that "the medical student of Upper Canada, if he have no opportunities beyond those offered him in the Province, must pursue his studies without a library, without a museum, without a botanic garden, without a hospital, without a dissecting room, in fact without public instruction in any branch of the profession, and it must be remembered that few indeed have the means of seeking academical instruction in the Mother Country."[8]

Although Widmer had been most constant in his efforts to bring about the establishment of the medical school and was at this time the chief surgeon at the Toronto General Hospital, he was not included in the list of appointments to the Faculty of Medicine. In all likelihood this may have been his own desire. John King became Professor of Medicine; William R. Beaumont, who had recently come to Toronto, was appointed Professor of Surgery; George Herrick became Professor of Midwifery, and Dr. Gwynne, Professor of Anatomy and Physiology. It was announced that the requisites for the degree of M.D. should include a degree in Arts, attainment of the age of twenty-one and certification of medical studies of not less than four years, including anatomy with dissection, anatomy and physiology, the principles of the practices of medicine and of surgery, and six-month courses in materia medica, pharmacy, chemistry, midwifery and diseases of women, and medical jurisprudence. During that time, the student was also required to attend the medical and surgical practice of a recognized hospital for eighteen months and medical as well as surgical clinical lectures for six months. In addition to a fee of four pounds for each major subject and two pounds for the minor subjects of materia medica and midwifery, hospital attendance cost fifteen pounds sterling for eighteen months. In 1844 the school was located in a new building, to be known

[8]*Ibid.*, p. 159.

later as Moss Hall, situated on the site to be occupied later by the Biology Building and now by the new Medical Sciences Building.

Christopher Widmer, at this time Chairman of the Board of Trustees of the hospital, made an offer to surrender the whole upper floor to the medical faculty for their exclusive use, on the payment of a hundred pounds sterling plus three shillings per diem for each patient under the care of a member of the faculty. This attempt to link the hospital directly with the Medical School was not accepted, however, as the medical faculty did not feel that it could stand the financial strain that would have been imposed upon it.

Through his work with the Medical Board, Widmer did much to increase the status of the medical profession in the province. But he gained his greatest recognition in the practice of his profession and his service to the hospital. Unfortunately, he did not leave any record of his professional experiences, but all who knew him spoke of his surgical skill and his direct approach to the problems to be faced. Dr. W. B. Geikie, recalling his trim figure and erect soldierly bearing, remembered him as being quick and active in all his movements:

> I fancy I can see him now as he often dressed in summer with his swallow-tailed blue coat with its black velvet collar, a light coloured vest, nankeen trousers and well-fitting low shoes, neatly tied with black silk ribbon. When looking after a patient for the first time, or at whatever might be going on that interested him, he always stood with his two or three fingers in his trousers pocket.

Dr. Arthur Jukes Johnson supplies the following story:

> One day an Indian was brought in to have a cataract removed from his eye. The Indian could speak no English but had an interpreter with him. Dr. Beaumont, one of the most patient and painstaking men, tried for over an hour to get the Indian to keep still while he attempted to cut out the cataract, but it was of no use; every time the knife approached the eye the man would either turn his head or close his eyes or do something which made it impossible for the doctor to operate. And all Beaumont would do was remove his spectacles, take his handkerchief out, wipe the right glass of it—he had only one eye himself although no one would ever suspect it.
>
> Presently we heard Dr. Widmer coming down the corrider dressed as usual in his riding breeches, top boots and riding crop. "What's this you have here, Beaumont?" he asked as soon as he entered the room. Dr. Beaumont explained the situation whereupon Dr. Widmer turned to the interpreter and said "Do you speak English?" "Yes, sir," answered the man. "Well," said Widmer, "You can just tell this man that if he does not keep his head still and his eyes open he'll go to the

> Happy Hunting Ground so d—— blind that he will never be able to find his way about." This was interpreted in the usual stolid Indian manner, word for word, after which the operation went on without the patient moving a muscle.[9]

Dr. F. C. Mewburn knew Widmer when he attended the old King Street hospital in the early 1830s. Half a century later he recalled the impact of the older surgeon's personality on his colleagues and contemporaries:

> He was notorious for two things, his awful swearing and his good surgery. But he was an amazing favourite with the ladies and I also believe with old Dr. Strachan. That only proves that both ladies and parsons rather prefer their doctor to have a certain quantity of the devil in him; and old Widmer had it fully developed. However, he was kind and attentive to the sick poor, never neglecting them; and no doubt this covered a multitude of sins.[10]

An incident that took place in September 1841 shows the surprising stamina of the old army surgeon. Lord Sydenham, the Governor-in-Chief of the reunited two Canadas, had been thrown from his horse and had sustained a compound fracture of his right femur. As his condition was very serious, a messenger was sent post-haste to Toronto from the capital at Kingston to seek Christopher Widmer's aid. Widmer set out immediately, and by means of relays of horses he reached Kingston non-stop in record time. In spite of his best services, the Governor's condition worsened and he died a few days later, but the patient's family appreciated Widmer's outstanding service and presented him with a gold watch in token of their gratitude.[11]

Even in his more advanced years Widmer was held in high regard. It was to him that Bovell turned for approval when he, with Hodder, undertook to treat cholera by intravenous milk, receiving the sage advice not to undertake this drastic treatment unless death appeared imminent.

Long after his retirement from general practice he was every day to be seen passing to and from the hospital on King Street in his well-known cabriolet, guiding with his own hands the reins conducted through the front window of the vehicle. He had now attained a great age but his slender form continued erect; the hat was worn jauntily as in other days and the dress was scrupulously exact; the expression of

[9]Clarke, *A History of the T.G.H.*, p. 62.
[10]Canniff, *The Medical Profession in Upper Canada*, p. 515.
[11]Harris, "Cholera—1832."

the face in repose was somewhat abstract and sad but a quick smile appeared at the recognition of friends. The ordinary engraving of Harvey, the discoverer of the circulation of the blood, recalls to some degree the countenance of Dr. Widmer.[12]

Outstanding among his many honours was Fellowship in the Royal College of Surgeons of England, conferred upon him by election on August 26, 1844. He became Chancellor of the University of Toronto in 1853 and held this high office until his death in 1858. He was the only medical practitioner ever to be Chairman of the Board of Trustees of the Toronto General Hospital, which office he held from 1844 until his death in 1858. And although he was defeated in an aldermanic election by the fiery William Lyon Mackenzie, he was appointed to the Legislative Council of the province in 1843.

His only son, Christopher Rolph Widmer, had died in 1857 at the early age of twenty-three. On a Sunday afternoon in May 1858 Widmer went to the cemetery to stand alone at the graveside. While there he was seized with a convulsion and some passers-by found him lying on the ground. He died that night. Following his funeral on Thursday, May 7, a group of prominent members of the medical profession decided that a full-length portrait of the deceased should be painted and placed temporarily in the Board Room of the Toronto General Hospital. It now hangs in the front hall of the hospital to link the memory of this distinguished surgeon to the institution to which he had contributed so much.

There is no question of the high regard and friendship which Widmer and Rolph had for one another. They were closely associated during the cholera epidemics of 1832 and 1834 and must have met frequently over the years as they went their rounds in the hospital attended by their students. Widmer also had many opportunities after Rolph joined the Medical Board to judge his ability and knowledge of medicine. But something more than this must have prompted Widmer to name his son Christopher Rolph; in a reciprocal action Rolph called his first-born George Widmer and his second son John Widmer Rolph after the first died in infancy. When Rolph was spending his enforced exile in Rochester, following the rebellion of 1837, Widmer wrote to him that "there are no dissections going on now, there or anywhere else. In you we have lost our Hunter!"

After his return to Toronto following the amnesty, Rolph avoided

[12]Canniff, *The Medical Profession in Upper Canada*, p. 660.

politics for the time being and resumed his practice and the teaching of medicine. It was then that he ushered in the era of the proprietary self-supporting schools of medicine, which followed a kaleidoscopic course for the next ten or twelve years until they became absorbed as faculties of medicine in the three universities in Toronto.

In primitive quarters at the rear of his home on Lot Street, shared by his horse and a cow, Rolph and his associates lectured and directed anatomical dissections. In spite of this accommodation the "Rolph School" prospered. One of his students, W. B. Geikie, claimed that "its tickets were received everywhere and its students were exceptionally successful in passing their examinations before the Medical Board." In 1851 this school was incorporated as the Toronto School of Medicine, but Rolph soon succumbed to what was always a tempting desire and became a member of the Hincks-Morin government, leaving the school under the direction of an old student and now his partner, W. T. Aikens.

Rolph also built at this time, at his own expense, a brick house to accommodate the growing number of students, but competition was keen, as the Faculty of Medicine of the University of Toronto had about sixty students and another school had been organized, the Upper Canada School of Medicine, which during its broken career became associated with the Rev. John Strachan's Trinity College. All these schools shared the clinical teaching facilities at the Toronto General Hospital, not always on a friendly basis.

In 1853 the Hincks-Morin government, with encouragement from Rolph, it is said, passed the University Bill to abolish teaching rights for the university faculty. In 1854, viewing with some concern the association between the Upper Canada School and Trinity, which permitted the granting of a degree on graduation, Rolph effected the transformation of the Toronto school into the Medical Department of Victoria University, which was then located in Cobourg. Rolph's interest in politics and his strongly held opinions made it impossible for his associates to continue very long in any organization dominated by him, and so within two years Aikens led a group of rebels out of the Faculty to re-establish the Toronto school once more. An announcement by Victoria College attempted to remove the resulting confusion:

> The Medical Department was lately, also "The Toronto School of Medicine," which was founded by the Hon. Dr. Rolph, in 1843, incorporated in 1851, and constituted the Medical Department of the University of Victoria College in 1854. But this style was dropped in 1856; and the name now appertains to the Richmond Street School.

> This Department, however, is still commonly known as Rolph's School, by which name "The Toronto School of Medicine" was also generally known, so long as Dr. Rolph was connected with it.
>
> The Department continues to enjoy a prosperity, which has been increasing every year; and this practical guarantee of public confidence, is a matter which claims, and receives, a grateful acknowledgement.[13]

John Rolph continued as the Dean of the Faculty at Victoria, in spite of growing opposition, until shortly before his death in 1870. His devotion to his self-appointed mission to teach medicine was the stimulus that allowed him to muster all his energies to maintain his position. But the peregrinations of this stormy petrel finally came to an end when Rolph died at seventy-seven years of age in the town of Mitchell, having been, one might say, active to the end. In tribute to their great teacher, the students of Victoria wore mourning bands for a period of thirty days, and concluded an address to his widow with these words: "Dear Madam, accept our deepest sympathy and heartfelt condolence on your present sad bereavement and we hope that when the cares of this life are over you may meet your dear husband in that brighter land that knows no parting."[14]

[13]Academy of Medicine, Toronto, *Miscellaneous Letters*, etc.
[14]*Canadian Lancet*, III (November 1970).

IV

The Rival Medical Schools

ON JULY 28, 1847, AN ACT OF THE GOVERNMENT OF THE Province of Canada incorporated the Trustees of the Toronto General Hospital. They were to comprise the Mayor, the President of the Board of Trade, three residents of the city appointed by the Governor-in-Council and the two Senior Professors of any medical school established in the city (or, lacking such a school, any medical men resident in the city, nominated by the City Council).

The trustees were empowered to have a Common Seal and to have and to hold all land and premises assigned to any former trustees. They were authorized to make by-laws, to appoint a clerk, secretary or agent, to invest money belonging to the hospital, to sue for the collection of debts and to have the right to sell land; finally, it was enacted "that it shall and may be lawful for any Medical Student in the said City of Toronto to visit the Wards of the said Hospital and attend them upon the payment of such fees, and under such regulations and restrictions, as the said Trustees shall and may by any By-Law from time to time direct and appoint."

By this Act the responsibilities originally invested on April 26, 1819, in the Hon. William Dummer Powell, the Hon. James Baby and the Hon. and Rev. John Strachan and their heirs and successors forever, came to an end. John Strachan, the sole survivor of the trustees, was now freed from all responsibility and could look back on twenty-eight eventful years. For no one could have possibly foreseen the tremendous problems which had been faced in maintaining the hospital and providing for the care of the sick and destitute who repeatedly overcrowded its meagre accommodation. The flood of penniless immigrants, bringing with them recurrent devastating epidemics, and the lack of adequate financial support from either the city or the provincial government had forced the sale of most of the land grants originally planned to support the hospital. Now, however, it was indicated by the new act that both the government and the city were recognizing their responsibility for the maintenance of an institution that had proved its value not only to Toronto but to its neighbouring areas. Of equal importance was the recognition of the hospital as a teaching centre, emphasized by a clear definition of its close relationship with the local medical schools.

The new Board of Trustees, consisting as it did of the Mayor and the President of the Board of Trade ex-officio, included Clarke Gamble, Esq., John King, M.D., and the Rev. H. J. Grasett, M.A., all appointed by the government, as well as the city appointees, the Hon. Christopher Widmer, M.D., and Lucius O'Brien, M.D. To fulfil its first responsibility, the board appointed Dr. Widmer consulting physician and surgeon, and Doctors Telfer, Herrick, Beaumont, Hodder, Bovell, Aikens and Wright to the hospital staff; and so a new generation of physicians and surgeons came to play a more prominent role in the work of the hospital and for the first time young Canadians would take their places with their longer-established British-trained colleagues.

The names of three of these men have become closely related. Sir William Osler, comparing them with Harvey and Sydenham, said that "they, by exemplifying those graces of life and refinements of heart which make up character . . . have left a most enduring mark—Beaumont, Bovell and Hodder . . . and men like unto them have been the leaven which raised our profession above the dead level of business."[1] This was high praise indeed from the greatest of Canadian physicians. It is possible that even the great Osler may have been a little prejudiced, if one bears in mind his own background, and the fact that for some years these three constituted the Trinity College medical hierarchy. Nevertheless, it cannot be denied that their contribution to medical practice in Toronto was outstanding.

William Rawling Beaumont, M.D., F.R.C.S., was born in London, England, in 1803. He received his medical education at St. Bartholomew's Hospital under John Abernethy and later spent ten months working under the distinguished anatomist Amussat in Paris. His progress was marked by becoming an M.R.C.S. in England in 1826, a

[1]Harvey Cushing, *The Life of Sir William Osler*, vol. I (London: Oxford University Press, 1925), p. 459.

Fellow of the Royal Medical and Chirurgical Society in 1836 and an F.R.C.S. of England by election in 1844. He finally received his M.D. from the University of Toronto in 1850.

After practising in London for a few years, during which time he was said to have the high regard of Astley Cooper, Herbert Mayo and Marshall Hall, he came to Toronto in 1841 and became the first Professor of Surgery at the University of Toronto (then King's College) when the medical faculty was established in 1848. He held this post for ten years up to the time of the abolition of the Faculty of Medicine, of which he had become Dean. He continued his clinical teaching, however, at the Toronto General Hospital and served as an examiner on the Medical Board under Widmer, also delivering a course of lectures on ophthalmic surgery to the students of the Toronto School of Medicine. In 1871 he was appointed Professor of Surgery in the Faculty of Medicine of Trinity College and continued in that capacity until his years of activity came to an end with the loss of his sight. In recognition of his great service he was appointed Professor Emeritus.

His good judgment and surgical skill were of a high order, and after Widmer's death in 1858 he became consulting surgeon to the Toronto General Hospital. Evidently he took Widmer's place, as well, in the respect and regard of the medical community of Toronto and of Canada West. He had an ingenious mind, and designed several surgical instruments, including one for passing continuous sutures which, it is claimed, became the principle involved in the original Singer Sewing Machine.[2] He wrote extensively, including papers on the treatment of fractures of the leg and forearm by plaster of Paris (1831), on polypi (1838), on a case of large cartilaginous tumour of the lower jaw (1850), on traumatic carotid aneurism (1854), and on several forms of lithotomy (1857). He died in October 1875, at the age of seventy-two.

The second of Osler's triad was James Bovell, whose example undoubtedly set Osler in the direction he should go. The extraordinary influence of this man prompted the young student, while at McGill, to scribble "James Bovell, M.D." repeatedly on the margin of his lecture notes.

Bovell was born in Barbados in 1817 and he received his medical education at Guy's Hospital, where he worked under Astley Cooper, Bright and Addison, and after two years spent in Edinburgh and Glasgow, having been too young to receive his London degree, he went

[2]*Medical Gazette*, 1836, and *Lancet*, March 1866.

as an M.D. (Glasgow) to work under Stokes and Graves in Dublin. He returned to practise in Antigua, coming to Toronto in 1848. He was instrumental in organizing the Upper Canada School of Medicine, which became the Faculty of Trinity College, of which he was Dean and Professor of the Institute of Medicine. His teaching of physiology and pathology was always flavoured by a theological association. He carried on a very large and active practice, with hospital appointments at the Toronto General Hospital and the Burnside Lying-In Hospital, and his contribution to medical literature was based on a wide knowledge of contemporary reports and scientific investigation. His most important medical paper was published in the *Canadian Journal* in 1855: "On the Transfusion of Milk as Practised in Cholera at the Cholera Sheds, Toronto, July, 1854." In this publication he presented a lucid and convincing argument for the theoretical efficiency of milk transfusion in lieu of blood. After analysing the constituents of milk and comparing it with blood, Bovell described the cases in which he personally administered cow's milk intravenously with the co-operation of Dr. E. M. Hodder. In his words,

> Hodder kindly undertook to introduce the tube and to inject while I superintended the procuration of the milk. An ordinary glazed earthenware bowl was placed in warm water at the temperature of the blood. A cow which was grazing close at hand was brought up to the shed, and the nurse with great care, keeping the teat against the side of the vessel to prevent frothing, drew off the milk.

Two patients, apparently moribund, showed immediate and dramatic improvement and both survived. However, five subsequent patients did not have such a satisfactory result from the treatment.

After the disruption of the Faculty of Medicine in Trinity College in 1856 he continued to teach in the Toronto School of Medicine, but decided to return to Barbados in 1870, where he gave up the practice of medicine and became a clergyman in the Church of England.

Edward Mulberry Hodder had a more varied career than either of his great associates. He was born in England in 1810, and after serving as a midshipman on his father's ship in the Royal Navy he received his medical education under a well-known surgeon, Joseph Amesbury, also acquiring a special interest in obstetrics from the teaching of James Blundell of Guy's Hospital. After he became an M.R.C.S. he continued his studies in Paris and in Edinburgh. He practised in London for a short time and later in the little town of St. Servans, in France, where he had gone to school as a boy. He came to Canada in 1838 and after five years of practice in Queenston he moved to Toronto in 1843. He was one of the founders of the Upper Canada School of Medicine, serving as Professor of Midwifery and Diseases of Women, and from 1870 until his death in 1878 as Dean of the reorganized Faculty of Trinity College.

He was elected a Fellow of the Royal College of Surgeons in 1854 and a Fellow of the Obstetrical Society of London in 1865. He was the only one ever to receive the Master of Surgery degree of King's College (University of Toronto) and in 1853 he received his M.D. from Trinity College. With Beaumont and Bovell he was an editor of the first medical journal published in Upper Canada. He also served as President of the Upper Canada Medical Board and President of the Canadian Medical Association in 1875.

Although his special interest was obstetrics and gynaecology, his surgical skill and practice covered a broad field, from amputation of the thigh to thyroidectomy and removal of a parotid tumour. He was an experienced ovariotomist and was reputed to have conducted 7,000 confinements, including a successful post-mortem caesarean section, which he reported in great detail. He was a senior member of the staff of the Toronto General Hospital and the Burnside Lying-In Hospital for over twenty years.

These three men conformed to an accepted pattern: British-trained, well educated, and with proven skills, they were capable of contributing greatly to any institution with which they were associated. But now a new era was developing and the educational efforts of John Rolph were producing Canadian doctors who were equal to the opportunities now available to them.

Typical of the new order was Henry Hoover Wright, son of a Canadian itinerant Methodist minister, who came to study under John Rolph in 1832. It was Wright who rode Rolph's horse along Queen Street to Dundas Road while Rolph walked unobserved from the city to meet him on that perilous night in 1837 when Rolph was forced to flee from Toronto, and it was Wright who later spent the years of exile with him in Rochester and, when his education was completed, taught in the Rolph School. It was as a representative of the Rolph School that he first became an active member of the staff of the Toronto General Hospital. With increasing experience he came to confine himself to non-surgical practice and in his mature years was the outstanding medical consultant in the city and Professor of Medicine at the University of Toronto.

J. H. Richardson, another second-generation Canadian, began his medical education under Rolph while he was living in Rochester, and he was the first matriculated student to enter the medical faculty of King's College. After graduation he continued his studies at Guy's Hospital, London, obtained his M.R.C.S. and returned to practise in Toronto, where he became the Professor of Anatomy, a post that he held in the University and the Toronto School of Medicine for over forty years. He also served on the staff of the General Hospital and as a surgeon to the jail, earning a reputation not only as a resourceful surgeon but also as a good citizen contributing much to the benefit of the city in which he lived.

William Thomas Aikens, the youngest of these inspired students of Rolph, was destined to be the most distinguished of all. After spending two years in the Toronto School of Medicine from 1847 to 1849, he continued his training, on Rolph's advice, at Jefferson Medical College in Philadelphia, where he obtained his M.D. in 1850. He then returned to Toronto to become Rolph's partner in practice, and when Rolph's interests again became political, he became Dean of the School of Medicine and, with Wright, its representative on the staff of the General Hospital. He became Professor of Surgery at the Toronto school and contributed so greatly to the school's high reputation that almost as a natural result he became Professor of Surgery when the Faculty of Medicine was re-established in the University, later winning appointment as Dean of the Faculty. Aikens combined a steadily progressing surgical skill with outstanding ability as a teacher. In later years George Peters, Herbert A. Bruce and F. N. G. Starr all bore tribute to his great ability.

The last years of the old hospital were fraught with constant criticism and acrimonious discussion. The building was not only inadequate but falling into bad repair, and the bitter rivalries of the medical schools, whether known as Upper Canada and Toronto or Trinity College and Victoria, spread down from the teachers to their students. Moreover, the lay and professional press seldom tempered criticism of the institution with even modest approval of its work.

In 1853 two editorials presented in detail the faults of the building and the organization which controlled its activity. The first appeared in the *Upper Canada Journal*, whose editor, S. J. Stratford, M.R.C.S., had been forbidden visiting privileges in the hospital after a protest from Dr. Beaumont as to the manner in which he had published Beaumont's lecture on the treatment of carotid aneurysm without Beaumont's permission. The second article was published on March 22 in the *Semi-Weekly Leader*, prompted no doubt by complaints of students and others impatient of the delay in building a new hospital.

In the first place, the critics pointed out, there was no reception room for new patients. More important, the lack of ventilation resulted in "a foulness of the air extremely dangerous to the patients, medical officers, students, attendants and others whose duty is frequently to visit the wards." How could it be otherwise, demanded the *Leader*,

> with perhaps a dozen persons taking medicine with nothing but a closed stool to resort to placed at their bedsides. . . . There is not a water closet in the whole building nor within at least eighty yards of it. . . . The odour which remains in the building is but too perceptible . . . the very walls being corrupt by it. . . . It is almost impossible for a patient to escape this noxious influence as is shown by the constant attacks of erysipelas and . . . other complaints that indiscriminately affect them after residing a short time in the hospital. . . . The poor patient . . . admitted for some surgical complaint, having obtained all the relief which the present advanced state of science could afford him . . . suddenly finds he has contracted a more deadly complaint from the hospital air which is even more likely to destroy him.

There was an almost endless tale of dirt and discomfort:

> The greater part of the blankets used would be rejected by any spirited stableboy if offered as a horse rug. Except for a dozen sent by the Mayor during the last cholera epidemic, not a new blanket has entered the institution in the last six years. . . . There is no bathhouse in the building unless one old tin concern can be dignified with that name. To reach this the patient has to wander through the basement to a rickety temporary wash-house, otherwise the solitary tin bath may be hauled up two pairs of stairs by main force and the water carried after it in pails which has at least the advantage of security against scalding the patient as the water has ample time to cool off.

There was no operating room in the hospital, the operations being performed in an ordinary hospital ward or at the end of a corridor and "the cries of the patient being heard by all the invalids no matter how injurious such a disturbance may be to them." The same ward was used for lectures twice a week.

Conditions in the lower wards were even worse:

> The ceilings are mottled with damp as water percolated through the upper floor in washing where the floors were worn and broken and the floor in proximity to the stove has holes three inches wide and a foot or two long.

The criticism of staff accommodation was equally biting:

> The Matron is stored away in a sort of cell of most scant dimensions in the basement and that dreary solitary underground room serves her for eating, sleeping and even other purposes. The outside wall is without plaster and an inch board separates the other side from the basement corridor. . . . The Resident Physician and Surgeon receive the munificent sum of £100 a year and an unfurnished room without board or servant for unremitting attention to from sixty to seventy patients.

Even the reorganization of the Board of Trustees was criticized, as the new system of medical men serving in the dual capacities of trustees and visiting physicians prevented any satisfactory investigation of the shortcomings of the visiting staff.

The medical students found many faults in the teaching that they received; as a matter of fact it was stated that only 57 of 137 students in training in the city had attended clinical lectures in the hospital. The student paid a fee of two pounds for six months or £2 10s. for a year. His routine was to meet the attending physician for the week in the surgery where the out-patients were seen and treated and then to accompany the physician on his rounds of the hospital to see the patients under his care. But as each week brought a different physician for routine duty the continued observation of interesting cases was not possible, and even the hospital records were not available as the students were only permitted to leave the surgery under the guidance of the visiting physician.

A crisis finally developed in 1855 as the result of a particularly scathing letter from "A Medical Student" published in the *Colonist* of March 24, 1855. It told the same old story, namely the indifference of some of the visiting physicians to their students, but it went into greater detail with regard to the preference given to students from Trinity over those of the Rolph school, the cruelty of the hospital staff to some of the patients, and the filthy conditions under which they were maintained in the hospital.

By this time the new hospital building had been erected on Gerrard Street, and although there were as yet no patients in the hospital the boardroom was available for the meeting of the hospital trustees to investigate the charges that had been made against them and the institution.

On March 29 the boardroom was crowded with students and "professional gentlemen" who had come to hear the trustees begin an investigation which was to last for three days.[3] H. G. Bowes, M.P.P., took the chair and Dr. Widmer and James Beattie were the other trustees present. J. W. Brent, the Secretary to the Trustees, read the letter. It cited the brutal treatment of a coloured patient by an orderly named Burns. The offence had resulted in a one-pound fine from a police magistrate, but in spite of this Burns continued to be employed by the hospital. The resident surgeon was said to have refused a student the use of dental forceps for tooth extractions, insisting that the patient should go to a dentist—which could cost the poor man two and six-pence, which he could not afford. The matron, Mrs. Donnelly, was frequently "in liquor" and used threatening language to patients whom she disliked. It was also claimed that the hospital was so filthy that the students referred to it as "the Lousy Hospital" and it was also known to be "the fountain of moral pollution." Time spent in it was worthless to the students, and the money spent on fees squandered. The investigation showed, however, that the author of the letter had never had a hospital ticket and had only studied medicine for about eight months. Consideration was given to the question of resuscitation of a patient, who was bled on the order of Dr. Bovell, by throwing a pail of water on him and then dragging him out into the open air, and it was stated that the water was not thrown on the man in a Christian spirit.

Students of Victoria were treated "as dirt." A patient under the care of Dr. Aikens was advised by Nurse Donnelly that he should have Dr. Beaumont or Dr. Hodder operate on him or else he might die. Dr. Aikens also referred to a patient under his care who was taken from the hospital and maintained in a nearby tavern where Dr. Hodder and Dr. Philbrick removed his leg. Dr. Wright complained of the lack of proper lances, leeches and brandy, but Dr. Widmer stated that the provision of leeches was beyond the financial capacity of the hospital; however, he had ordered some new instruments. Mr. Bowes, the chairman, said that available funds did not warrant the provision of brandy, but admitted that the quality of the whisky available was not very good.

The lines of contention were sharply drawn. A letter was produced signed "Veritas," and another from a group of students, both contradicting most of the original criticisms. Before the investigation was completed, Dr. Beaumont cast considerable doubt on the ability of Aikens and Wright because their training had been mostly acquired

[3] *Trustees' Report on an Investigation in Certain Charges Against the Management of the Trustees* (Rare Book Room, University of Toronto Library), 1855.

locally, and added that he would not desire to assist in any operation performed by either of them. Dr. Edward Clarke, the resident surgeon, strove to justify his preference for the Trinity School. He admitted that the medical officers were not chosen on account of their professional standing but because they were representatives of the different medical schools, and concluded: "I consider the medical staff of Trinity College the most efficient in Upper Canada; I consider it the most perfect staff in Upper Canada. . . . Every chair is filled by a professor who is admitted by students of all schools to be a very able man."

Finally, a letter was presented to the trustees signed by Telfer, Herrick, Beaumont, Hodder and Bovell saying that they believed great credit should go to Dr. Clarke, the resident medical officer, for the general good order and cleanliness of the hospital and for his zeal and attention and ability. Dr. Beaumont also answered the criticism that teachers were not present more often for the instruction of the students by saying that he had tried to be on time as far as possible, and reminded the meeting that his services were provided gratuitously. Dr. Aikens and Dr. Wright were very definite in their criticism of Nurse Donnelly, the occasional insobriety of Dr. Clarke, the filthy state of the bedclothes and the constant verminous infestation of the patients.

Eventually the tempest subsided. Dr. Aikens and Dr. Wright were rewarded for stirring it too vigorously by receiving letters from the board of the hospital on April 14 dispensing with their services as medical officers. To this Aikens and Wright entered a formal protest to the legislature, repeating their criticism of the hospital and claiming that seventy of their students were now left without instruction. As the decision of the board had not been unanimous it was overruled by the legislature early in the following year, and they were reinstated in their appointments to the hospital staff. The board, however, concluded the whole matter to its satisfaction with a resolution stating that

> from our personal knowledge of the Toronto General Hospital, as well as from the evidence which has been adduced during the prolonged investigation into the charges contained in a letter signed "A Medical Student," we feel bound in justice to add our testimony to the statements made in the communication, exculpating the Hospital from those false charges.
>
> (Signed) John Scott, M.D., M.R.C.S.L.
> John Grand, L. & P.S.G.
> W. Hallowell, M.D., M.R.C.S.(Ed.)
> F. M. Russell, M.D., M.R.C.S.(Eng.)
> J. Richardson, M.D., M.R.C.S.(Eng.)
> N. Bethune, M.D., M.R.C.S.(Eng.)
> Cornelius Jas. Philbrick, F.R.C.S.

The proceedings closed at nine o'clock on Saturday night, having occupied three days. Through all the turmoil it was more than obvious that the old hospital had had its day, and that the opening of the new hospital was long overdue.

V

The Critical Years

THE HOSPITAL TRUSTEES WERE WELL AWARE OF THE INADEquacies of the old hospital on King Street. They were faced, however, with the problem of procuring the large amount of money necessary to provide the features essential in a new hospital building. It was also true that the years of the great epidemics had impressed the Board of Health with the growing need for a permanent hospital of sufficient size so that no sick person should ever be refused admission.

As a result, on September 3, 1847, a special meeting of the trustees discussed a letter received from the President of the Board of Health asking that they should consider with as little delay as possible the necessity of preparing a more extensive and permanent hospital, and the Mayor and the President of the Board of Trade were authorized by the trustees to approach the government asking for assistance in erecting a general hospital on the security of the properties at present held in the name of the Toronto General Hospital.

The government replied that it did not have the power to loan money for the erection of a new hospital, and the trustees and the Board of Health were forced to continue to provide temporary accommodation in time of need in cholera sheds, immigrant sheds and various buildings in the general neighbourhood of the hospital. The temporary quarters, for that matter, did not compare unfavourably with the conditions in the old hospital, as the following description of a building at Wellington and John streets indicates:

> Notwithstanding its external appearance this building is admirably adapted for the use to which it has been put. It is very large and

capable of holding more patients than the old hosiptal on King Street. We believe we are correct in stating that 70 patients can find ample accommodation in the Wellington Street Hospital, which was far from being the case in the other. The arrangements of the rooms in the building are very advantageous. The nurses are now accommodated with rooms in a wing of the building, separated from the patients but still on the same floor. In the King Street hospital the nurses were obliged to sleep in the basement of the building, which was both inconvenient and unhealthy. The ventilation is very good and far superior to the other building which was scarcely ventilated at all. There is a very good supply of water on the premises, and gas will be shortly introduced into the building. The chief drawbacks to the comfort of the building are a want of planking before the entrance and a gas lamp at the gate, both amendments are very much needed. We cannot conclude this notice without remarking on the clean state in which the hospital is kept. The different wards are as neat and clean as it is possible to make them. This very gratifying state of affairs will doubtless contribute much to making the institution sufficiently useful and efficient until the new hospital shall have been completed.[1]

Frequent meetings of the trustees were held to find a solution to the problem, and finally in September 1853 a decision was reached to abandon the old hospital and build a new one. The chosen site was in the city's east end in a block in the Park Reserve bounded by Spruce, Sumach, Gerrard and Pine streets. Arguments in favour of this site stated that with the increase in population in the west end, property was becoming very valuable and that it was not desirable to maintain the hospital, admitting as it did many patients with highly infectious diseases, in a growing residential section of the city.[2]

From the beginning the hospital trustees must have realized the tremendous financial problems which faced them in building and administering the work of the new hospital. On September 14 a public auction was held to sell on perpetual lease the grounds surrounding the old hospital. Lots on King Street brought only from 3s. 6d. to 8s. per foot and on Peter Street from 3s. 9d. to 7s. 6d.: the total sum realized

[1]*Daily Leader*, September 20, 1855.

[2]*A Brief Historical Sketch of the Toronto General Hospital, Its Origin and Progress during the Period from 1818–1911 by A. F. Miller*. This history of the hospital, written at the request of the Board of Trustees by Mr. A. F. Miller, long-time secretary of the hospital, was found in a sealed copper box in the cornerstone of the College Street Building, placed there in 1913, and found again in 1963 when remodelling of the front entrance was undertaken.

was a little over £10,000. The small amount of money coming from this sale and the disposal over the years of so much of the original land grants left the trustees with no alternative but to offer the sale of debentures. This was advertised in the *Leader* of September 19, 1854:

> TORONTO GENERAL HOSPITAL DEBENTURES
>
> Tenders will be received at the office of the Secretary of the TGH until the Tenth Day of September for the purchase of debentures to the extent of £5,000 bearing interest at the rate of 6% per annum, payable one-half yearly at the Bank of Upper Canada, redeemable within a period of twenty years in sums of £500 each and issued under an Act of the Provincial Parliament, the Twentieth.
>
> August 11, 1854 (Signed) J. W. BRENT
> Secretary-Treasurer

There was a good deal of controversy regarding the site chosen for the new hospital. The *Upper Canada Journal*, prompted by medical sectionalism, claimed that the old menace of the miasma from the Don would be a serious threat to the patients, but it was contradicted by an article in the *Leader* of August 10, 1853:

> Our readers are aware that the site chosen for the new hospital lies a little east of Parliament Street, north of the Don and Danforth Road. The situation is elevated far above the Bay and the extent of the ground attached, several acres, secures the new building from the injurious effects of overcrowding and gives it all the advantages which are to be derived from an airy and unconfined position. The selection of this site has met the general approbation of the public. The allegation is made that the ague has prevailed almost universally during the past summer in that neighbourhood. Of the prevalence of ague in the city during the autumn few need to be informed for most persons have heard, seen or felt something of it but the statement of the *Journal* which goes to confine its range to the eastern part of the city is at once invidious and untrue. If the editor of the *Journal* will make a reference to the number of applicants for a remedy for ague at the Toronto Hospital he will find that the western and central portions have supplied as many cases in proportion to the quality of the inhabitants as the eastern. The latter population, as one knows, is composed of the labouring class which is miserably housed or rather "hutted" in tenements pervious to the night air and in a constant state of dampness, and the reader does not need to be told that the habits of this class render them more susceptible of receiving and being affected by the poison of ague from their want of that scrupulous attention to cleanliness which is so great a preservative of health, and their more general addiction to intemperance. When the *Journal* drew such terrible pictures of the effects to be dreaded from the miasmata

of the neighbourhood of the Don it showed a strange forgetfulness of the condition of the Bay in the front of the City.

It is hardly short of a miracle that so little disease occurs in the central portions of the City when it is considered what a deposit of filth rests in the waters of the Bay, and that the disgusting mixture is constantly agitated, during the warm season, by the action of steam paddles, which rake up the deposits of preceeding days, and by exposing them to the air produces a most fertile source of menace. The delicious mixture of feculent matter and bay water is served up through pipes and distributed through the City to be swallowed by the citizens.

The *Journal* admits that the situation of the new hospital grounds is comparatively a high one and afterwards it lays it down as an ascertained fact that a situation immediately on a level with the marsh would experience the most intense influence of the poison and that a more elevated position would not be so likely to suffer. If this be true then the new hospital grounds are more secure from miasmata than King Street inasmuch as they are elevated far above the level of King Street or any other densely settled portions of the City.

The next objection raised is that the proposed location of the Toronto General Hospital would render it extremely inconvenient for medical students to attend and that those at Trinity College would in consequence suffer the positive injustice of "almost" being prevented from attending the medical classes of the hospital. The editor of the Journal ought to be aware, and doubtless is aware that the medical lectures at Trinity College are not now nor are they in the future intended to be delivered in the College buildings. At present a house on Spadina Avenue is occupied by the class of Trinity College. The building is unsuited for the purpose and we learn that it is intended to vacate it and obtain another in a suitable location when the new hospital has been erected.

It may be, as the *Journal* suggests, that there are many other sites in the City that would serve for a general hospital, but it is the business of the Trustees to have a due regard to economy in their movements. If the rents of the hospital bring over £800 a year the change is, in fact, so much gain to the revenue of the Trust for the grounds now selected for a site which have hitherto yielded no revenue whatever.

The *Leader* then went on to discuss a question raised by the *Journal* regarding the union of all the medical schools in Toronto:

As this would be a matter of purely private arrangement the public will feel little concern regarding it, but when the suggestion of amalgamation is put forward as a preliminary to a union between the medical schools and the hospital there is reason to fear that the jealousies, suspicions and the prejudice of the public would be aroused. There exists in most minds a morbid idea of horror at the

> prospect of having their own bodies or those of their friends submitted to the dissecting-knife and an open and approved union between a medical school and a general hospital would be apt to be regarded as placing the dissecting-knife in too close familiarity with the bodies of the patients who might die in the institution.[3]

William Hay of Edinburgh, who was at that time resident in Toronto, was chosen to be the architect for the new building. He was a man of outstanding ability and while in Toronto also designed St. Basil's Church at St. Michael's College, the Yorkville Town Hall, and the House of Providence which was to be erected on Power Street. On his return to Edinburgh he became responsible for the renovations at St. Giles Cathedral, a major undertaking which required his services for a period of eleven years.

The building that he planned was of a French Provincial type; of three storeys with a central tower a hundred feet in height and smaller towers at the angles of the building. With three wings running back from the central block it covered a space of 170 feet by 120 feet. A stone stairway led through the front door into a spacious entrance hall, on which were located a boardroom and some consulting rooms. There were two wards on this floor for acute surgical cases. The dispensary, some private wards, quarters for the resident surgeon, the nurses and the hospital steward were located in the wings on this floor. A broad central stairway led up to the operating theatre in a central wing. With sky-lighting and commodious galleries for spectators it was in keeping with the times, and below it was the mortuary. There were twenty hospital wards, the largest accommodating twelve patients, and on both the second and third floors large sitting-rooms were provided for convalescents. It was claimed that there was a liberal supply of baths, washrooms, water closets and other sanitary conveniences. The kitchens were located in the basement, reservoirs for water were placed in the towers, and a room was provided in the central tower for a museum. Finally, special features to provide a flow of fresh air throughout the building, with air vents and flues in the walls and ceilings, were a source of satisfaction to all who beheld them.

Construction of the new building began in the spring of 1854 and was completed early in 1855. The first patients, however, were not admitted until October 1, 1856, when twelve patients were transferred to the hospital. Dr. Edward Clarke was re-appointed as the Resident Physician and Surgeon, but his years of service came to an end suddenly

[3]*Leader*, August 10, 1853.

when he was found lying dead in his room during the morning of December 18. An inquest held under the chairmanship of Dr. E. M. Hodder attributed his death to poisoning by prussic acid, and the evidence indicated that for some time he had suffered from spells of marked depression, particularly on the day of his death. Although he lacked diplomacy in his relations with the partisan groups of doctors working in the hospital, those who knew him best paid tribute to his keen interest and loyalty to the institution during years that had thrown unceasing responsibility on the Resident Physician.

So in 1856, as the doors were opened, the trustees faced all the tribulations of a new Pandora's Box. Fundamentally the trouble was due to two factors, the inadequacy of the fixed annual grants from the provincial government and the refusal of the city authorities to provide for the maintenance of the large number of indigent patients constantly in hospital. In fairness, however, it should be realized that this latter reaction was prompted by the considerable number of such patients who came into the hospital from the surrounding countryside.

An account of one meeting of the City Council shows the difficulties that faced the hospital trustees. At this meeting the Committee on Finance and Assessment reported a communication from the Toronto General Hospital stating that

> as the funds of the Hospital are only equal to the support of 80 patients, until the number is reduced below 80 no patient can be admitted except in cases of accidents but by the payment of .25¢ per diem and recommend that the Council appropriate the sum of $1,000.00 for 1859 to be applied to the payment of city patients only, admitted to the hospital if the number exceeds 80, to be charged at the rate proposed and to be admitted upon certificate of the mayor and police magistrate. The said amount of $1,000.00 or any such portions of it ought to be chargeful to the City, to be paid quarterly upon a proper certified return being made of city patients admitted beyond the number of 80, and not being cases derived from accidents.

This report brought a mixed response. One alderman felt the thousand-dollar grant was excessive "without an exhibit of its affairs," and pointed out that the by-law prevented them from appropriating funds out of the next year's taxes. He recommended that the decision be postponed until a new council took over.

One of the councillors spoke in favour of the report, though he believed there was a good deal of property belonging to the Hospital Trust which might be made productive. Another alderman agreed to the necessity for a public report of the hospital's affairs, adding that it was a disgrace to "this Christian city that it never yet appropriated funds toward this charitable institution. There were funds at hand out of which an appropriation could be made and the only question was should they give it." The alderman who had tendered the original objection pointed out that the surrounding country might send in the whole eighty and the city would therefore have to pay for every patient they sent in over that. He therefore moved an amendment that the proposed payment of twenty-five cents per head should only be paid for patients over the number of eighty sent in by the city authorities. This amendment was seconded and, after some further discussion, carried.

Some time later, when the provincial government had reduced its grant by $3,000, the Hon. Mr. Howland, Receiver General, inspected the hospital in company with a member of Parliament. They hoped to be able to discuss its requirements from personal experience when the subject of appropriation to charitable institutions should come up for discussion in the House at the next session. Mr. Howland was gratified to discover that nearly seven-eighths of the patients were from outside the city—Parliament had been reluctant to grant aid to the hospital on the assumption that it was a purely local institution. He promised the trustees that he would enlighten the legislature on this point as soon as it reconvened.

As each year went by, the increasingly critical financial situation of the hospital became more widely known. Finally, at the request of a number of ratepayers, the mayor convened a public meeting in the St. Lawrence Hall in December 1865. At this meeting the Hon. G. W. Allen moved "that this meeting learns with regret that owing to the reduction of the Government grant the Toronto Hospital had a deficiency in funds and that many patients are refused admission and that those who are received are not provided with some of the comforts necessary." Mr. Allen then presented a detailed report, as summarized here by the *Leader*:

> The hospital derived its income principally, indeed he might say altogether, from two sources, the first was the rent and interest from its endowment and the other was the annual grant from the Government. The rent and interest which the hospital received last year amounted to $4,945.00. There was another item of revenue alongside of this which he blushed to be compelled to read—private charities—$15.00. Then there was paid by patients $1,175.00 and students' fees $721.00, which with the Government grant of $11,200 made a total

> income of $18,058.00. The expenditures as against that were as follows: repayment of the debt and interest, $4,180.00. This he explained was what the hospital Trustees had to pay on their debentures which had been issued to pay for the construction of the present building. Then the other items were rent, taxes, repairs and insurance, $277.00, salaries and wages $2,683.00, medical comforts and medicine, $2,302.00, food for patients, $9,017.00 and other expenditures $1,607 making a total of $20,168 as against the income of $18,058. In addition to all this not only was the hospital suffering from a deficiency in its funds but it was also as the resolution stated "unable to provide even the necessary accommodation for the patients within its walls." The hospital had not the means to supply a sufficient supply of bed linen, bedding, blankets and other clothing of that kind necessary for the comfort and resoration of health to the patients. The Trustees had a very considerable debt amounting to something like $23,000.00. A good deal of additional expense was imposed upon the Trust in consequent of the state of the new building which when they entered upon the discharge of their duties was found to be badly constructed, so ill ventilated and lighted and so difficult to heat in the winter that the Trustees had to go to considerable expense in order to obviate the inconvenience.

In analysing the causes of the situation, a number of old wounds were re-opened, and the report ended with an emotional appeal to the charity of the whole community:

> Now it might very naturally be asked by some what had brought the hospital to its present embarrassed state; of course the cutting down of the Government grant which was originally $15,000.00 but was now only a little over $10,000.00. This was the main cause of the embarrassment of the Trustees. But in addition to this, exception had unquestionably been taken to the former management of the hospital. The wisdom of putting up the very expensive building on the site which was now occupied had been very much questioned and they all knew, who knew anything about the affairs of the Trust that complaints had been from time to time made with regard to the domestic and financial management of the institution. A communication had been received from Bishop Lynch offering to maintain the 120 patients now in the institution for the same expense as was now incurred in taking 85, that is maintaining 35 free patients in consideration of obtaining the Government grant. But the offer of Bishop Lynch had been turned down by the Trustees, he thought quite rightly. He thought that the hospital should be a general institution supported by the general public. It would not meet the approval of other denominations if the charge were given to one particular denomination. He thought an appeal should be made to the citizens when they recollected that this Toronto Hospital was the only institution of its kind, the only refuge of the sick in the whole of

> Upper Canada they would surely never admit for a moment that it ought to languish for want of funds or run the risk of having its doors closed to the sick and distressed for the sake of a few paltry dollars necessary to support it. It would be a disgrace to this wealthy community for it was a wealthy community, notwithstanding all they had heard about hard times. Not only were the sick poor of Toronto relieved there but they must remember that there was not a single place of the kind in the country except this hospital where a poor unfortunate being, suffering from the effects of accident or disease could seek a refuge and obtain medical and other assistance necessary to his relief and even here in this city what were the facts? Why time after time poor, sick, miserable creatures borne down by the weight of disease and distress had applied and they were obliged to refuse them admission and they went home to die perhaps in some miserable hole without any of those comforts which tend to alleviate distress and make the pains of disease more endurable.

The Rev. Alexander Torre, who seconded the motion, went on to say that he had inspected the accounts of the hospital and found them accurate. Despite reports that only fifty patients were supported annually in the institution, he had found that the average was often closer to ninety. He recommended that the hospital be regarded as a provincial rather than a local institution, and pointed out that its training facilities were ultimately serving the whole country rather than just the city and is environs. His sentiments were shared by Mr. A. P. McCord, who advocated a resumption of the government's hospital grant in addition to a small appropriation from the taxes of the city.

One proposal that met with little enthusiasm was the suggestion of Bishop Lynch that the domestic management of the hospital be entrusted to the Sisters of Charity—which, he said, would save $7,000 and provide for at least thirty more patients. But the objection was raised that this would turn the hospital into a "proselytizing institution," and the Bishop's resolution was turned down despite his insistence that Protestants would continue to form the majority on the Board of Trustees as well as among the nurses and visiting clergymen.

Following this meeting a committee was appointed to consider the problems of hospital finance. After consultation with the trustees, they failed to reach any conclusion regarding ultimate plans for the hospital, but they did manage to propose measures to meet its immediate needs and increase the number of patients to one hundred:

> An initial sum of $2,000.00 will be required immediately and as it has been ascertained that its internal furnishings generally are very much impaired by time and constant use and would require in many

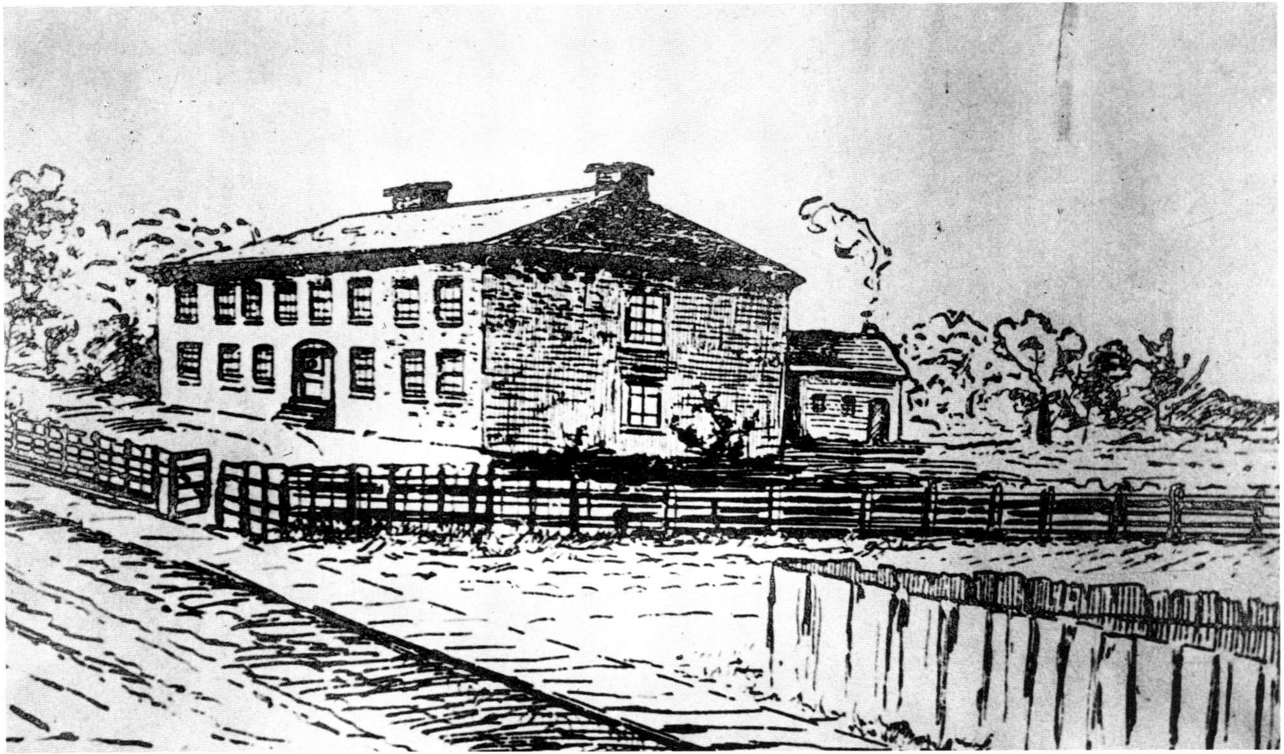

York General Hospital, 1820.
Occupied as temporary Parliament Buildings, 1825–28; used as a hospital, 1829–56.

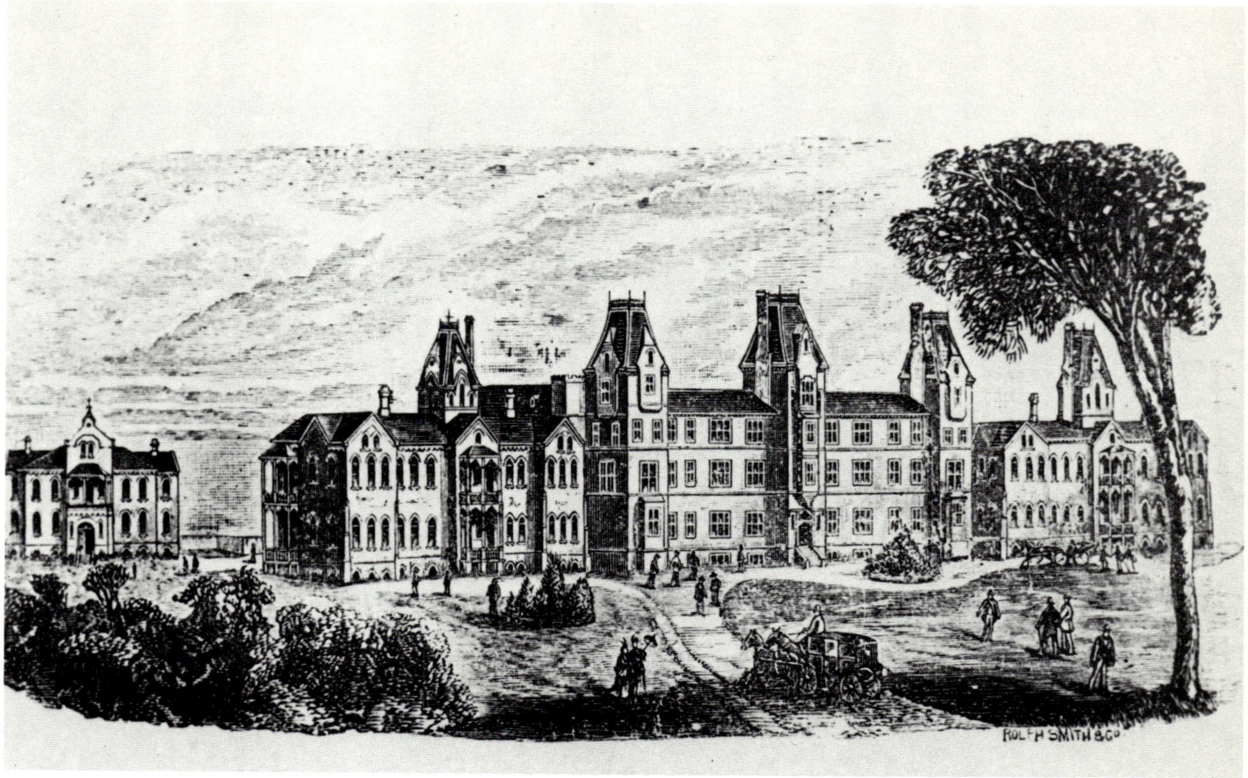

Toronto General Hospital, 1878.

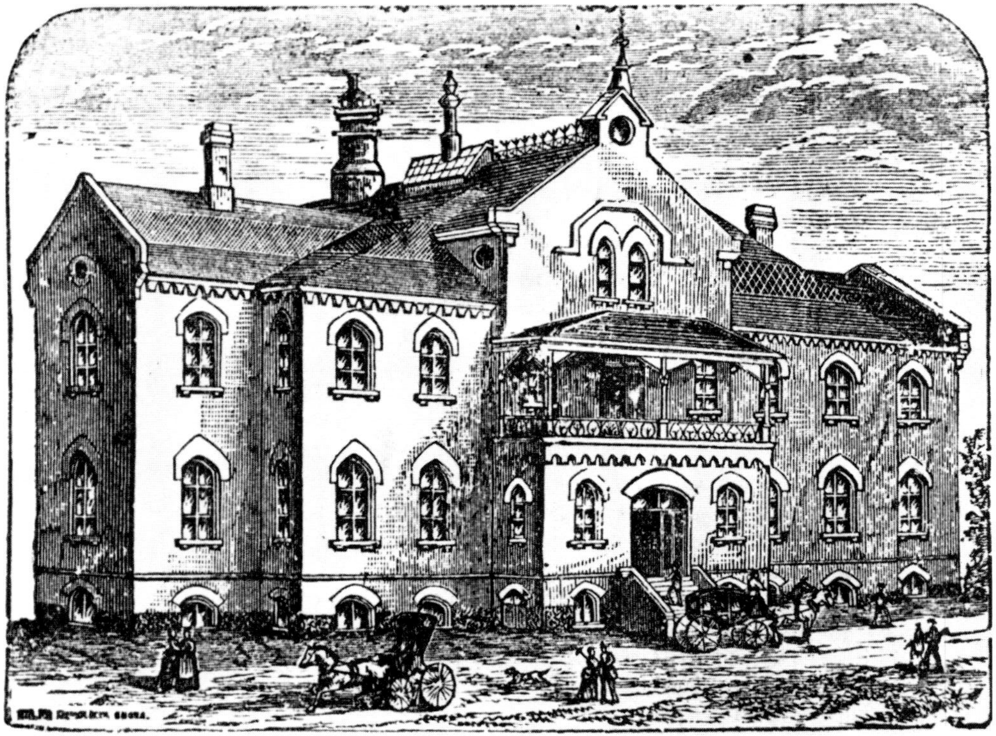

The Burnside Hospital, 1878.

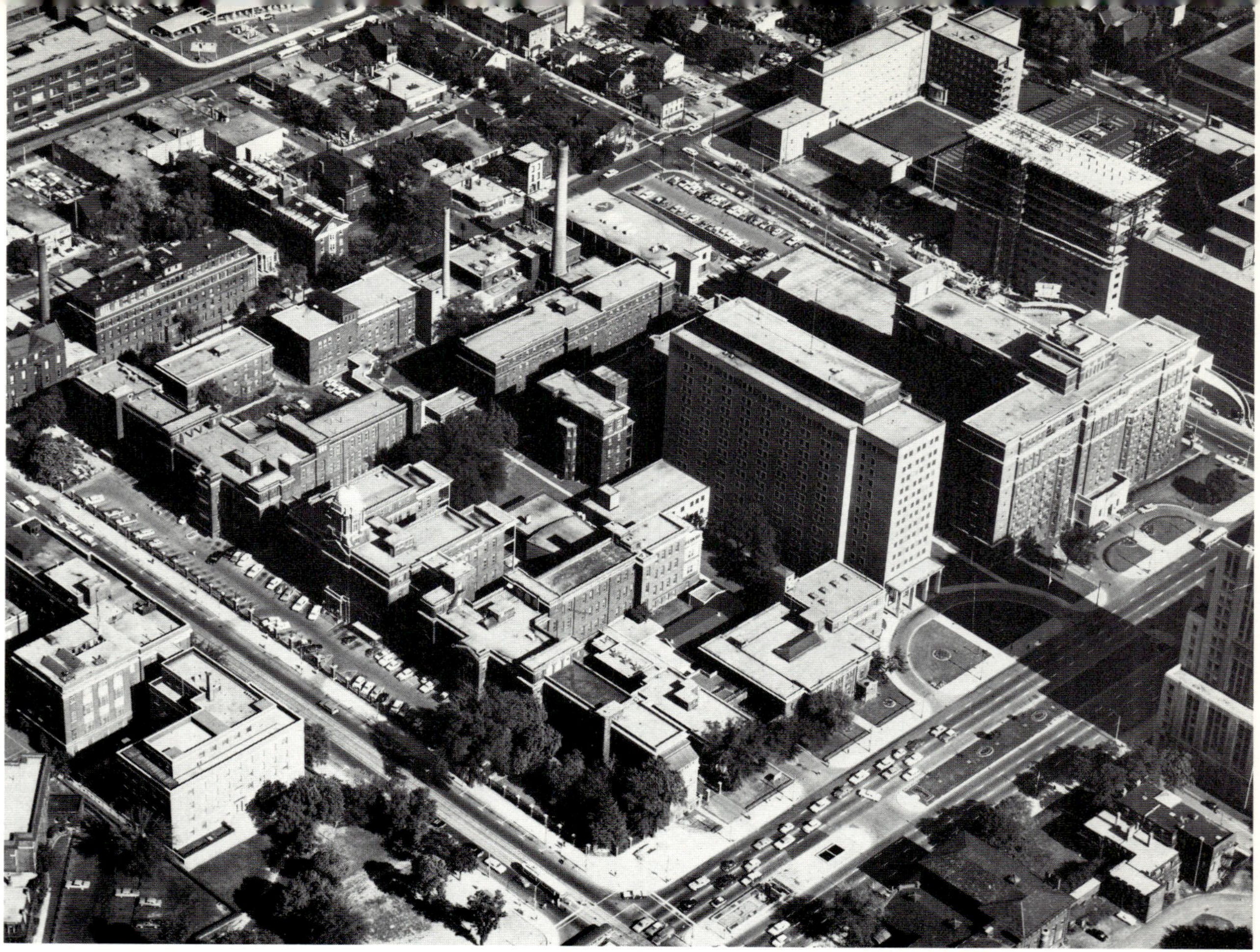

Aerial view of Toronto General Hospital, 1960s.

> cases to be entirely renewed, especially in the matter of bedding. A considerable portion of it may be regarded as altogether unfit to be used. Indeed almost the whole furnishings of the beds will require to be provided anew in order to ensure anything like proper comfort and warmth of the patients and this will involve another $2,000.00.

They then stated that an appeal was being made to fellow-citizens for $4,000 to meet these urgent needs, adding that "it is to be distinctly understood that this appeal is not to be repeated."

As a result of the generous response of the citizens to this appeal, Mr. Allen was able to report to the trustees of the General Hospital that $7,443 had been collected. The trustees now requested that Dr. Joseph Workman, Superintendent of the Lunatic Asylum, and Messrs. Gundy and Langley, architects of this city, visit the hospital and advise them with regard to obvious faults in the internal structure of the building. The ventilation system, which had in the beginning received such approbation, had proved of no value, and the sewage disposal into cesspools beneath the building required immediate correction.

It is not clear how far the work on the renovations proceeded at this time. For in spite of the constant efforts of the trustees in seeking help wherever they thought it might be found, the financial situation deteriorated markedly. After much discussion, City Council offered to pay fifty cents per day for city patients but demurred when the trustees requested that this should apply to a constant number of forty patients. Then, in February 1867, the council discussed a by-law to raise $10,000 to support the hospital. After prolonged debate the motion was finally passed, but nothing ever came of it.

By the spring of 1867 the trustees warned all and sundry that the closure of the hospital was inevitable. In July a notice was sent to the mayor and aldermen informing them that, as the debts of the hospital had reached the sum of $5,000, it had been resolved to close the hospital for the reception of patients, on the first of August. Dr. Hampton, the Resident Medical Officer, was also directed to consult with the medical staff with regard to dismissing the patients at present in the hospital as soon as possible. In order to justify this drastic decision to the citizens, the secretary was instructed to have the following notice inserted three times in the *Leader* and the *Globe*:

> TO THE PUBLIC
>
> It is the painful duty of the Trustees of the TGH to announce that from the want of funds they are compelled to close the hospital for the reception of patients from the first day of August next.

Previous to this, the trustees reported to a meeting in the mayor's office that they had visited the building occupied as a branch asylum in the Queen's Park and had formed the opinion that it was suited for a hospital. A telegram sent to the government asking permission to remove the patients from the hospital to this building was immediately turned down. A letter was then sent to Dr. Workman, Superintendent of the Asylum, with the same request. He replied that it would be quite impossible to turn over the accommodation, as it was urgently required for the admission of numerous lunatics lying in the various county jails throughout the province or confined by their friends at home in quarters hardly better than those afforded by the jails and much less secure. He proceeded to point out that there were two hospitals under construction and that, on inspection, he had found the county jail utterly unfit for the comfortable lodging of lunatics. He had checked the list of the patients in the chief asylum and also at the branch, and had concluded that there was more than a fair share of the accommodation taken up by patients from the city of Toronto.

By October 14 the hospital was entirely empty of patients, and the only employees retained were the secretary, J. W. Brent, the steward and one orderly. The trustees, however, met frequently, seeking a solution to their problems. During the months that the closure of the hospital was threatened and while it was not occupied, the Officer Commanding the Garrison, Lt.-Col. Sir Henry Havelock, approached the city authorities and the trustees to see whether it would be possible to use the hospital as a barracks, but the answer to this request was diplomatically delayed. At the same time, after the use of the Queen's Park Asylum was refused, the old jail and the House of Refuge were both inspected but neither was considered suitable for use as a temporary hospital.

The provincial government debated the closure of the hospital in January 1868. Mr. J. C. Rykert, the Member for Lincoln, moved that the provincial importance of the hospital warranted a full investigation by committee. The Prime Minister, Sandfield Macdonald, intimated finally that the government had lost confidence in the board under John Sterling. As a result an entirely new board was appointed in April under the chairmanship of Judge Adam Wilson, consisting of three trustees appointed by the government, the mayor of Toronto and one trustee elected by subscribers to the hospital funds. On June 8 the new chairman presented a long report to the Lieutenant-Governor-in-Council, reviewing the whole question of the financial failure of the hospital and presenting sound advice as to the future management of the institution:

> The Trustees of the TGH beg leave to report that when they met in the month of July last for the purpose of re-organization after the appointment of three new Government members, the affairs of the hospital were in the following condition: the hospital was closed, the steward alone being in charge as caretaker. From that time the patients were removed from it last fall. The unpaid debts for groceries and other necessities, medicines, wages, firing repairs and insurance were $4,872.00 and the arrears of interest on debentures amounted to $2,640.00 making a total of $7,512.00.

He went on to say that their assets, including a half-yearly allowance of $5,600 from the Dominion legislature, should have amounted to $18,237 but the Dominion allowance had not been paid. It was necessary to expend over $2,000 to make the hospital fit for re-occupation and after all the expenses had been met they had actually in hand for strictly hospital purposes only $3,825.

He proceeded to point out some of the many changes that should be made in connection with the hospital. The first was that it should be regarded as a public institution and supported by taxes which bore equally upon everyone. No incurable cases should be received or retained by the hospital, as it was strictly a curative establishment, and there should be a separate institution built for these. There should be an isolation building for the treatment of smallpox and other contagious complaints, under the care of servants and others who should not, while engaged there, have any communication with the General Hospital. To these recommendations he added:

> It is a reproach that such an establishment with ample accommodation in which all classes are interested cannot be maintained in such a country for the want of a few thousand dollars. The conclusion is forced upon us that there is something radically wrong in the present system of hospital management, and that a different scheme must be provided for their future maintenance. The sick, as a class, are entitled to quite as much consideration as the insane or the deaf and dumb, and it is very plain that if it be worthwhile to educate people at enormous public cost, it is worthwhile to take care of them when they are educated and struck down by sickness. It is a duty we owe to the community not to suffer dangerous infectious diseases to remain amongst the healthy. Their removal and treatment should, in most cases, be at the public expense. The basis of such a system must be public support continuing, regular, always ready for the emergency, and bearing equally upon all—not private alms, inconstant or

> irregular—too late for the occasion and pressing too heavily on the liberal, while many who are able to give go free.

He went on to deal with what should be done with the hospital properties and the arguments pro and con regarding selling them or maintaining them at the present rental, in order that they should be re-rented, when the leases ran out, at a much greater income. And having dealt again with the possible sources of income, he concluded with the following paragraph:

> The Trustees sincerely hope that this may be the last year that such an establishment will have to appeal for relief in this manner and that all the hospitals of the Province may be ranked hereafter amongst those public charities which it is considered to be an honour as well as a duty to maintain.

So, after a period of ten months, the Toronto General Hospital opened its doors once again on August 7, 1868. As there was only $3,800 available to meet the expenses for the rest of the year, it was decided to restrict the number of public patients to twenty-five and demand payment of forty cents per day from any seeking hospital care beyond this number. At the same time, out-patient services were re-established and Dr. W. B. Hampton resumed his position as Resident Physician and Surgeon. Re-establishment of the medical staff followed and as a result teaching was resumed by the professors of the Toronto School of Medicine and the Victoria School, using their own patients or those under the care of other members of their schools.

The hospital was now launched upon a period of recovery during which its financial security became less doubtful, but the road was long and tortuous. In an act passed by the provincial legislature in 1868 entitled "Prison and Asylum Inspection Act," Mr. J. W. Langmuir was empowered to inspect, among other institutions receiving government grants, the Toronto General Hospital. Following his inspection in December 1869, he was highly critical of the hospital with regard to the cost of maintenance, the lack of cleanliness in the wards and the indifferent management of the institution by the trustees. In a reply submitted to the government, the trustees repudiated his criticisms and pointed to obvious inaccuracies in his comparison of the Toronto hospital with those of Hamilton and Kingston.

During the year ending October 1 there had been 632 patients admitted to the hospital, and when comparisons were made on a basis of patient-day occupancy the discrepancies between the hospitals became much less marked and were further influenced by the types of patients accommodated in the different hospitals. A major factor, however, was the expenditure for beer, wine, spirits, medicine and medical comforts, which was nearly three times greater than the amount spent in the other two hospitals, on the same patient-day basis. At this time milk cost 12½¢, beer 25¢ and whisky 85¢ a gallon.[4] The trustees claimed that the expenditure on these commodities and medicines was not their responsibility for "they have obtained the best medical advice and skill to be had in the city . . . and they must trust that these gentlemen will order that which is right and not more of anything than is necessary." They included in their report a comparison of the orders of the eight medical officers of the hospital, which showed considerable variation in practice and liberality. They agreed with the inspector's criticism of irregular attendance by the medical staff, suggesting that their jurisdiction with regard to the staff should be strengthened and that the patients would probably receive better care if the medical staff carried out their duties on a joint rotational basis.

The staff responded with a resolution of their own:

> We are of the opinion that a plan proposed of transferring the patients from one medical officer to another would be objectionable to both of these gentlemen and injurious to the welfare of the patients and their treatment. That the daily duty which would necessarily result would be so prolonged and inconstant as to interfere seriously with the private practice of the medical officers and could not be discharged faithfully without entailing upon them great loss and inconvenience.[5]

The charge of uncleanliness was indignantly repudiated by the trustees. The inspection had been made in the absence of the Lady Superintendent, although she was available in the building. The discoloration and dirty condition of sheets, blankets and coverlids was not unreasonable, as the inspection was made on Thursday and the bedding was always changed on Saturday. It was felt that the sheets must not be tested by the standards of a private family or even of a jail or a lunatic asylum, "because they were often stained by blood and ulcerous matter." The Inspector had criticized particularly the bedding in the Male Ward, but actually he was referring to the Blind Ward in which "the most uncleanly and troublesome of the male patients are put and in which the worst of the bedding is used."

[4]*Leader*, February 4, 1871.
[5]*Canadian Medical Journal*, April 1870.

Finally, it was a matter of great concern to the trustees that the Resident Medical Superintendent, Dr. Hampton, and the Lady Superintendent "who are so adequately performing their duties should be charged without just cause with neglect in matters of cleanliness and order in this institution."

There is no doubt that the trustees showed by the detail of their answer that they were well aware of their responsibilities and anxious to maintain the good name of the hospital. The inspector's report itself showed, above all, the desire of the government to establish controlled support for the provincial hospital. A direct result of this was the Charity Aid Act of 1874, by which the government undertook to provide from the public funds systematic support for charitable institutions in the province, and suggested at the same time that municipal and other corporations as well as private individuals were to be encouraged to give liberal support to such institutions. The hospitals mentioned by name included the Toronto General Hospital, the Burnside Lying-In Hospital, and the Toronto Eye and Ear Infirmary, all of which were to receive twenty cents a day for every patient admitted, with an additional ten cents available providing that this did not bring the government grant in excess of one-quarter of the entire income of the hospital. In accepting this responsibility, the government established jurisdiction for regular inspection of the institutions and also requested the hospital directors to enact by-laws governing the duties and salaries of all "officers and servants, the by-laws to receive approval only after the report of the visiting inspector." The Act approved the payment of $11,200 to the Toronto General Hospital, $480 to Burnside and $1000 to the Toronto Eye and Ear Infirmary for the current year.

The minutes of the meetings of the Board of Trustees indicate very clearly the conscientious and diligent manner in which they conducted the business of the hospital. In spite of their best efforts, however, they were repeatedly criticized, often on pure hearsay, for their management of the hospital.

At a meeting on March 4, 1873, they discussed a circular letter which had been addressed to the trustees of the hospital by His Grace, the Rt. Rev. John Joseph Lynch, now the Roman Catholic Archbishop of Toronto. The Archbishop had suggested that the Roman Catholic Church should take over the Toronto General Hospital, and repeated his proposal that the employment of the Sisters of Charity would greatly reduce the cost and enable the hospital to look after a greater number of the needy poor. On March 5 a long reply was prepared by the secretary, Mr. Brent, pointing out that the Archbishop's communication was based upon two false assumptions. The first was that the hospital was in embarrassed circumstances: it was pointed out that since the reorganization and re-opening of the hospital in 1868, it had lived strictly within its budget without increasing its debts. The only debt facing the institution at this time was for the debentures that had been sold to build the hospital. It was accepted that if the Sisters of Charity were to replace the paid nurses there would be a saving of $1,042 per year, but against this the statement was made that in the city the majority of the citizens would not be in favour of having any church jurisdiction over the hospital, either Protestant or Roman Catholic. The trustees were also willing to make way for any others who "will undertake the labours and the responsibilities of the Trust. It is neither a place of profit nor of ease. We do not covet the office nor shall we envy the position of our successors." Mr. J. D. Merrick, one of the trustees, dissociated himself from the stand the other trustees had taken.

At the same time, a new controversy developed with the City Council regarding the support of indigent patients who were residents of Toronto. The council had already passed an order whereby payment would only be made for a period of two weeks, a longer stay in hospital requiring repeated authorization. As a result of this ruling the trustees protested indignantly when a deduction of $1,375 was made from a bill which they had submitted to the Finance Committee for $3,217. The trustees considered it "preposterous that a patient with a broken leg could be expected, even by his Worship, to be able to walk in two weeks or that they should discharge a patient hovering between life and death," adding that the length of hospitalization of patients was the province of the medical officers of the hospital. In spite of their best arguments, the discussion continued from May to October 1873 and there never was a definite settlement.

Undoubtedly the turning point in the fortunes of the hospital might be dated from March 2, 1875, when the executors of the late Erland Erlandson of Port Hope, a gentleman long associated with the Hudson's Bay Company, announced a bequest of $15,000. This and another legacy of $5,000 coming from the estate of James F. Gentle of Montreal provided sufficient money to allow major alterations and repairs. During the summer a new steam heating system was installed to replace the old coal or wood stoves, new water closets were put in, and, by a new allocation, twenty-four more patient beds became available and much better quarters were provided for the nurses. The room beneath the theatre was changed to facilitate out-patient accommodation and a new entrance and stairway provided for the students so that they could enter the theatre without passing through the front of the hospital or coming near the patients' accommodation. The hospital also undertook to build its own sewer to empty into the Don River.

The minutes of the regular meetings of the trustees following the re-opening of the hospital are evidence of an increasing efficiency on the part of the Trust. Under the new trustees and the chairmanship of Adam Wilson, John Macdonald, C. S. Ross and W. H. Howland, order came from near-chaos. The change was clearly evident in the manner in which the debenture debt of the hospital was arranged. In January, 1869, a letter was sent to the Lieutenant-Governor-in-Council which showed that the original issue of $40,000 in 1855 had been increased by $24,000 in 1857 and as a result of default in repayment the interest rate had had to be raised from six to eight per cent. At the time of writing the debt stood at $58,000 but the Board felt that the value of hospital properties, including the hospital itself, could be estimated at $200,000, which was felt to be ample security. A short time later it was ruled that no further property sales should be made except for retirement of the debenture debt, and in January 1877 the chairman, W. H. Howland, reported on a very satisfactory year and stated that the outstanding debentures now overdue amounted to only $35,000. To meet this situation the Board accepted an offer from the financial house of Pellatt and Osler to underwrite a new issue of debentures for $40,000 bearing six per cent interest at 93. This provided the hospital with sufficient funds to retire the previously issued debentures and represented a saving of approximately 1½% on interest payments.

Early in 1875 it was decided that a per diem charge of fifty cents or $3.50 a week was to be made for the patients in the general wards of the hospital and ten dollars a week for private patients. But when the annual report for 1876 showed a favourable balance on the maintenance account of $1,237, it was decided to reduce the per diem charge to forty cents and increase the number of free beds in the hospital from twenty-five to fifty. A news item in the Toronto papers, referring to Mr. Howland's report, went on to say:

> It is perhaps not as well known as it might be that in the private wards sick persons have all the advantages of the best medical attendants coupled with as much comfort and privacy as they could enjoy at home while the cost is much less than in their own houses.

> An offer has also been made by the Trustees designed to meet the wishes of the benevolent and the requirement of county municipalities and small towns, namely the granting of permission to subscribers of $50.00 per annum to send four patients, whose cases are not chronic, to the hospital during the year without further expense. This should materially assist small corporations who find it difficult to maintain their sick at home as by becoming subscribers to the hospital they will have it in their power to relieve several cases of suffering during the year at a very moderate cost. Many charitable persons, we doubt not, will gladly avail themselves of the same offer as will open to them a ready method of procuring medical attendance and care for deserving applicants upon their bounty.

J. W. Brent had been appointed Secretary-Treasurer to the hospital in 1848, and there is no doubt of the good service he rendered to the institution. He carried on his work in an office located on King Street East, near Church Street, and although this situation may have been justified in the early years it forced unusual responsibilities on both the Resident Medical Officer and the Steward.

Before the financial collapse, the sale and lease of hospital property was the chief source of income for maintaining the hospital. The Steward bought meat, vegetables and provisions at the market with the money received directly from patients, or else he obtained his supplies from storekeepers on credit when funds ran short. Likewise, the Resident Medical Officer bought medical supplies and even firewood with money that he received from patients. The accounting in both cases must have depended largely on their honesty.

With the closer supervision of the trustees this situation became entirely unacceptable, and considerable friction developed between Brent and the board. He was loath to move his office into the hospital and, as a matter of fact, did not do so until 1874. Finally, in February 1876, the Board considered a memorandum which stated that from want of system, delay, and loss in not collecting promptly amounts due to the hospital, and the unsatisfactory arrangements of the office work generally, the "Trustees have decided to appoint an Assistant Secretary who shall have charge of the greater part of the secretary's duties." It was decided that Mr. Brent was now to have charge of the lands and rent books and to receive the payments of rents, paying over amounts to the assistant secretary "as may be afterwards ordered." He was ordered to have a report in the hands of the hospital's solicitor by the third day of each month as to the state of these finances: it would then be possible for the chairman and the solicitor to go over the arrears and see what course of action should be adopted. The solicitor would notify each debtor that the "claims are in his hands for recovery," following which he and the chairman would report to the board their opinion of the requirements of each special case.

The assistant secretary was to take charge of all the books, accounts and money transactions (except those related to the properties of the Trust), including the monthly wages of employees. He would also receive deposits and pay from private patients, but he would not allow any money to remain in his hands in excess of fifty dollars. It was to be promptly deposited in the bank. No accounts against the hospital were to be paid until passed by the board in its regular sessions.

The Medical Superintendent would certfiy all the accounts which applied to his jurisdiction and the Lady Superintendent those which applied to hers, and strict regulations governed them both:

> No articles or work shall be ordered without the authority of the Trustees, but it is understood that there will be some urgent requirements which can be dealt with on an emergency basis. The Medical Superintendent, the Lady Superintendent and the Steward are ordered to each have a book containing their requirements on which the decision of the Board is desirable. These books will be available at the weekly meetings of the Board. The Assistant Secretary will have available on the first of each month the outstanding accounts against the City Corporation and other municipalities or individuals guaranteeing patients covering the previous month so that the Board may decide what action will be taken in each case.

As the result of these decisions, Mr. A. F. Miller was appointed Assistant Secretary in May of 1876 at a salary of $600 per year. Brent promptly submitted his resignation, but continued with his limited duties until May 1879, when he retired. In appreciation of his faithful services over a period of more than thirty years, the trustees provided a moderate annuity for the rest of his life.

A new era dawned in 1877. It was obvious to the board that the land occupied by the hospital was not sufficient to take care of any future extension that they might plan. Therefore, they purchased land to the north and west of the hospital area. Then, in March, a meeting was held with Stewart and Strickland, the architects, and tenders were invited through the daily press for the erection of a brick building at the rear of the hospital which would contain a laundry, boiler, and cold room, a post-mortem room and a mortuary. At the same time the architects and the Medical Superintendent were instructed to procure the best laundry machinery possible. On completion it was claimed that the General Hospital now had the best equipped and most modern laundry in the Dominion.[6]

A very favourable reaction to the appeal for subscriptions to the hospital resulted in the decision to have one of the trustees elected by the subscribers each year, and as an example to others it was noted that William Gooderham, Sr., James Worts and William Cawthra had each subscribed $4,500 to the hospital. The favourable publicity that the hospital was now receiving prompted the board to send a circular letter to the clergy of all the city churches, suggesting that they might have a hospital Sunday when an appeal might be made for the subscription of funds for the Toronto General Hospital.

[6]*Globe*, August 16, 1878.

VI

A New Era and the Centralization of Hospital Services

During the twenty years when the old hospital was coming to an end and the new hospital was struggling for existence, two new developments completely altered the age-old practice of surgery.

Prior to the development of anaesthesia in 1846, the surgeon had to remain oblivious to the appalling suffering of his patient while he hastened to complete his operation. Now, with the conquest of pain, it became possible for him to undertake procedures of a scope hitherto denied him. But, in the absence of the control of infection, it seemed almost as if the gain only intensified the problems of curing disease, and surgical operations too frequently hastened death, rather than delaying it. With Lister's triumph in the Glasgow Infirmary, where he established in 1865 the principle of antisepsis, the door finally opened to a new era of modern surgery.

Unfortunately, there are no detailed records available regarding the work of the hospital at this time. But a report published in the *Canadian Lancet* for the year ending September 1871 showed that there had been 703 admissions to the hospital, the most frequent diagnoses being:

Typhoid Fever	38	Dipsomania & Delirium Tremens	25
Smallpox	15	Cancer	17
Phthisis	25	Tumours	18
Pneumonia	24	Enlarged Liver	13
Venereal Diseases	24	Constipation	28
Rheumatism	36	Urethral Stricture	27
Hemiplegia & Paralysis	43	Cystitis	6
Nephritis	17	Calculus	7
Heart Disease	8	Fractures & Dislocations	54

Cholera was no longer epidemic, there being only six cases admitted. While there were only four cases of diabetes, there were seven patients with epilepsy. Twenty-six were admitted because of ulcers; sixteen with necrosis and seven with caries, but the anatomical location of the new lesions was not tabulated. Two patients had tapeworms, three were masturbators and one was an opium eater. The cancers included four epitheliomas and three cancers of the stomach. Most of the surgical operations were for fractures and dislocations, but twenty-seven were to relieve urethral strictures and twenty-three for the treatment of caries or necrosis.

One of the last operations performed in the Toronto General Hospital without the benefit of anaesthesia has been described by a student of J. H. Richardson:

> Old Tom was the janitor; he had been a sailor, was wounded at the Battle of Trafalgar and had his leg amputated at the hip and suffered from the most horrible attacks of sciatica. He was not a very satisfactory janitor. He was gruff, and very deaf. On fine days he spent his time on the lawn under the trees with a long clay pipe in his mouth and in foul weather he retired to his room or somewhere out of sight and presumably continued to smoke. He eventually developed cancer of the tongue. Dr. James H. Richardson operated, removing the tongue with the ecraseur. Old Tom refused an anaesthetic. He said with a nail between his teeth he stood the amputation of his leg and so he could stand this. And he did, giving a responsive groan at each tightening twist of the instrument till the tongue came off, when Dr. Richardson, placing it on the table, turned to the students and said "You see of what our sailors are composed." The next morning Old Tom was under the trees smoking his pipe as usual.[1]

At a meeting of the Academy of Medicine, Toronto, at the time of Lister's death in 1912, those who contributed to the evening vied with one another in presenting the impact of Lister's work on practice at the General Hospital. Dr. George A. Bingham recalled that in the pre-Listerian era it was routine after the amputation of a limb to place a tourniquet higher up, which could be promptly tightened when, almost invariably, the dreaded secondary haemorrhage occurred as a result of suppuration of the stump:

> I can remember when a clinic consisted of a rabble of students following a professor about the foetid smelling ward while he examined unhealed wounds with unwashed hands; then after lower-

[1]Clarke, *A History of the T.G.H.*, p. 84.

> ing his olfactory organ to the reeking stump he would straighten himself up and declare to the class "gentlemen, this pus is laudable." Yet the patients died just the same. I remember the preparation of a fashionable surgeon for a major operation consisted in turning back the cuffs of his Prince Albert coat, which was preferably an old one, and washing his hands in a very perfunctory way at the tap. The usual treatment for compound fracture was an amputation, otherwise the patient would die, as he often did anyway. I recollect that during one whole winter session the abdominal cavity was opened on only three occasions, with two deaths.

Dr. R. B. Nevitt recalled his service as an interne in the Hospital:

> As yet there was no official recognition of the surgeon as distinct from the physician. Hodder, Aikens and Bethune admitted and attended medical cases just as Geikie, Henry Wright, and Thorburn did surgical work.
>
> The operations consisted principally of amputations or the removal of tumours from accessible parts. Sometimes soap and water were used timidly. Most often the patient with a suppurating wound, inflamed, poisonous and gangrenous, was brought down and on the table the vast stinking poultice was removed with its stench and ordure and the limb was amputated. Instruments and basins were cleaned after the operation in the manner of a camper washing his dinner dishes, and then put away for the next operation. The silk and linen thread used for ligatures was cut to convenient lengths as it came from the shop and often passed through the buttonhole of my coat to be reached for use by the operating surgeon when required to tie a vessel or put in a suture. Scissors and probes were wiped on a towel or bandage and used again without special preparation. I carried in the upper pocket of my vest a probe, a pair of scissors, a pair of dissecting forceps and a scalpel and would only wash them in water if it was handy. Dr. Bethune had a case which I now recognize as being one of appendiceal abscess, and who was desperately ill. The belly wall was tight and protuberant, the skin slightly oedematous in the region of the superior spine of the ilium. "Pus there, ought to let it out." Without a word I put my hand in my vest pocket and pulled out a scalpel and Dr. Bethune cut down upon the abscess and gave vent with explosive violence to a vast quantity of stinking pus, gas and faecal matter. And this patient got well. During an operation the favourite place for the knife when it was out of use was in the surgeon's mouth to prevent the danger of its edge being dulled by contact with the table.[2]

The memories of these distressing situations possibly had such a dramatic appeal to those who had viewed them in their earlier days that, comparing them with a lifetime experience of steadily improving

[2]*Canadian Journal of Medicine and Surgery*, May 1912.

conditions, they did not modify the story with any recognition of successful work done by some surgeons who must have appreciated to a real degree the value of aseptic cleanliness. Beaumont, Hodder, and Aikens were not successful by pure chance.

At any rate it did not take very long for Lister's teaching to begin to affect surgical practice at the Toronto General Hospital. Although it may not have been the first operation performed with this routine, the first available record describes the removal of a large fibrocystic tumour of the parotid gland by E. M. Hodder on October 17, 1868, with the following details:

> A female patient, 59 years of age, gave a history of tumour developing over a period of 16 years. The removal of the tumour was comparatively easy and after haemostatic control was established the cut surfaces were wiped over with carbolic acid in oil . . . and a strip of lint soaked in a similar solution was laid over the cut edges and kept in place by a few strips of plaster and a bandage. A week later it was noted that "there has not been any suppuration, even in the course of the ligatures." This patient left hospital in a month with a well healed wound but with facial paralysis.[3]

From all accounts the early days of anaesthesia were fraught with great uncertainty and constant risk. On January 15, 1863, the *Evening Leader* reported an inquest held in the Toronto General Hospital on the body of Richard Humphries, who had died while under the influence of chloroform. This was said to have been the first fatality of its kind in the hospital in a period of over fifteen years, occurring when Hodder, with the assistance of Beaumont, was removing a tumour of undefined nature and location, of which the patient said "As soon as he attempted to walk it became painful and inflamed." The fatalistic reaction to anaesthesia prompted the patient to remark as he faced the operation that he was "prepared to die as all should be who got operated under the influence of chloroform." Dr. Bovell, who gave the anaesthetic, described the efforts made to resuscitate the patient, which included applying the poles of a galvanic battery to the neck and to the pit of the stomach to stimulate the phrenic nerve. Section of the jugular vein was performed to relieve cerebral congestion, which was thought to be a factor in the patient's condition. This only removed two ounces of blood, because by this time the patient was dead. The verdict exonerated "the medical gentlemen from any blame as it was obvious that

[3]*Dominion Medical Journal*, I (1869). See also C. G. Roland in *Journal of the History of Medical and Allied Sciences*, XX (1967).

the greatest care and skill had been exercised in this case."

As has already been indicated, specialization was largely nominal, and it was therefore natural that a competent surgeon like Hodder should treat many patients suffering from conditions beyond his particular specialty. He reported a successful operation performed in the General Hospital for traumatic epilepsy on a boy of seventeen, who had suffered a markedly depressed fracture of the skull from the kick of a horse when he was eight years old. After trephining, the depressed bone was forced outward and partly broken off. The patient recovered promptly and was sent home "entirely cured of his trouble."

In those days ovariotomy was the most frequently performed abdominal operation. Hodder, the Professor of Midwifery and Diseases of Women in a succession of local medical schools and a senior member of the staffs of both the General Hospital and the Burnside Lying-In Hospital, had considerable experience with this procedure and reported a series of ovariotomies performed between 1869 and 1871. Some of these operations were performed in the General Hospital, but he evidently preferred to operate in the Matron's private room in the Lying-In Hospital or in a private home. He took a conservative approach to operative treatment, saying that he had seen many cases in which medical treatment had kept a tumour in a chronic state for years. He reported an operating time of twenty minutes in a favourable case. Several tumours of tremendous size were successfully removed, drainage of the cystic content being routine with little regard to spillage into the abdominal cavity. It is remarkable that so many patients survived in spite of shock, dehydration, post-operative distension and very inefficient attempts to control pain with huge doses of opium and brandy. Anaesthesia was frequently unreliable and several operations were completed on semi-conscious patients receiving brandy when chloroform had caused severe dyspnoea and a very livid patient.[4]

William Beaumont's practice covered a wide range of surgery. In 1851 he reported a series of successful operations for cataract,[5] performed chiefly in the old King Street Hospital, and almost at the other extreme he reported three patients treated by lithotrity for large bladder calculi,[6] one of whom required fifteen repetitions of the procedure, eventually resulting in the removal of about a hundred fragments, this being the only patient who required chloroform anaesthesia. By com-

[4]*Canadian Lancet*, IV (1871).
[5]*Upper Canada Journal*, I (1851–52).
[6]*Canadian Lancet*, III (1870).

parison, Canniff, who at this time was Professor of Surgery at Victoria Medical School, and who was just beginning to develop his surgical practice, described the extreme difficulty he experienced in performing perineal lithotomy for a stone the size of a billiard ball. The patient, suffering from haemorrhage and shock, died post-operatively and to justify his experience Canniff quoted the mortality rate reported from London in the removal of stones of a similar size as being 1:1.57.

Canniff also reported a case of extensive cancer of the tongue, which he removed using an ecraseur applied through the floor of the mouth. It was the old story of a clay pipe smoker who had been treated by local applications until the tumour had grown to involve the whole side of the tongue, causing great pain. After removal of the tongue there was very little haemorrhage, and this was easily controlled by ice placed in the mouth. The patient was discharged within a month with the ability to utter words so as to be distinctly understood. As might be expected he returned seven months later with massive recurrence, and refusing further treatment, he went home again. In the final appraisal of this case it was claimed that intolerable pain had not recurred and some months of "perfect health had followed the operation."[7]

About this time W. T. Aikens was beginning to develop an ever-increasing surgical practice and had already given evidence of great competence and skill. He performed an operation on a seventy-year-old patient with evidence of ossification of the arteries, for a tumour that caused marked swelling of his face and which was found to involve the maxillary antrum, the floor of the orbit and also the "ethmoid bone." The superior maxilla was removed and the "whole diseased mass was carefully scooped out and the cavity filled with cotton and sutures applied to the flaps." On examination, the tumour "presented many of the features of incipient encephaloid disease." The patient was reported later to be "doing very well."[8]

Assisted by Dr. Beaumont, he removed a tumour the size of a man's fist from the orbit of an eight-year-old child. This required "scooping out the whole cavity." Microscopically this tumour was also described as encephaloid, and "although the boy is relieved of an offensive mass it is altogether likely that it will return in all virulence and ultimately secure its victim."[9]

[7]Canniff, *The Medical Profession in Upper Canada*, p. 203.
[8]*Canadian Lancet*, IV (1874).
[9]Charles Harris, "William Thomas Aikens," *Canadian Journal of Surgery*, V (April 1962).

About this time he also reported a scirrhus carcinoma of the breast which he removed by mastectomy with axillary gland dissection and a satisfactory primary result.[10]

Aikens made many contributions to newer methods of traumatic surgery, and the types of splints which he developed were still in use thirty or forty years later.[11] Among his pupils were several who were to be outstanding members of the surgical staff of the hospital long after the conclusion of the First Great War.

Dr. Herbert A. Bruce in later years described his experience when Aikens, still appreciating the lingering danger of the hospital operating room, undertook an osteoplastic operation in a patient's home. The operation, which was performed on the kitchen table, began early in the morning:

> The surgeon removed his coat, turned up the cuffs of his shirt, washed his hands and dipped them in a solution of bichloride, put his instruments in a solution of carbolic acid and after a few minutes transferred them to a dish of boiled water. He then proceeded to operate. My student friend and I took turns holding up the arm. He made a vertical incision over the projecting elbow joint and then with a small saw carefully removed the end of the humerus and the ulna which constituted the bony joint, afterwards dissecting out the remaining synovial membranes, all of which were involved. When this was completed he closed the skin and covered it with a dressing.
>
> Although observing some of the Listerian measures of antisepsis, whenever Dr. Aikens wanted to "park" his knife he put it between his teeth!
>
> From the length of time taken it is obvious that he worked with great deliberation. At 1:00 o'clock the mother of the patient called to say that lunch was ready. So after instructions to the anaesthetist to "keep her under" the 3 of us went and had a hearty meal, returning later to relieve the anaesthetist. After about an hour's delay the operation proceeded and it was finished about 4:00 o'clock.

Dr. Bruce reported with satisfaction that the patient, as a result of the operation, had a movable elbow joint.[12]

Dislocations were reduced by manipulations which had become standardized and simple fractures of the lower limb were treated by suspension and continuous traction. With Lister's technique, compound fractures healed slowly but many useful limbs resulted, which would have been sacrificed by amputation a few years before.

There was an unique association between the invention of the

[10] *Ibid.*

[11] *Ibid.*

[12] Herbert A. Bruce, *Varied Operations* (Toronto: Longmans, Green, 1958).

ophthalmoscope and the birth of the first pure specialty in medical practice. With this instrument and his knowledge of the physiology and anatomy of the eye and ear, Helmholtz gave a scientific basis for the work of physicians in a highly technical field of practice. Up to this time general surgeons removed cataracts and treated traumatic lesions of the eye, but now ophthalmologists and aurists took over the care of patients suffering from all conditions affecting both the eye and the ear. In 1875 R. A. Reeve, a medical graduate of Queen's University, Kingston, and later trained in Britain, became the first specialist in this field to be appointed to the staff of the Toronto General Hospital. He had already served as an assistant surgeon at the Toronto Eye and Ear Infirmary and he demonstrated his considerable experience when he published accounts of the surgical treatment of glaucoma,[13] showing a surprising recognition of the proper approach to the problems of this disease. Many patients with a chronic state of this lesion were benefited for considerable periods of time by operative treatment.

The medical treatment of patients did not change so dramatically. It was obvious, however, that the diagnosis of disease had markedly improved. The primitive sphygmograph presented pulse tracings indicating cardiovascular disease, hitherto only recognized by palpation, percussion and auscultation. While specific therapy was still a long way off, cause and effect were being increasingly recognized.

A lecture by Dr. W. B. Geikie, Professor of the Practice of Physick and Clinical Medicine at Victoria University and a medical officer of the hospital, indicated clearly the change toward more rational treatment. Its title was "A few observations on the Past and Present Employment of Bleeding in the Treatment of Fever and Inflammatory Disease." "Coming to our own times," said Geikie, "the most modern authorities differ widely as to the value and necessity of the lancet in acute diseases," and quoted Dr. Aikens "that we should so bleed as to secure the advantages of the remedy and avoid its disadvantages." His final conclusion was that "full and recent observations prove that measures tending to reduce the general strength in disease are, as a rule, more injurious while appropriate medicine and sufficient support with or without stimulation as may be required will secure all that skill can accomplish and show a far lower mortality than 'King Lancet could ever boast'."[14]

[13]*Canadian Lancet*, IV (1871–1872).

[14]W. B. Geikie, "A Few Observations on the Past and Present Employment of Bleeding in the Treatment of Fever and Inflammatory Disease," *Lancet* (1857).

Physical agents were a dominant factor in the treatment of most diseases. R. B. Nevitt recalled the treatment of pneumonia when he was a house physician:

> When the respirations were 45 and the temperature 104 and 105, the patients were raised up in a sitting posture to enable the nurse to properly apply the poultice, and what was still worse, the weaker the patient got the oftener the poultice was applied. If the patient survived for five or six days, the next thing to be done was to sponge him with soap and water and then apply a fly blister. After the blister was on from six to eight hours it was removed. A poultice was again applied and, as soon as the part was healed another blister was applied. On the other hand, if the patient lingered for a long time and did not respond to this treatment there were a few physicians who would introduce a seton and have it turned round daily, to the great discomfort of the sufferer.[15]

The segregation of patients with infectious diseases was haphazard, and it was only in 1868 that a letter was written to the mayor offering the services of the medical staff if the old House of Refuge could be prepared to receive patients with small-pox, which was epidemic in the city that year. Up to this time they had been admitted to a ward in the hospital with no isolation routine, and as very few patients would submit to vaccination, patients frequently contracted the disease in hospital, some with fatal results.

Sanitary conditions in the city continued to be very bad. Various articles in the *Leader* of 1871 showed that little improvement had occurred in twenty years. In October Mr. Carr, the recently appointed City Commissioner, recommended that scavenger carts should be employed to remove garbage from the lanes and streets, and he reported that

> contractors for night soil have emptied upward of thirty water closets from premises complained of. A number of piggeries have been disposed of and a number of parties have been allowed time by the City Commissioner to dispose of their animals. Between five hundred and six hundred head of cattle have been impounded. The suppression of slaughter houses and butcher shops requires a great deal of time and attention.[16]

A long editorial entitled "Imperfect Drainage" appealed for the provision of pure water and better drainage facilities: "It is next to

[15]Clarke, *A History of the T.G.H.*, p. 83.
[16]*Leader*, November 10, 1871.

impossible to over-estimate the great importance of proper drainage, more especially in this neighbourhood, for most of the people obtain the water from dug wells and the earth being impregnated with the foul sewers must necessarily contaminate the water in this vicinity."[17] The alternative to well water was Toronto Bay, into which all the main sewers of the city emptied. It was no wonder, therefore, that typhoid fever had a seasonal recurrence and was becoming the major epidemic disease.

Hospital records show that service to the patients improved steadily, if slowly. In the first place, the duties and responsibilities of the Resident Physician and Surgeon were becoming clearly defined. Originally, with poor roads and lack of communication, his most urgent service had been to meet the crises that beset many of the patients, and his co-operation was often the major factor in their survival, considering the rather infrequent visits of the attending physicians.

There are no records regarding the service of Dr. J. Gardiner, who became the Resident Physician after the death of Dr. Edward Clarke, but he trained his nephew, W. B. Hampton, to succeed him in 1863 and this very young man served the hospital with faithful industry during the years of the closure and the reopening of the hospital. Reference has already been made to the manner in which he shouldered considerable responsibility when Mr. Brent's office was some miles away from the hospital. He died in August 1871—almost literally, according to the *Leader* obituary, from overwork—and the tribute paid to him showed that many were aware of the important services rendered by the Resident Physician.

Following Hampton's death, Dr. J. H. McCollum was chosen from nine applicants for the position of Resident Medical Officer, and he received his appointment on a yearly basis. He had been a student at the Toronto School of Medicine, graduating from the University of Toronto with honours and the silver medal in 1869. He practised in the country before coming to the hospital, and the trustees soon came to rely on his judgment regarding many phases of their own responsibilities. Although he only held the appointment for five years, he succeeded in organizing the medical and nursing services on a very satisfactory basis.

After considerable discussion, more regular service to the hospital developed on the part of the active attending staff, which at that time

[17]*Ibid.*, December 2, 1871.

consisted of Edward Hodder, Norman Bethune, W. B. Geikie, William Canniff, James Thorburn, James Richardson, I. Cassidy and J. E. Graham. The clinical lectures at the hospital were consequently well attended and relations between the hospital and the faculties of the Toronto School of Medicine and Victoria and Trinity universities became reasonably satisfactory. The trustees, however, maintained that appointments to the staff of the hospital was their sole jurisdiction, refusing to be influenced by the frequent changes which took place in the faculties of the medical schools. The trustees and not the medical schools controlled the sale of tickets permitting students to receive clinical instruction at the hospital.

In 1872 Mr. J. T. Abbott was appointed as assistant to Dr. McCollum and two years later it was decided to hold competitive examinations for three annual appointments, the candidates sponsored by the three schools having had at least three years' training. Dr. McCollum, now designated Medical Superintendent, was authorized to lay down rules governing the behaviour of these medical assistants, who were to be entirely under his jurisdiction. The assistants were to carry out his orders and to report on the condition of patients day and night. All intimacies or familiarities with patients, nurses or servants were strictly forbidden and any infraction of this rule would be punished by instant dismissal. They were warned that they must keep in mind that the great object of the institution they served is "the relief of your sick and suffering fellow creatures." The steward was also made responsible to the medical superintendent and ordered to report to the visiting trustee for the week. He was also responsible for the time and wages of nurses and servants as directed by the lady superintendent. The medical superintendent was finally relieved of the responsibility of collecting debts of pay patients, as by this time the secretary had moved his office to the hospital building.

From the account given by R. B. Nevitt, the interns spent busy days and nights. He recalled making up eighty or ninety prescriptions daily, and although clinical reports were non-existent he made complete rounds of the patients morning and night, saw all new admissions, kept himself available to join the attending physicians on their rounds in hospital and also kept the daily list of the student attendance. It was during Dr. McCollum's time that the first pathologist, Dr. M. Hilary, was appointed, and he also became curator of the hospital museum. A new mortuary was built to the north of the main building and the space beneath the operating theatre was renovated to provide for the reception of out-patients and a new entrance for the students attending the hospital. Also, with Dr. Reeve's appointment to the staff special rooms were set apart for the reception and examination of patients suffering from eye and ear conditions.

Probably the most important change that took place affected the status and service of nurses. Miss Mary Hay was appointed as Matron in January 1869 at a salary of forty pounds per annum with board, lodging and fuel, and with her arrival the rising tide of "Nightingalism" began to show itself at the hospital. Within six months she was promoted to Lady Superintendent with an increase in her salary, and during the McCollum period of service the cooperation of Miss Hay and the Medical Superintendent laid the foundation which would culminate in the Training School for Nurses a few years later.

When the hospital re-opened in 1868, the cook and the washer-woman received nine dollars per month while the nurses only received eight, and in 1872 McCollum warned that two of his best nurses would resign because of their poor pay, which was then raised to nine dollars per month. R. B. Nevitt said that there were only two or three nurses with any experience and "they were the terror of the patients, the rest were raw and uncultured and many could do little more than write their names. Old Eliza was the senior and was on night duty. She was utterly useless, but she kept the patients in order and they would let her sleep all night."[18]

Up to this time the nurses' room had been below stairs but to improve their condition a ward was set aside for "the maids, scullions and nurses. Occasionally they became noisy and at times furiously quarrelling and on one occasion had to be threatened with the police."

The whole atmosphere of the hospital was changing and it is possible that the presence of good young assistants, interested in the clinical aspects of disease, encouraged a more intelligent nursing service. In December 1875 the board decided to purchase clinical thermometers for use in all the wards and about the same time articles began to appear in the current medical journals, often the work of the assistant house physicians, presenting the successes and failures of the attending staff of the hospital in the treatment of their patients, which did not suffer by comparison with other articles in the journals.

The Charity Aid Act which was passed by the Legislative Assembly of the Province of Ontario in 1874 was responsible for the great

[18]Clarke, *A History of the T.G.H.*, p. 87.

expansion of the Toronto General Hospital. No matter how arbitrary J. W. Langmuir's annual reports may appear to have been, there is no doubt of the ability and the over-all satisfactory manner with which he carried out his duties as the Inspector of Prisons, Asylums and Public Charities. It was he who recommended in 1876 the amalgamation of the several hospital charities of the city under one management, and this prompted the boards of the General Hospital, the Burnside Lying-In Hospital and the Toronto Eye and Ear Infirmary to start the discussion that led to the union of the three institutions.

The origin of the Burnside Hospital goes back to the early days of York, when the care of women in childbirth was a primary consideration. At a meeting of the Governesses of the Society for the Relief of Women during their Confinement, held at the Government House November 12, 1821, the following report was read and adopted:

> 12 months have elapsed since the establishment of the Society for the Relief of Women during their Confinement. The Governesses report their proceedings to the subscribers as the best means of declaring their continued patronage to so excellent a charity, a charity which was first suggested by several applications having been made to different ladies by women strangers without comforts or even a home when they expected to be confined. Their deplorable situation excited the powerful sympathy of the persons to whom they applied; and so it was resolved to form a general association for that purpose under the special patronage of Lady Sara Maitland. Upwards of thirty-four ladies signed the subscription paper and many gave sums which entitled them to become Governesses. Hardly were the requisite preparations finished when applications for relief were made by several women under circumstances of peculiar affliction. During November, the first month, three cases were relieved; one, a woman whose husband had been accidentally drowned a few months before leaving her with an infant and near her confinement with the second. To all these one of the Governesses (for each lady in turn discharges the duties of the Society during one month) sent comfortable clothing of all kinds, a midwife and a physician (if required) and the best nourishment. Proper dresses were likewise provided for the child. The consequence of this humane treatment was that the patient recovered rapidly. In December two women solicited and obtained from the Governess of the month, the benevolence of the Society and were frequently visited by her during their illness to see that everything was as comfortable as the situation of the patients would admit. The case of one woman who required assistance during the month was very distressing: her husband had died four months before her confinement leaving her with five young children. Applications were made almost every month; and during the year seventeen women

> have experienced the benevolence of the Society and what is a matter of grateful praise is that not one of the patients has died or experienced a tedious confinement. All this good has been accomplished with very little expense for the greater part of the subscription is laid out for such articles of clothing as were necessary for the mothers and children; some of which were given and some lent during the confinement. The economy practised by the Society has been, however, liberal and not parsimonious for the relieved will most willingly attest that no comfort was wanting that could contribute to their recovery.[19]

With the increasing number of poor immigrants arriving year after year and existing under appalling living conditions, the problem was ever-present. Although a number of women were admitted to the General Hospital for their confinements, these represented only a small percentage whose needs were very great. In 1832 the Medical Board of the hospital brought the situation to the notice of the Lieutenant-Governor:

> . . . The destitute condition in which many arrive and the unavoidable publicity of their scanty and crowded lodgings in which they are sometimes, inevitably exposed at an hour so critical and delicate, often rend their situation during their sufferings most distressing to their feelings and unpropitious to their recovery—
>
> Besides the benefits which would be afforded by such an institution to destitute strangers, it might be subservient to the instruction to students and midwives, being an object of pressing importance to the Province at large. . . .[20]

Considering the condition of the hospital in those days and the frequency with which even well-established lying-in hospitals were affected by apparently uncontrollable epidemics of puerperal fever, it was customary for women whose circumstances permitted to remain at home during their confinements. This preference also applied to physicians, even when faced with major complications of childbirth. A good example of this practice was reported in the first number of the *Upper Canada Journal of Medical, Surgical and Physical Science*, published in 1851, in which E. M. Hodder described "A Case of Apoplexy Terminating Fatally in which a Caesarean Section was Performed with a Favourable Result to the Child." The unconscious patient was obviously suffering from the effects of a major eclamptic

[19]Firth, *Town of York, 1815–1834*, p. 226.
[20]*Ibid.*, p. 236.

seizure, and failed to survive after bleeding, purging, blistering and poulticing, but Hodder, arriving at her home a few minutes after her death, delivered a living child by a prompt post-mortem section.

There were, however, a sufficient number of women going into the General Hospital to provide a nucleus for the teaching of midwifery, and in 1845 the Registrar of King's College wrote to the trustees complaining that the hospital did not provide accommodation for the students. In the discussion that followed it was proposed to remove the lying-in patients from the hospital and admit them to a specially equipped house where they would have the benefits of visits from the Professor of Midwifery and a resident pupil could be in constant attendance. On this basis the first lying-in hospital in Toronto was opened on June 1, 1848, on the northwest corner of Richmond and Victoria streets in a large two-storey house, which for many years was considered the best frame house in the town. The attending staff of this lying-in hospital consisted of E. M. Hodder, Lucius O'Brien and James Bovell and the first matron was Mrs. Jane Winter. Since it was entirely dependent upon public charity, this hospital was forced to close because of lack of financial support in 1865.

There was also for a time a maternity hospital on Adelaide Street West, associated with the Toronto School of Medicine. But it was the Provincial Lying-In Hospital and Vaccine Institute, located at Richmond and Shepherd streets, which continued in service over many years. Here G. S. Herrick, the Professor of Midwifery at the University of Toronto, gave lectures three days a week on Anatomy, Physiology, etc., and Natural and Unnatural Labour, and Diseases of Women and Children.

With the passage of time and the variations in the fortunes of the individual hospitals, the medical staffs finally became sorted out and associated with the surviving institution. When the question of amalgamation arose, the staff of what had come to be known as the Burnside Lying-In Hospital consisted of Doctors Hodder, Russell, Temple, Bethune and Grasett.

Various articles in the medical and lay press indicate the work that was being done in the Burnside Hospital. In 1869, eighty-eight patients were admitted and only one died, and the hospital showed a favourable financial statement with a balance of $670.

The year 1871 was an outstanding one. In the previous two years over two hundred patients had been admitted without a single death. The increase in numbers was attributed to the opening of a free ward in which sixteen patients had been cared for, these being so destitute as to require clothing before they could take their infants home. Investigation showed that whereas there had only been three newborn infant deaths in hospital, 65 of 112 infants who were taken home had died within the year. Maintenance cost at this time was twenty-two cents per day.

The next year the good record of the hospital was broken by an epidemic of puerperal fever. There were three deaths, forcing a temporary closure of the hospital.

In 1874, in addition to the bill which was passed by the legislature to govern the appropriation of funds to charitable institutions, another bill was passed to legalize the incorporation of the trustees or managing officers of benevolent societies which would be receiving funds for the support of their institutions. Edward Hodder, M.D., Sarah Grasett, the Directress, Frances Hodder and ten other ladies were empowered by this act to be a "Body Politic," to be known as the "Burnside Lying-In Hospital of Toronto," and the women involved with the hospital could trace their organization back over a period of fifty years.

It was undoubtedly through the benevolence of Dr. Alexander Burnside that the financial security of the hospital had been established. He was an enigmatic figure. There is no record suggesting that he had any particular interest in midwifery. But it is altogether likely that his generosity was influenced by his nearby neighbour on Adelaide Street, Dean H. J. Grasett of St. James Cathedral, who held a responsible post on the governing body of the Lying-In Hospital, and by Burnside's personal appreciation of the work of the Ladies' Benevolent Society.

Born in New Hampshire in 1779, Burnside had come to York and appeared before the Upper Canada Medical Board in January 1820. The board found him unfit to practise and recommended further study. Two years later he was found qualified to practise and obtained his licence. The medical historian Canniff wrote:

> A trustworthy informant says of him "an American by birth, of no education and one considered by all medical men of standing a Yankee quack. The country people seemed to think that he had a knowledge of local fevers, etc., and employed him. His practice was never large at any time but he acquired considerable property. During the first cholera epidemic he was the outstanding witness for the defendants upon an indictment for nuisances; always proving to the satisfaction of the jurors that the stench complained of, whether it arose from stables, tanneries, privy vaults or any other abomination, was conducive to health. At least he found it so in his practice.

Another said of him that he had for a time a large practice up Yonge Street. He was capable of selling water at a penny a pail; an ignorant man, but a money maker. Fine looking, portly, neat, tidy, he always wore a large gold seal.

Dr. Scadding has described him in a more attractive form:

> a New England medical man, of tall figure, upright carriage and bluff, benevolent countenance. An early promoter of the Mechanics Institute movement and an encourager of church music, vocal and instrumental. Dying without a family dependent upon him, he bequeathed his property, partly to charity in the town and partly to the University of Trinity College, where two scholarships perpetuate his memory; in fact, he donated the greater portion of his property to Trinity College.
>
> Notwithstanding all animadversions, the fact remains that Dr. Burnside's benevolence and charitable bequests entitle his memory to the greatest respect. The relief which has been and will continue to be afforded at the Burnside Lying-In Department of the General Hospital is beyond human estimation and can only be weighed by an Almighty Hand. He died December 13th, 1854 in his seventy-fifth year.[21]

The students of Trinity College attended his funeral as a group and on his monument in St. James' Cemetery this tribute is engraved:

> Beneath this pillar rest the mortal
> remains of Alexander Burnside, Esquire,
> A sincere christian and a faithful
> member of the Church of England.
> Born in the United States while yet
> Colonies he rejoiced in being a
> British subject and on completing
> his medical education hastened to
> Canada to claim and enjoy his
> privileges. In this city he followed
> the practice of medicine for nearly
> forty years and by frugal industry
> and patient assiduity acquired a
> considerable fortune which notwith-
> standing his strict exactness in
> business he distributed with a
> generosity rarely equalled in any
> community, devoting nearly the whole
> to charitable and religious purposes.

During the summer of 1877 arrangements for the amalgamation of

[21]Canniff, *The Medical Profession in Upper Canada*, pp. 273–274.

the Burnside Hospital with the Toronto General proceeded without delay. Dean H. J. Grasett, at this time the chief trustee of the Burnside Hospital, gave a deed for the Burnside property to the trustees of the General Hospital, who agreed, on assuming the assets of the Burnside Hospital with their nominal value of $11,500, to erect a suitable hospital in connection with the General Hospital, having forty beds and with proper provision for isolation in case of infectious diseases. The building was to be called the "Burnside Lying-In Hospital" and the entire economic and medical control was to be in the hands of the trustees of the Toronto General Hospital. The present medical staff was to continue its service under the new management and the lady managers of the Burnside, who up to this time had been the governing body of that hospital, were empowered to organize a visiting committee to impart "moral and religious instruction to the patients to their full satisfaction."

It was decided to erect the new building in the northwest part of the hospital grounds on land repurchased by the Hospital Trust. The new building had an external appearance in keeping with the main building and the accepted tenders amounted to $10,587. The trustees authorized an issue of debentures through Pellatt and Osler for $10,000 to cover this expense, and the new Burnside Hospital was opened on October 2, 1878. By this time the trustees had rented the old building and land on Shepherd Street to the Mechanics Institute to provide a temperance restaurant, library, reading room and coffee room, the object being "to entice young men away from the snares of the bar-room and give them in its place the means of spending a pleasant and profitable evening."

With the amalgamation of the Burnside Hospital two distinguished surgeons were granted the unusual appointment of a lifetime membership on the active staff of the Toronto General Hospital without any designated service. Frederick Le Maitre Grasett, a Torontonian, had received his medical degree in Edinburgh and was the first Canadian to be a house surgeon under Joseph Lister. He had served on the staff of both Trinity College and the Burnside Lying-In Hospital, and during his long and active career he taught the principles which he had learned under Lister and also the great J. Y. Simpson. James Algernon Temple had graduated from McGill in 1865. After postgraduate training in England, where he received his M.R.C.S., he returned to practise with Dr. Edward M. Hodder, whom he succeeded as Professor of Obstetrics and Gynaecology at Trinity University in 1878. When Geikie resigned as Dean of the Medical Faculty, Temple served in this post at the time of the union of the faculties of Trinity and the University of Toronto.

A second development was the establishment of the Mercer Eye and Ear Infirmary. This took the form of a major extension of the main building towards the east. It was two storeys in height and provided waiting, examining and operating rooms for eye and ear patients and, on the floor above, a dining room and wards.

S. J. Stratford was the first ophthalmologist in Toronto, announcing his practice in 1850 as a surgeon, an accoucheur and an oculist. He established the first eye and ear infirmary at King and Church streets, but through lack of funds his venture failed in 1863. Shortly after this he gave up his practice and left the city.

Stratford was followed by a man who profited by the newly recognized status of ophthalmology. Abner Roseburgh, a graduate of Victoria College Medical School, with postgraduate training in New York and London, was not only a well-trained opthalmologist but had increased his knowledge by animal and mechanical research. He taught at both the Toronto School of Medicine and Victoria University. In 1865 he invented an ophthalmoscope with which he could photograph the fundus of the eye. Produced locally in Toronto, it sold for $10. Later he became interested in electrotherapeutics and designed various original forms of equipment for use in this field.

In 1865 he opened the Toronto Eye and Ear Dispensary at Yonge and Adelaide streets, announcing that "the poor will receive gratuitous treatment every Tuesday and Friday."[22] In 1867 he was joined by his brother-in-law, R. A. Reeve, and the report in the *Dominion Medical Journal* showed that 224 patients had been admitted in the first two years and that an appreciable number of patients described as "quite blind" benefited from the treatment they received.[23] In 1870 this institution was moved to Adelaide Street and accommodation was provided for sixteen intern patients as the result of an annual grant from the provincial legislature of $1,000. In the previous two years 108 operations had been performed: 39 for iridectomy and 20 for cataract. The charge for intern patients was three dollars per week, private patients not being admitted as "the institution is for the poor only."

The infirmary was constantly overcrowded, and Inspector John Langmuir drew this to the attention of the government. Although Roseburgh continued to claim that diseases of the eye and ear were

[22]*Leader*, February 3, 1865.
[23]*Dominion Medical Journal*, II (1870).

more likely to be successfully treated in special institutions rather than in general hospitals, the trustees of the Toronto General Hospital were approached and asked to consider building a new infirmary in connection with the hospital. Naturally this led to a request for a special building grant, which was approved by the legislature on condition that the new building should be known as the Andrew Mercer Infirmary in memory of the man whose estate would provide the money necessary for this extension to the General Hospital.

Andrew Mercer was a Scotsman who had come to Canada with Chief Justice Scott. He received a Crown grant of considerable land, living in a cottage on the southeast corner of what are now Wellington and Bay streets. In 1810 he ran a small general store in partnership with Samuel Ridout, and for some time towards the end of the War of 1812 the *York Gazette and Oracle* was printed in his cottage. In 1830 he was appointed a "Marrying Agent" and became a Justice of the Peace in 1833. For many of his later years he kept as a housekeeper Bridget O'Reilly by whom he had a son about twenty years before his death. When he died in 1871 he left an estate valued at $150,000, but being intestate and without recognized heirs, this was escheated to the Crown. Some time later, however, his son, Andrew Mercer, Jr., together with a law student named Reynolds, claimed to have found in the leaves of an old book in the cottage a scrap of paper six inches long and two inches wide on which was inscribed in the shaky hand of old age:

> June 7th, 1871. In case I should die before my son should return or before I have time to make my will, I wish James Smyth and Charles Unwin to have my estate divided between my wife and son.
>
> ANDREW MERCER

This claim came before the Surrogate Court and besides Andrew Mercer, Jr., being represented, a Mr. McGregor appeared for the housekeeper who claimed to have been married to Andrew Mercer on June 25, 1851, by the Rev. Father O'Reilly, the parish priest of the Gore of Toronto, a month before her son was born. As Father O'Reilly was now dead Bishop Lynch was called to verify the marriage record in the parish registry, which he did, recognizing the handwriting. Nevertheless the Court discredited the validity of the will and the case was finally taken to the Privy Council in England, who ruled that the province had complete right to the Mercer estate. The Crown, however, made a grant to the housekeeper of $12,000 and a further $30,000 was given to her son and his family.

The satisfactory result of this contentious matter was expressed in a resolution of the trustees of the Toronto General Hospital on May 14, 1878:

> That the Trustees of the Toronto General Hospital gratefully accept the donation of $10,000.00 made by the Government of the Province of Ontario out of the Estate of the late Andrew Mercer to be applied towards the construction of an eye and ear Infirmary on the grounds belonging to the said General Hospital. The above donation to be subject to the conditions attached thereto by the Legislature, providing amongst other things that the Infirmary shall be called "The Andrew Mercer Eye and Ear Infirmary."

The tenders, when received, showed that the cost of this extensive addition to the hospital containing examining, reception and operating rooms, with a dining room and wards for the eye and ear patients, would amount to $17,500. Fortunately the hospital's finances were in a satisfactory state, and building proceeded to completion about a year after the Burnside Hospital.

The establishment of the Mercer Infirmary marked the parting of the ways for the brothers-in-law, Roseburgh and Reeve. While the latter as a result of his appointment two years previously to the staff of the General Hospital became the senior member of the staff of the Mercer Infirmary as it developed, Roseburgh continued his work for many years at the Toronto Eye and Ear Infirmary. During a long lifetime his interest broadened, and in addition to electrotherapy he took an active part in prison reform and founded The Ontario Society for the Reformation of Inebriates.

The third major addition to the hospital undertaken at this time was the so-called "Fever Hospital," an addition to the west of the main block comparable in size to the Mercer Infirmary. The contributions of William Gooderham, Sr., James Worts and William Cawthra, amounting in all to $13,500, were more than sufficient to cover the expense entailed, and the wards provided in this two-storey building allowed ample room for the segregation of patients suffering from infectious diseases. The over-all result more than doubled the front of the main building as it faced Gerrard Street, and at the east end quarters were erected for the Medical Superintendent, with an entrance from Sumach Street. As an added satisfaction, a trolley was installed running the full length of the basement for the transportation of food and supplies.

On May 3, 1879, the trustees, well satisfied with all that had been accomplished, made a final payment to the architects, Stewart and Strickland, of $650 for their good services in planning and supervising the building of the new laundry, the fever hospital, the Burnside Hospital and the Eye and Ear Infirmary. Consideration was also given to raising the salaries of the Medical Superintendent, the Lady Superintendent and the Secretary in view of their added responsibilities. The trustees also agreed to allow the Mechanics Institute to sell ale and lager beer in their club, located in the old Burnside building on Shepherd Street, to bona fide members, as an added defence against the temptations of strong drink. About the same time, and probably prompted by the same motive, the trustees directed that in lieu of the pint of beer available to nurses and servants each day, those who chose to give it up should receive one dollar per month in addition to their usual wages.

VII

A Good Triumvirate

WHEN DR. J. H. MCCOLLUM AND MISS MARY HAY, THE LADY Superintendent, resigned at the end of 1875 the trustees were faced with the replacement of two highly efficient administrators. In the case of Dr. McCollum there was no delay, as the board offered the post of Medical Superintendent to Dr. Charles O'Reilly of Hamilton, who accepted promptly.

This appointment received the approval of the Inspector of Hospitals and many of the medical practitioners in the city, but met with a vigorous protest from the Chairman of the Board, the Hon. John Macdonald, who claimed that the decision had been made too hastily and should have followed a public request for applications. Since this brought into question the legality of Dr. O'Reilly's appointment, the whole procedure was referred to the hospital's solicitor, Mr. Clarke Gamble. Mr. Gamble endorsed the action of the board, but recommended that the appointment of the medical superintendent, the lady superintendent, the secretary and the steward should be considered on a different basis from the hiring of servants and other employees. To avoid both public criticism and the real danger of favouritism, the vacancy should be advertised and applications invited, and such an appointment should only be made after special consideration by the board. Following this advice, the board amended the by-laws of the General Hospital accordingly, and henceforth, appointments were considered only at special meetings of the board.

There was no question regarding the qualifications of Dr. O'Reilly, for he had established an outstanding reputation after nine years' service at the Hamilton City Hospital. He was the son of a medical practitioner in Hamilton and an 1867 graduate of McGill University and it was felt, therefore, that he would not have any inherent prejudice regarding the merits of the staffs of the various Schools of Medicine in Toronto. He was appointed for a period of one year at a salary of $1,000 per annum with apartments and subsistence allowance, though the garden which up to that time had been for the use of the superintendent and the lady superintendent was now to become a vegetable garden to supply the hospital. Within three years he thoroughly vindicated the choice which had been made, and received a permanent appointment at a yearly salary of $1,500.

At one of the first meetings which Dr. O'Reilly attended, the board requested that the gentlemen now composing the medical staff should constitute themselves an organized deliberating body under a suitable name, with a presiding officer and secretary to be elected annually. All the members of the medical staff were to be members of this body and no other. Stated meetings were to be held to consider matters connected with the medical management of the hospital, and the result forwarded to the trustees in the form of recommendations for adoption by the board. This association was to be permanent and so available all the time. The board would not pledge itself to adopt all or any of the recommendations, but would give them "respectful consideration." The board requested that they should give their opinion at the present time on:

1) The number of medical officers required for the institution;
2) the classification thereof;
3) the mode and time of attendance;
4) the classification of the patients and wards;
5) the development of a pharmacopeia;
6) the adoption of a system of written instructions to the nurses for every patient so that the matron might see that they were carried out.
7) the desirability of having the students, other than resident clinical clerks, receive all their clinical instruction in the theatre instead of the present system of going through the wards.

This was the first authorization of a medical advisory board, and became the basis for a much closer association between the lay Board of Trustees and the medical staff. It also brought the teaching function of the hospital more clearly into focus.

At this time the pharmacopoeia of the General Hospital was published. In spite of its modest size, it was not only of great importance to the hospital but became the vade-mecum of successive classes of students and of graduate physicians. It purported to contain "the prescriptions in use in the various Departments and an epitome of surgical and obstetrical techniques and tables of foods, doses and poisons." In those days before the time when the great pharmaceutical houses provided all-embracing preparations to treat every disease, the most important room, next to the doctor's consulting room, was his dispensary, with its bottle-laden walls and mortar and pestle in which he produced the "medicines" that were largely the basis for his local reputation. It followed as a matter of course that the pharmacopoeia in his pocket, soon joined by Osler's *Principles and Practice of Medicine* on his book-shelf, brought comfort and reassurance in time of doubt to many a troubled physician.

In accordance with the recently amended by-laws an advertisement was published in the newspapers for a lady superintendent to replace Miss Hay. The notice stated that the duties of the lady superintendent were defined by the by-laws, subject to such modification as the trustees might order from time to time, but added that they involved chiefly the supervision of the domestic economy of the hospital ("the Steward has charge of stores and provisions"). The salary of $320 per annum was to be paid monthly, and separate apartment, board, etc., would be provided.

Miss Harriet Goldie, the successful applicant, was appointed Lady Superintendent early in 1876. During the interval before she took over her duties Miss Mary Mulkins, one of the senior nurses of the hospital, took on the responsibilities and had the opportunity to advise the trustees that a head nurse should be appointed to serve under the lady superintendent and to be responsible for the management of the wards and nurses. She recommended Miss Eliza Storie, who had been trained in King's College Hospital, London, England, and suggested that her wages should begin at ten dollars per month. Miss Mulkins' experience also prompted her to recommend that each patient should have a towel to himself instead of having to use one of the two long roller towels now available in the wards. Miss Storie's service was so satisfactory that two months later she was appointed deputy matron and head nurse, with a salary increase of two dollars per month.

Miss Goldie was without any hospital experience, but she had considerable administrative ability and was well aware of the quality of nursing service required at the Toronto General Hospital. Her first innovation was to require all the nurses to wear uniform dresses while on duty, and the following year she asked the trustees to establish a nurses' training school. The trustees were duly impressed, and, to study the question, set up a committee consisting of W. H. Howland, the Chairman of the Board, W. T. O'Reilly and Mr. John Gillespie. A few months later Dr. Charles O'Reilly was sent to visit the principal schools for nurses in the U.S.A. and on his return plans for the development of the school proceeded steadily. The board approved a set of by-laws to govern the school and an advertisement was placed in the daily papers announcing that the school would open on February 1, 1879, and inviting applications from prospective pupils.

It was not an easy matter to change from a system of nursing that had depended on many untrained individuals to the discipline of a training school. By this time, however, there were an increasing number of nurses on duty in the hospital who had previously received training in British or American hospitals, and a training school had already been established in the General and Marine Hospital of St. Catharines.

It took two years to organize the new school, which was officially opened on April 1, 1881. The Chairman of the Board of Trustees, now Mr. Justice C. S. Patterson, and Dr. Charles O'Reilly made the final arrangements which provided that the cost of furnishings must not exceed $600. Miss Goldie and Miss Storie were each to receive $100 a year for their extra responsibilities, and nurses already on duty at the hospital were invited to receive instruction provided they were willing to enrol for two years. The nurses were to receive five dollars a month, with uniform, caps and aprons, and nine dollars a month during the second year when they would receive a certificate and a silver badge after passing an oral examination. Certificated nurses remaining on duty in the hospital were to receive twelve dollars a month with their uniforms.

By the end of the year Miss Goldie presented her report to the Board of Trustees on the work done by the nurses and probationers during the previous seven months:

> Since the first of April a thorough system of instruction has been given to the nurses in the wards by Miss Storie and lectures twice a week on the most important points in nursing. On that date the nurses numbered 17. Since then 2 have married, 2 have left on account of insubordination, 2 through incapacity and 1 from ill health, 1 to return to her family, leaving at the present time 9 who are giving entire satisfaction. Each nurse has been changed from medical to surgical wards, remaining on each not less than a period of 3 months, also taking her time on night duty. They all had a fortnight's

holiday. Six have been present at 6 cases each at the Burnside, 3 were nursing in private families altogether for 7 weeks, where their attention and care of the patients were highly spoken of by the attending physicians. Ten probationers have entered since June 1st, 6 are still in the hospital, intelligent, competent women who are likely to prove valuable nurses. Two left through ill-health and one was unable to perform the duties required of her. A large number of pupils is much needed for though many apply few are found suitable and the demand for skilful trained nurses is daily increasing. Sincere thanks are returned by Miss Storie and myself for the kind help and co-operation given, not only by the medical staff, but by several of the attending physicians who have taken much trouble to explain to the nurses the different cases and treatments required.

November 18, 1881 (Signed) HARRIET GOLDIE
Lady Superintendent

The uniform that was adopted at this time consisted of a princess-style dress of washable material made with a long train worn in the morning, and a dress of gray lustre with a bow of blue ribbon at the throat for the afternoon. The nurse's headdress at this time was a large muslin mob-cap.

The nurses served the meals in the wards and washed the dishes as well. They were allowed one hour off duty each day, one afternoon each week and one half of every alternate Sabbath. Their dining-room was in the hospital basement and the sleeping rooms were scattered throughout the hospital, some in the west wing, some in the attic, and some in the Eye and Ear Department. A few years later a large room was furnished and set aside as a sitting-room, and by means of contributions from the nurses a piano was rented for the next two years.

Miss Goldie, whose health was not good, retired as Lady Superintendent at midsummer, 1883, and was succeeded by her assistant, Miss Storie, who by this time had become Mrs. Fulford. But difficulty in the arrangements to provide accommodation for her husband prompted her resignation. In March 1884, Miss Lucy Pickett, a graduate of the Massachusetts General Hospital, was appointed. During Miss Pickett's short term of office the duties and responsibilities of the Lady Superintendent were more clearly defined. She was to have the supervision of domestic arrangements, including servants and nurses—her supervision extending, in fact, to everything appertaining to the nurses, wards, housework and supplies, including the enforcement of discipline among all who came under her supervision. She was to superintend and sit at the table with the medical assistants. In all matters she was to be directly responsible to the Medical Superintendent. At this time it was also decided that "a proper man" should be appointed to assist in the wards and to be under the orders of the Lady Superintendent. This was, in effect, the appointment of the first orderly at the Toronto General Hospital.

The short tenure of office of Mrs. Fulford and Miss Pickett must have caused the trustees and medical staff considerable concern. But this situation came to an end when Miss Mary Snively took up her duties towards the end of 1884. Born in St. Catharines, she began her career as a school teacher, but was influenced towards nursing by friends on the staff of the General and Marine Hospital in St. Catharines. She trained at the Bellevue Hospital in New York, graduating in 1884, and only a few months later she was appointed Lady Superintendent to the Toronto General Hospital. From the first, her dominant personality was to make her a tradition in the training school of the hospital. Unsparing of herself, she was an inspiration to her nurses and a constant challenge to the medical staff to co-operate with her in providing the practical and theoretical training essential to the knowledge of a professional nurse.

In 1887 the new Nurses' Residence was opened. The building was erected on the west front of the main hospital and connected to it by a covered bridge. It contained double bedrooms, a dining-room, "two prettily furnished parlours with a piano" (the gift of some benevolent friends of the school) and a medical and general library. This building was the outward and visible sign of the important place the Training School had taken in the function of the General Hospital.

Four years later the trustees published the first regular Annual Report from the hospital, giving medical and statistical information of interest to the public, including news of the great progress of the Training School. In the last year there had been 600 applicants for training, of whom 67 were accepted on probation; 38 of these proved satisfactory and were admitted to the school. Compared with 16 nurses in the school in 1881, there were now two permanent nurses, 55 nurses in training and 5 probationers—a total of 62. In ten years 131 nurses had graduated, of whom 29 held positions on hospital staffs and 5 were foreign missionaries. Members of the medical staff were giving lectures in anatomy, surgery, diseases of the lungs, eye and ear, throat and nose, obstetrics, gynaecology, dermatology, materia medica and therapeutics, the problems of nursing phthisis as well as typhoid fever and other contagious diseases. Demonstrations were given in bandaging, surgical appliances and urinalysis. At the end of this course of instruction and after two years' experience on the wards, a Board of Examiners judged the competence of the nurses before they received their certificates and badges of graduation. It was not surprising that graduates of this school were sought by hospitals throughout Canada and that many held senior appointments in hospitals in the U.S.A. Discipline was strict and the days full—from 6:00 a.m. until lights out at 10:30 p.m.—but the record showed an ever-increasing esprit de corps. The Medical Superintendent, in addressing the graduating class, referred to their experience in their final year. They had nursed 3,374 indoor patients, including 459 cases of typhoid fever, 139 cases of diphtheria and 34 of scarlet fever and "you have stood at the death beds of 255 human beings and have witnessed scenes of suffering as harrowing and depressing as those found on battlefields."

By 1894 the Training School for Nurses had become the largest in the Dominion, and Miss Snively was constantly sought as a speaker to keep the public informed of the progress of the nursing profession. In 1895, recognizing the importance of dietetics, especially when a great deal of nursing service was carried on in patients' homes, a "competent party" was engaged to carry on cooking classes in two rooms in the hospital basement which were equipped with a coal range, a refrigerator and a sink. By 1896 the course in the Training School was increased to three years and a nine-month curriculum was organized. In 1901 twenty-eight hospitals applied for graduates of the General Hospital to fill administrative positions.

By 1905 it became obvious that the duties of Miss Snively were too demanding in her dual role as Lady Superintendent of the hospital and Superintendent of the School of Nurses. A matron was appointed to supervise the routine nursing services and housekeeping while Miss Snively, as Lady Superintendent, concentrated her activities on the work of the Training School. At this time monthly payment of student nurses was discontinued and an appeal from them for an eight-hour day was refused. Miss Snively's long and distinguished association with the hospital came to an end in 1910, but even to the present day nurses in this Training School revere the memory of a very great lady.

In 1874 the trustees decided that the graduating students who were appointed to assist the Resident Medical Officer should be chosen on merit, and they asked the faculties of the three medical schools, namely the Toronto School of Medicine, and those of Victoria and Trinity colleges, to recommend one candidate each on this basis. It was suggested that fifteen dollars a year might be a proper reimbursement for their services, but on this the board appears to have had a change of heart as some time later graduate appointees complained that they received no monetary reward.

Within a year the growing importance of the resident appointments became obvious. In 1875 rules were adopted to govern the behaviour of young graduate physicians who were accepted for duty, and they were asked to sign a formal agreement to abide by them. They were completely under the jurisdiction of the Medical Superintendent, carrying out his orders in their daily routine, responsible day and night for the care of their patients, warned against any familiarity with patients, nurses or servants, and having neither the right to give orders to the Lady Superintendent nor the right to prescribe or compound drugs for patients except under special orders.

This same year the trustees appointed a Mr. William Honeywell as assistant to Mr. W. G. Stark, who was then in charge of the hospital dispensary. Stark was licensed under the Pharmacy Act of 1871 but there is no record of Honeywell's receiving such recognition. The records show the appointment of W. G. Stark as Resident Medical Assistant in 1876 and Honeywell a year later, so that it would appear that during their undergraduate years they were employed as pharmacists in the hospital, obviously very valuable training for their future careers. At this time an inventory of the drugs in the dispensary showed a valuation of only $202.84.

There is a report of an inspection of the hospital in January 1882. Mayor McMurrick, accompanied by his wife and daughter-in-law, Alderman Boswell and Mr. Reddy, the City Clerk, visited the hospital and they reported that "a better managed charity would be difficult to find; in fact it is a credit to Toronto. Its cheerful exterior appearance is prepossessing and the interior more than fulfils the expectation which a stranger visiting it for the first time would be disposed to entertain." The *Globe* report continues:

> The party was met by the Medical Superintendent, Dr. O'Reilly, in the lobby, from which the tasteful decorations of the Christmas holidays had not been removed and was conducted through almost every room in the building. The doctor appears to be admirably fitted for a position in which executive ability, suavity, kindness and cheerfulness and contagious enthusiasm are so much required. The hospital is found in as good a condition as it well could be, and far from beyond what those who have never visited it could imagine. The

> spacious corridors and large airy rooms in themselves tend to impart cheerfulness to patients, but there is much more visible of so pleasing a character that the hospital is as bright a place as a luxuriantly furnished home could well be. Everything is neat and attractive; nothing old and dilapidated. The key to the cleanliness everywhere apparent is furnished in one of the instructions given in a circular for the information of nurses in training. This instruction reads "there is no part of the hospital clean if it cannot be made cleaner." That this injunction is carried out to the letter, the spotless coverlets, floors and walls testify. No housekeeper could keep a kitchen in better order and no engineer could have an engine room more free from grease or dirt of any description.
>
> However, there is a convalescent ward needed. There is no separate department for convalescents though it is very much needed and their recovery would be more rapid were they excluded from sick rooms and furnished with cheerful occupation to while away their hours.[1]

Plans were developed for the convalescent building shortly after this, and the building and its furnishings were completed by July 1883. Generous donations from William Gooderham, Jr., John Macdonald, Albert Nordheimer and several others helped to meet the expenses. The official opening of the building was timed to coincide with the presentation of certificates and badges to the first five nurses who completed their training in the Training School for Nurses. Mr. Justice Patterson occupied the chair and Mr. William Gooderham, Mr. Goldwin Smith, Mr. Christie the Inspector of Hospitals and Asylums, John Gillespie and Walter Lee were on the platform. The building was described as a "neat structure situated at the north-west corner of the main hospital, its architectural features being that it is of the domestic gothic type." It was a two-room, two-storey structure surrounded by a verandah on both floors. A conservatory at the west end was filled with beautiful plants in full bloom. One floor was intended for female and the other for male patients, and a large number of games had been provided for recreation purposes, with a billiard table planned for the lower room. The building was entirely separate from the hospital, but a covered gallery was to be erected before winter so that the patients could go back and forth without being exposed to the weather.

In 1883 the number of resident medical assistants was increased to four yearly appointments, and in 1888 this was further increased to six. Then in 1893 the Medical Superintendent informed the board that

[1]*Globe*, January 30, 1882.

the Medical Colleges wished to have the appointments recognized as rewards of merit. The Colleges were then asked to submit the names of at least eight men in their graduating classes from which the house staff could be chosen. During these years the list of resident physicians and surgeons included many who would later become prominent in the practice of medicine: George Langstaff, J. F. W. Ross, T. H. Stark, W. J. Charlton, George Peters, Crawford Scadding, W. P. Caven, Charles Trow, Llewellys Barker, Thomas Cullen, Geoffrey Boyd, J. A. Amyot, C. B. Shuttleworth, Donald Armour, Gilbert Royce, A. A. Beattie, W. J. O. Malloch and Donald McGillivray.

The most important change that took place in the organization of the medical staff of the hospital came as a result of a meeting of the trustees in June 1888, when the by-laws were amended to recognize physicians separately from surgeons. Various specialist groups were designated, and in response to obvious needs a dental surgeon was appointed and an extern staff was organized to be responsible for the daily clinics held for out-door patients.

At the same time it was considered advisable to classify diseases so that the patients on admission might be assigned to particular members of the staff. A weekly rotation of the surgeons and physicians was suggested in order that individual members of the attending staff should have continuing responsibility for the treatment of patients from the time of their admission.

The extern staff and the pathologists were largely young men for whom the appointments were a stepping stone to the senior staff. Formal recognition of the value of their services came a few years later when the board decided that members of the extern staff who had served for three years would be allowed to attend non-charity patients in hospital, limiting the number at any time to two patients who must not have had previous treatment in the out-patient department. In addition, a closer relationship with the hospital was established when the trustees appointed members of the extern staff as assistants to various members of the attending staff of the hospital.

About the same time, the board accepted a growing demand from many physicians who were not on the staff to be permitted to attend their own patients when they were admitted to private wards. The proviso governing this privilege was that the physician must be a member in good standing of the Dominion Medical Association, the Ontario Medical Association, the Toronto Medical Society or the Toronto Clinical Society.

Specialization was becoming more and more a feature of the staff of the hospital. In 1882, through the generosity of John Macdonald, William Gooderham, Jr., and several others, funds were provided to erect a pavilion for the special diseases of women. This was a two-storey building situated just east of the Burnside Lying-In Hospital. It was a self-contained unit with examining and operating rooms and had accommodation in public and private wards for forty patients. By this time several members of the staff of the Lying-In department had had special training in gynaecology, and so the out-patient clinics and teaching in the new building came under their jurisdiction.

Development of the special study and treatment of patients suffering from dermatological conditions may be attributed to the work of one man: Dr. James E. Graham. He was born in Brampton, Ontario, and spent much of his boyhood on his grandfather's farm that was located on the site of what is now the Toronto International Airport. He was educated locally and at Upper Canada College and received his medical education in the Toronto School of Medicine, graduating from the University of Toronto in 1869 with the Gold Medal. He was a close friend of William Osler, the result of the time they spent on their Saturday mornings studying microscopy under James Bovell. Upon graduation he became a resident in the Brooklyn City Hospital, later serving in Germany during the Franco-Prussian War as a physician with the Prussian army. After continuing his postgraduate studies in Vienna and in London, where he obtained his L.R.C.P., he returned to Toronto where he began to teach at the Toronto School of Medicine, and was appointed to the staff of the Toronto General Hospital in 1873. When the Faculty of Medicine at the University of Toronto was re-organized in 1887, he became Professor of Clinical Medicine and Medical Pathology and Lecturer in Dermatology. He was the first Canadian to specialize in dermatology and acquired international recognition in this field, serving as President of the American Dermatological Society in 1888 and winning election as a member of the Royal College of Physicians of London in 1893. He was also President of the Canadian Medical Association and a member of the Senate of the University of Toronto. Unfortunately in his later years he developed diabetes, which led to his death in 1899. He was not only a good physician but an outstanding teacher and a productive student of disease, as was evident in his many publications, particularly his presidential address in 1888 which dealt with Public Health Measures in the Prevention of Scabies, Taenia Tonsurans, Syphilis and Leprosy.

In May 1889, on the request of Dr. A. A. MacDonald and Dr. Graham, the Board of Trustees authorized the purchase of "some electrical apparatus at a cost not exceeding $100.00," and Dr. C. R. Dickson was appointed to the staff as specialist in electrotherapeutics. A room was put at his disposal on the ground floor of the building. This was the first recognition of a department of physiotherapy.

Electrotherapy as practised at this time had no scientific basis, but it had a broad use in the treatment of many unrelated conditions such as neuralgia, gout, angina pectoris, migraine, general paralysis, bladder paralysis, locomotor ataxia, torticollis, infantile paralysis, uterine fibroids, aneurisms and the treatment of some malignant tumours. Some of its advocates considered it to be of such value that one authority, in closing his address before the Hunterian Society of London, England, said, "I hope that a knowledge of medical electricity may soon be considered an indispensable part of the education of every medical practitioner."[2] Experience modified this opinion, and even the most enthusiastic came to look upon it as largely a treatment of the last resort, which prompted a local therapist of good repute to state "electricity is one of the most powerful agents you can employ in the treatment of disease but it is useless or mischievous according to the manner in which it is applied."[3] In the year ending September 30, 1891, 767 patients received electrotherapy at the Toronto General Hospital.

When Dr. Charles O'Reilly presented the annual report in 1891 it showed the progress which had taken place during his tenure of office. In the sixteen years from 1876 to 1891, there had been an increase in the hospital beds from 150 to 400 available in the main building, the Mercer Infirmary, the Burnside and the Pavilion, with thirty-three being set aside for private patients. As a result, annual admissions had increased from 810 to 2,995.

Senior students, in addition to being appointed surgical dressers in the various parts of the hospital, were helping to maintain records as clinical clerks, and young physicians not on the active staff of the hospital were appointed annually as registrars responsible for the compilation of medical and scientific data. These eventually became much-sought-after appointments. The number engaged in the work

[2]Herbert Tibbets, "Diathermy—How to use a Galvanic Battery in Medicine and Surgery." An Address delivered before the Hunterian Society, November 8, 1876 (London: J. A. Churchill, 1877).

[3]A. M. Roseburgh, "The Apostoli Treatment of Uterine Fibroids," *Canadian Practitioner*, XIII (1888).

increased yearly until in 1896 there were thirty-one registrars appointed by the trustees. By this time the list included J. T. Fotheringham, J. A. Amyot, W. B. Thistle, Graham Chambers, F. N. G. Starr, D. J. G. Wishart, B. L. Riordan, C. A. Temple, H. C. Scadding, Harold Parsons, H. J. Hamilton and J. O. Orr.

Out-patient clinics were held at 1.00 p.m. daily except Saturday and Sunday, with special clinics for eye and ear, throat and nose, dermatology, electrology and diseases of women. There were no antenatal clinics, but arrangements were available so that senior students might attend certain out-patients during their confinements in their own homes. As a result of all these services, in the previous year 10,929 patients, including 577 emergencies, received free medical advice and medicines—though it was stipulated that they must provide their own clean bottles and gallipots.

The most serious problem was the increasing number of patients with typhoid fever, with 385 admissions and 49 deaths. The reason was not hard to find, as the daily press in editorials and news items constantly drew attention to the appalling state of the water supply and the sewage disposal. The new Isolation Hospital had been opened, but the General Hospital still reported 135 cases of diphtheria with 28 deaths and 30 cases of scarlet fever.

Twenty-six patients died in the hospital from pulmonary tuberculosis, and pneumonia, "the old man's friend," accounted for another 20 deaths. With improving methods of diagnosis, 45 cases of cardiac disease were recognized, of whom 19 died, and, as might be expected, its frequent precursor, acute rheumatic fever, accounted for 92 admissions. Sixty-three psychiatric patients were admitted and the age-old problem of alcoholism resulted in 95 sufferers being admitted for hospital control; perhaps as an end result of the latter, twelve patients were admitted with cirrhosis of the liver, of whom five died.

Sixty-five patients were admitted with cancer, including twenty-four involving the skin, ten cancers of the breast, three of the uterus and six of the rectum. Nine patients died of cancer, the sites being the face, neck, oesophagus, pancreas, stomach and rectum. During the year twelve mastectomies were performed and eight patients were operated upon for epitheliomata, one of whom required an excision of the inferior maxilla. There were also thirty patients admitted with "ovarian disease," which was not differentiated as being either benign or malignant. Even in those days there was a sympathetic reaction to cancer, as in 1890 a Mr. E. M. Peel left $2,000 to endow a bed for a cancer patient.

The special departments were constantly busy. In 1889 the Burnside reached a peak with 192 deliveries, and during the year 1890–1891, 216 patients were admitted to the Mercer Infirmary, 47 requiring surgical treatment for cataract. In the new Women's Pavilion J. A. Temple, Uzziel Ogden and J. F. W. Ross maintained the tradition of E. M. Hodder and, at a time when abdominal surgery was limited in its scope and application, they performed 35 laparotomies for ovarian and uterine disease. There were also 11 operations performed for prolapse of the uterus.

The pride of the hospital was its central theatre, recently enlarged to seat five hundred students and said to be unsurpassed on the continent. Here operations were performed on Saturday afternoons and at any hour of the day or night in case of emergency. But its chief use was for daily clinical lectures and demonstrations, particularly for the third- and fourth-year students, though the floor of the theatre was reserved exclusively for the hospital medical staff.

The major interest in surgery was in the treatment of fractures and dislocations, which had improved greatly as a result of the increasing knowledge of the mechanics of splints and extension apparatus. Antisepsis had practically eliminated amputation in the treatment of compound fractures. Surgical treatment was undertaken for seventeen fistulae of the rectum or of the bladder and two wiring operations were performed for fractures, one of the patella and the other of the tibia. However, there was only one appendectomy during the year, and three other operations performed for peri-appendiceal abscess resulted in the deaths of two patients.

In all of its history the Toronto General Hospital was never served more conscientiously than by A. F. Miller.[4] Appointed nominally as Assistant Secretary in 1876, he progressed to recognition as a valuable officer of the hospital and in 1891 received a salary of $1,500 per annum. Under his supervision expenses were thoroughly scrutinized by the board, formal tenders were advertised for major purchases, and money was expended with care, so that the hospital retained its solvency through the years of constant expansion. How much he became an integral part of the hospital is seen in his 42 years' service in

[4]Clarke, *History of the T.G.H.*, p. 114.

association with seven chairmen of the board, four medical superintendents and six lady superintendents of nurses. Dr. C. K. Clarke, who knew him well, referred to him as the "Grand Old Man" who inspired the greatest confidence and admiration.

No longer were the members of the board under public criticism, but as they applied the same industry and business principles which made them outstanding citizens, they presented to the people of Toronto an institution that had become increasingly a source of civic pride. The satisfactory financial condition of the hospital reflected the efficiency of the boards which served under John Macdonald, C. S. Ross, W. H. Howland, C. S. Patterson, Walter Lee and John Blaikie.

Improvements in the facilities kept pace with the times. In 1876 steam heating replaced the old wooden stoves. In 1885 the Bell Telephone Company installed the first telephone, costing thirty dollars per annum, and it was not until 1898 that the rate was increased to forty-five. During this time house phones had been installed at a very reasonable rental. In 1892 Otis Brothers erected an electric elevator in the main building for $3,200 and power was supplied by the Toronto Electric Light Company at a cost of fourteen dollars a month. The major development came in 1898, when gas illumination was replaced by electric light, the new installation costing $2,000 and maintenance and power only $1,200 annually.

Under ordinary circumstances the combined revenues of the hospital were sufficient to cover routine expenditures, but in 1900 an extensive addition to the Nurses' Residence and improvements to the Pavilion, including a new operating room, presented the board with an expense of $20,000. George Gooderham, a member of the board, promptly offered a personal loan of $14,000 to meet the situation and with this help and sound administration the board was able to meet its financial obligations. Mr. Gooderham's generosity was another example of the support available to the hospital in time of need, which had prompted the board in 1891 to have two marble tablets placed in the entrance hall on which were engraved the names of the Hospital Benefactors. The following year it bore these names:

1861	Alexander Sanderson	$ 400.00
1867	George Michie	$ 2,000.00
1869	John Walker	$ 400.00
1871	George Henry	$ 2,000.00
1875	James Ferrier Gentle	$ 500.00
1875	Erland Erlandson	$15,000.00

1878	William Gooderham, Sr.	$ 4,500.00
1878	James Worts	$ 4,500.00
1878	William Cawthra	$ 4,500.00
1882	William Gooderham, Jr.	$ 2,000.00
1882	John Macdonald	$ 500.00
1883	John Macdonald	$ 500.00
1884	Executors of John Michie	$ 5,000.00
1886	Executors of Margaret J. Rolph	$ 1,000.00
1886	The R. B. Butland Bequest (estimated)	$14,000.00
1887	Executors of Alexander McGregor	$ 500.00
1889	Executors of John B. Lloyd	$ 600.00
1890	Executors of James E. Drinkwater	$ 1,500.00
1891	Executors of George Davison	$ 2,000.00
1891	Executors of Hon. John Macdonald	$ 2,000.00
1891	Executors of The Rev. Father T. McMahon	$ 2,820.00
1884–1891	Grand Trunk Railway	$ 1,000.00
1892	Estate of Late A. F. Fulton	$ 5,000.00
1893	Estate of Late Henry Buck	$ 1,000.00

An endowment depending upon revenue from real estate was always a source of constant concern. Not only were many rentals in arrears, but the maintenance of old and often poorly constructed buildings demanded unrelenting supervision. A generous legacy, the Butland bequest, which came to the hospital in 1886, was particularly demanding in its administration. The trustees of the General Hospital were appointed executors for Richard Butland who, after providing liberally for his wife, had left his real estate with the residue of his personal effects to the hospital—requiring, however, the payment of annuities of $300 to his wife and to his daughter and $200 to Annie and to George Verral. The real estate included houses on King, Queen and Sackville streets and the total value of the bequest was estimated to be $14,000. The hospital appointed two members of the board, John Gillespie, Managing Director of the Dominion Lands Company, and Walter Lee, Manager of the Western Canada Loan and Savings Company, whom they designated "syndics," to administer the will. Over the years the minutes of the board meetings show the extra responsibility which was placed on A. F. Miller and a few years later he received $150 per annum in addition to his regular salary.

Many of the houses of the Butland Estate were much worse than those already maintained by the hospital—dilapidated, without proper heating, having no sewers, and often failing to meet the requirements of the Board of Health. More centrally located land was rented on the basis of a 21-year lease, the lessee being allowed to erect his own building, provided it met with the approval of the trustees. With such an arrangement, in 1893, the hospital received an annual rental of $4,045 for a property of 104 feet on King Street and 103 feet on York Street. Ten years later the proprietors of the Arlington Hotel, which was situated a short distance west of the present Royal Alexandra Theatre, signed a lease for their property with 117-foot frontage on King Street and $425 per annum for two years, increasing to $705 for the next twenty-one years. The returns were not very great, being in line with land values of the time, but at least the trustees were spared the worry of the day-to-day maintenance of the properties.

In the twenty-two years between 1880 and 1902, the financial condition of the hospital was constantly changing. In this time the admissions had increased from 1,703 to 3,290, with an average occupancy rising from 191 to 252 patients. At the same time the cost of maintenance rose from $48,163 to $87,172, which represented a per diem patient rate of 68¢, becoming 95¢ in the latter year. The number of employees increased from 47 to 166, and this resulted in a monthly wage bill of $706, rising to $2,100. Mr. Miller warned the board that the growth of expenditures was out of proportion to the increase in receipts and that at a rate of seven dollars a week semi-private patients could no longer be considered as self-supporting. At this time the income from house rents was about $1,400 per month, but he thought this might very easily decline in the future.

For several years the grants from the Ontario government had declined. In 1895 the Charity Aid Act had been amended so as to make grants to each hospital from a fixed sum on a per capita basis. This precipitated a serious problem, as the number of hospitals sharing the grants increased from 18 to 55 in the years 1897–1902. This precipitated a great controversy, the trustees consulting the governing bodies of St. Michael's, the Toronto Western and Grace hospitals about it, and the problem was the chief subject discussed at the first meeting of the Ontario Hospital Association held in 1904. A suggestion was made that the government should devote a larger proportion of the succession duties to aid the hospitals and also that the sale of cutting rights on timber lands might be devoted to the same purpose. Finally the government decided that it would consider fifty cents per day an acceptable rate for public ward patients for an indefinite stay in hospital, and here the matter rested.

Mr. Walter Lee died in January 1902, having been a Trustee of the hospital for twenty-five years and Chairman of the Board for the last thirteen, and Mr. Joseph Flavelle was elected to his place. Mr. John Blaikie, another faithful veteran, served as chairman for the next two years and on his retirement Mr. Flavelle began his long and productive tenure as chairman. Characteristically, he left nothing to chance. He accepted the responsibility of advising Mr. Miller on the daily problems of finance, and when he had made a tour of inspection of all the hospital properties he suggested that the other members of the board might well do likewise. Then he and Mr. P. C. Larkin, another recent appointee to the board, made a thorough inspection of the hospital buildings, reporting that the present buildings had become entirely inadequate for a great hospital in a growing city like Toronto. In the meantime it was realized that the sanitary conditions of the hospital required immediate renovation. They had found that the pantries where much of the food was prepared were inadequate, poorly equipped and generally inefficient. They recommended that all the drains leading to and through the hospital should be put in a thoroughly efficient condition, that all unsanitary closets, traps and pipes be replaced or renewed, and that the existing bath-tubs be replaced by new ones. The use of the bathrooms for emptying slops, washing bed-pans, etc., was to be discontinued and slop-rooms were to be provided for the various wards and furnished with suitable fittings. A new laboratory was also ordered for the Eye and Ear building, to be fitted and furnished as a clinical laboratory under the supervision of Dr. John Caven. When the final cost of this extensive work was estimated at $23,000, the board followed Mr. Flavelle's advice and sold lands on Eastern Avenue and Front Street to the Canadian Northern Railway for $47,500, thus providing for the last major expenditure on the Gerrard Street hospital.

Dr. Charles O'Reilly's value as the primary advisor to the board increased greatly over the years. It was over his signature that the students received their cards of admission for clinical instruction, and he prepared the certificates of clinical experience that they submitted to the Ontario College of Physicians and Surgeons in order to be licensed to practise in the province. For over eight years he was an examiner in clinical medicine for the University of Toronto. His outstanding ability as a hospital administrator was widely recognized, and when he retired in 1905 after twenty-nine years of service with the hospital he became the patron of the Postgraduate Society of Toronto, composed of members, house staff and ex-house staff of the hospitals of Toronto and of Ontario. Not only the Board of Trustees but the whole medical profession of Toronto tendered him complimentary dinners. His particular interest in the welfare of nurses and especially of patients suffering from tuberculosis resulted in his appointments to national and international boards, and his busy life did not come to an end as he took up fresh responsibilities and a renewed interest in the practice of medicine with his son, Dr. Brefney O'Reilly of Toronto.

It is impossible to exaggerate the value of the contributions which Charles O'Reilly, Mary Snively and A. F. Miller made to the General Hospital, for they established the broad basis on which this institution came to the forefront in Canadian medicine.

VIII

Various New Services

Over the years there had always been general dispensaries located in the industrial area of Toronto where victims of accidents and the nearby poor could receive treatment. When the General Hospital was moved to Gerrard Street in 1856 and out-patient services were organized, it did not answer the need for more conveniently located service, and many physicians and surgeons on the hospital staff still continued their association with the downtown clinics.

One of the best of these was the Toronto Dispensary, organized in 1854, located first on Adelaide Street West and later at 133 Simcoe Street. Here, in spite of inadequate quarters, in a small two-storey house where the hall served as a waiting-room, several thousand patients received treatment annually and home care was provided for a considerable number who were unable to attend the regular clinics. F. L. Grasett, James Thorburn, J. E. Graham, R. A. Reeve, Alexander McPhedran, A. H. Wright, I. H. Cameron, R. B. Nevitt, Allan Baines, J. F. W. Ross, A. C. Myers, D. J. G. Wishart and Goldwin Howland were among those who gave gratuitous service, while generous citizens supported an institution of inestimable value. The medical schools, appreciating what it meant to their students, advertised it as a feature in their yearly calendars.

It was becoming increasingly obvious, however, that something better than this purely voluntary service was required. In 1897 the Advisory Medical Board convinced the trustees that they should undertake the responsibility of maintaining an emergency branch hospital in a central location. At first it was thought the old Burnside Hospital building at Richmond and Shepherd streets, rented at that time by the Y.W.C.A. for use as a boarding house for working girls, might be suitable, but inspection proved otherwise. Finally a house on Bay Street, just south of the present National Club, was leased from the London and Canadian Loan and Agency Company in March 1898. A monthly rental of thirty dollars was increased somewhat, as considerable alterations were required to provide for waiting, examining and operating rooms, a dispensary, a kitchen and a small dining room. There were two wards for patients on the second floor and quarters for the staff, including two house surgeons, on the third floor. The staff appointed in 1898 to the Emergency Hospital consisted of Doctors Allan Baines, W. P. Caven, J. M. MacCallum, J. T. Fotheringham, Graham Chambers, E. E. King, N. A. Powell, Alexander Primrose, Bertram Spencer and George Bingham, and during the eight years that it remained in service there was only one change, when F. N. G. Starr replaced Dr. Spencer. The Emergency developed an active service, with a monthly attendance of between 250 and 300 patients. In the accident book, kept by the house surgeons in an old scribbler, are recorded the cases from November 19, 1900, to March 24, 1905. Here are presented the "short and simple annals of the poor," beginning with an old Irishman of eighty years, who was found at the Union Station in a state of collapse. He had come in from Caledon with a massive cancer of his face and mouth, from which he died a few days later. There were other patients so severely injured that they did not survive transfer to the main hospital and a nurse who served at the Emergency recalled how week-end celebrants provided a never-failing flow of patients.

There was, by this time, a well organized ambulance service. An anonymous female benefactor had presented the first ambulance built in Canada to the Hospital trustees, and after quite a number of years it was still in service for the use of patients with infectious diseases. Mr. John Ross Robertson presented a modern ambulance to the city in 1887, and a short time later the Manufacturers' Life Assurance Company gave a similar ambulance to the Police Commissioners, who at that time were responsible for this service, the ambulances being kept at the Court Street Station. The ambulances were so designed that they might be drawn by one horse or readily converted into two-horse vehicles, and they provided a patient comfort hitherto unknown, with a tubular rubber air bed and a supply of stimulants, emetics, antiseptics and surgical appliances, including a stomach pump, catheters, splints and dressings. In the rules governing their service it was stated that "in responding to a call the ambulance should always be driven at a rapid but not a dangerous rate and the gong kept sounding to warn other vehicles. In returning it must be driven moderately except when the case must be brought to the hospital without delay." No charge was made for this service, but while it was available to women in labour it was not to transport cases of erysipelas, delirium tremens or acute mania, such cases being referred to the Medical Board of Health physician who would provide special transportation for them.

Active though it was, this downtown branch of the hospital had a short career. In May 1906 the trustees decided that it was no longer possible to carry on the Emergency Hospital, faced as they were with the ever-increasing expenses of maintaining the Gerrard Street hospital and the problem of financing the new hospital on College Street. The property on Bay Street was sublet to the Printers' Club for the remainder of the lease.

When Dr. Charles O'Reilly retired as superintendent in 1905, Dr. J. N. E. Brown was appointed as his successor. Dr. Brown had graduated from Toronto in 1892 with the Silver Medal and had served as a house surgeon in the General Hospital, besides carrying on a private practice and simultaneously serving as an obstetrician on the staff of St. Michael's Hospital. The experience that primarily influenced his future career was the time he spent as Medical Health Officer in the Yukon during the gold rush. The many problems which he had faced in this rough and ready frontier produced the mature mind that he now applied to his new responsibility, reflected in his first report to the trustees:

> It is clear then that the efficient hospital has a double obligation to fulfill; first to relieve the necessities of the sick in its wards, and secondly to do all in its power to add to the general stock of medical knowledge. In order that a hospital may fulfill this part of its function it cannot be too strongly emphasized that its requirements will be much greater in the future. Suitable laboratory accommodation must be provided with the necessary equipment and apparatus for the scientific study of medicine. Use must be made of modern discoveries in physics and chemistry. Special attention must be given to the pathological department, as without efficiency here the work of the hospital would be deprived almost entirely of scientific value.

The report for the year ending September 30, 1905, showed that there had been 3,495 admissions during the year and that 172 children had been born in the Burnside Hospital. There were 10,639 out-patients treated. The largest disease entity was still typhoid fever, with 127 admissions of whom 12 died. Rheumatic fever and pneumonia also contributed a fairly large number of patients. In all there had been 1,671 medical patients and 2,068 surgical patients. There were 242 cases of appendicitis with 6 deaths, and of the patients with malignant disease there were 22 with cancer of the breast, 13 with cancer of the uterus, 12 with cancer of the stomach and 10 with cancer of the rectum. As this was before the hygienic control of milk supply, 32 patients with tuberculous glands were operated upon in the surgical department. There were 58 autopsies performed and only 101 surgical specimens were examined microscopically. The hospital pathologists at this time were John Caven, H. B. Anderson, H. C. Parsons, J. J. Mackenzie, H. J. Hamilton and A. H. W. Caulfield and the registrars responsible for the material in the annual report were F. W. Marlow and G. W. Howland.

The annual reports for the next five years showed a steady improvement in hospital services. In 1898 Dr. H. C. Scadding became the first to be designated as "hospital anaesthetist," responsible for the instruction in anaesthesia of the undergraduate students and the resident house staff. As the service developed, members of the extern surgical staff were appointed as his assistants. Finally, in 1904, the hospital invited applications for two paid anaesthetists and Dr. Samuel Johnston and Dr. Duncan Anderson were chosen. The hospital undertook to collect the fee for anaesthesia, the minimum to be five dollars of which two dollars was retained as a charge for chloroform. If the surgeon preferred to have other than an official anaesthetist, the payment of two dollars was then made directly to the hospital. In October 1905 this financial arrangement was reviewed, and it was reported that $64.00 had come to the hospital from 32 cases in the second category and that the 417 patients who had received service from Dr. Johnston and Dr. Anderson provided $1,654, which was divided between them. The board then decided that they would be permitted to collect their own fees from private and semi-private patients, while the hospital charged for operating services. The trustees felt that the volume of work warranted that a nurse should be appointed to supervise the operating theatre.

This was also a time of rapid improvement in the treatment of the mentally ill. Shortly after Dr. Brown's appointment alterations were made to the hospital lodge for his accommodation and the old quarters of the medical superintendent were made available to receive neurological patients. Dr. Campbell Myers was appointed to take charge, and at the end of the year he reported that sixty-nine patients had been under his care during that time. He also made the proud claim in the annual report that these wards were the first provided anywhere in Canada for the treatment of borderline psychoses.

The following year Dr. Myers became a member of Dr. W. P. Caven's service, with continuing responsibility for patients with "functional neuroses." In 1908 Dr. C. K. Clarke, at that time the Superintendent of the Toronto Asylum and Dean of the Medical Faculty, was appointed Psychiatrist to the General Hospital, with Dr. Gerald Fitzgerald as his assistant. The next year he organized an out-patient psychiatric clinic in a house on Chestnut Street, where Dr. J. F. W. Ross had organized an out-patient gynaecological clinic the year before. A distinguished British psychiatrist, Dr. Ernest Jones, became director of the clinic, and it was said that it was the first of its kind in Canada—showing the value of the early recognition and treatment of mental disease.

Dr. Clarke was constant in his efforts to establish a special hospital for psychiatric patients. In his report to the trustees he drew their attention to a serious situation, in that he had been surprised to find so many patients suffering from mental disease in the general wards of the hospital:

> The public must not understand, apparently, that the institution is not equipped to deal with these people satisfactorily or with safety to the patients and nurses. Apparently there is no adequate provision made for them in hospitals for the insane. It is a matter of regret that no psychiatric hospital has been provided either by the city or the Government. Meanwhile we must open our doors to patients suffering from various psychoses; we do so at very great risk, especially when patients are either homicidal or suicidal. No amount of foresight in buildings not specially equipped can provide against a tragedy occurring in some of these institutions.

For a while it was thought that a special hospital might be built on the new hospital site or in the immediate neighbourhood, but nothing came of the proposal. As a result, both the out-patient clinic and the in-patient service were discontinued, pending completion of the College Street hospital.

In 1911 Dr. Clarke was chosen to succeed Dr. J. N. E. Brown as the hospital superintendent. He had already established a distinguished record as administrator, psychiatrist and teacher. When he was a medical student in Toronto he came under the spell of Joseph Workman, under whom he had worked as clinical assistant. It might well be said that the "spirit of Elijah doth rest on Elisha," for following his great master, C. K. Clarke became recognized in America and Europe as a great protagonist of modern psychiatry. At the end of his career he paid this tribute to Workman:

> Dr. Workman not only showed how terrible the tragedy of mental disease is, but his wonderful sympathy and devotion taught a lesson never to be forgotten. Truly his was the life of a great man devoted to a great work. Even in the shadow of old age, I look back with love and admiration on the work of the greatest man I have ever known.[1]

Dr. Clarke served in posts of increasing importance in Hamilton and Kingston before he became Superintendent of the Asylum in Toronto in 1905, and he was Professor of Psychiatry at both Queen's and Toronto universities.

In 1914, taking advantage of the facilities of the Out-Patient Department of the new hospital on College Street, he established a psychiatry clinic with Dr. Clarence Hincks and Dr. O. J. C. Withrow as his assistants. At the same time Dr. Goldwin W. Howland, who had had special training in the Nettley Hospital in Queen Square, London, England, was appointed to the medical staff of the hospital under Dr. Graham Chambers, to be responsible for the care of neurological in-patients. The Psychiatric Clinic soon proved its worth and it became a veritable clearing house for the mentally ill. For the first time social agencies throughout the city could refer the feeble-minded to a well organized centre and it soon became evident that the nurses, Miss E. deV. Clarke (Dr. Clarke's daughter) and later Miss Marjory Keys, both nurses with a very special interest in social service, provided a link with outside conditions which was invaluable to the physicians responsible for the observation and treatment of the patients.

No one appreciated as much as Dr. Helen McMurchy the need for a social service organization for the hospital. In 1901 she had been the first woman appointed to the resident staff of the hospital and after postgraduate training under William Osler at Johns Hopkins Hospital she held a junior appointment in Obstetrics and Gynaecology at the hospital and at the University of Toronto. Her work in this department led her to her particular interest in maternal and child welfare and it was not long before her clear approach to these great problems resulted in her appointment as lecturer in the Social Service Department of the University. Fortunately for the hospital she enlisted the cooperation

[1]Clarke, *A History of the T.G.H.*, p. 9.

of an outstanding group of ladies and with their support she became Chairman of the Social Service Association which was organized in 1911. The time was opportune and in future years, when her career had led to nation-wide responsibilities, she must have looked back with increasing satisfaction on the ever-broadening field of service that developed from such a modest beginning.

The first professional appointment to the Social Service Department was Miss Norah Holman, who was originally known as the "Lady Almoner." She soon demonstrated the service that could extend to patients who were attending out-patient clinics or had been discharged from hospital. She was followed by Miss Jane Grant of Cleveland, who organized the department so that in 1918 it consisted of herself, five social service nurses and a secretary. From the beginning a steadily increasing number of ladies, led by Mrs. D. A. Dunlap, Mrs. J. F. W. Ross, Miss Eileen Larkin, Mrs. W. B. Hendry and Miss Clara Flavelle and members of the alumni of the Training School for Nurses, gave not only their unstinted service but also assumed the responsibility for the financial support of the department. Their good example and unfailing service has over the years provided a strong foundation for an efficient professional organization.

In 1906, on the advice of Dr. Alexander McPhedran, an out-patient clinic for patients suffering from pulmonary tuberculosis was organized under Dr. Harold Parsons with the consulting supervision of Doctors Harold Parfitt and Ephraim Elliott of Gravenhurst. The public as well as the profession were aware of the public health problem that this disease presented. Dr. J. L. Davidson, speaking to the Insurance Institute in Toronto in March, 1904, stated that tuberculosis was responsible for fourteen per cent of all mortality in all ages and in all social conditions of life, and he suggested that the public should be made more aware of the contagious nature of this disease, especially as it affected households and families.[2] Another phase of the problem was presented in a report from the Gravenhurst Sanitorium by Dr. Elliott, who expressed the hope that more patients would be sent for treatment in the earlier stages of the disease when there was a reasonable hope of cure.[3] The clinic was organized so that it could cooperate with the sanitoria, and Mrs. P. C. Larkin of the board offered to underwrite the

[2]John L. Davidson, "Some Points on Tuberculosis," *Canadian Practitioner and Review*, XXIX (1904).

[3]J. H. Elliott, "Report of the Physician-in-Chief at Muskoka Cottage Sanitarium," *Canadian Practitioner and Review*, XXVII (1902).

expenses entailed, including the salary of a social service nurse, Miss Christina Mitchell. Some idea of the work that was done is evident in a yearly report of 1910 which showed that there had been 157 new patients, 381 patients under prolonged supervision, 23 patients sent to the Gravenhurst Sanitorium and 48 to the Weston Sanitorium. At the same time there were 89 patients admitted to the General Hospital with tuberculosis, including pulmonary and various types of so-called "surgical" tuberculosis.

A department of immunization and medical research was organized in April 1907 under Dr. G. W. Ross. This was prompted by the work of Sir Almroth Wright, the pathologist of St. Mary's Hospital, London, England, one of those dedicated geniuses who knew no working hours. During the South African war (1899–1902) he had proved to his own satisfaction that immunity to typhoid fever could be achieved by means of dead typhoid culture, and he had developed a microscopic blood test to show the degree of natural or acquired immunity in the individual. One of his young associates said that his work was "the chief growing point of medicine for the next twenty years and represented a complete breakaway from the doctoring of the '90s which largely consisted, for the most part, of a 'mixture' prescribed perhaps with some art, but little or no science; the application of a leech or a counter-irritant, or an antiseptic, or resort to the knife." It was from the stimulating atmosphere of Wright's laboratory that G. W. Ross, and a little later A. H. W. Caulfield, came back to Toronto to establish immunology, and a laboratory was furnished for Dr. Ross at a cost of $775. This was the first time in the history of the hospital that the term "medical research" was applied to its activities. The reports of the next two years showed that laboratory investigations, new to the institution, were applied to a broad range of diseases, and the treatment of "microbic conditions" was undertaken, often, as might be expected, when all else had failed. Various tuberculous lesions and acute and chronic skin conditions were the most frequently treated and for a number of years extreme optimism dominated Dr. Ross's reports of the results of his treatment. Postgraduate students were accepted, a considerable number coming from the U.S.A., and Dr. Ross was permitted to lecture in the hospital theatre.

Vaccines were prepared and supplied to many physicians, even outside the city. But probably the most important contribution was the increasing use of anti-typhoid vaccine. This resulted finally in the inoculation of the nursing staff of the hospital in 1912, with the satisfactory result that no nurses developed typhoid fever—a great reassurance to the hospital authorities at a time when nurses were exposed to a large number of typhoid patients. In 1910 the Registrar, Dr. George Strathy, stated that the typhoid records of the hospital were "instructive if deplorable." In 1908 there had been 180 cases with 14 deaths; in 1909, 242 cases with 13 deaths; and in 1910, 304 cases with 32 deaths, 253 of these patients coming from within the city. The effect of water control showed the next year when Dr. Strathy and Dr. D. E. Robertson reported a decrease from 304 to 209 cases, remarking that "the effect of chlorination of the water was seen in a few weeks by the fall in typhoid admissions."

As Dr. J. N. E. Brown had informed the trustees, the basis for scientific treatment of disease depended fundamentally on good laboratory and pathological service. It was fortunate indeed that by this time John J. Mackenzie was available to organize the services which were required. His primary interest had been biological science and while he was an undergraduate in University College, Toronto, he came under the influence of Professors J. M. MacCallum and Ramsey Wright, both traditional figures in the Medical Faculty of Toronto. After graduating with honours he studied anatomy and physiology in Leipzig and Berlin. Ludwig, His, Koch and Virchow were his teachers and when he returned to Toronto he became bacteriologist to the Provincial Board of Health. After teaching comparative anatomy and bacteriology in both the Dental College and Medical Faculty he took his medical degree in 1899 and when Professor John Caven retired from the chair in 1901 was appointed Professor of Pathology. In the same year he was appointed to the pathological staff of the General Hospital and became Head of the Department in 1908.

From an insignificant service the department developed rapidly, even in the limited quarters available on Gerrard Street, and by 1914, when a report was available for the first full year in the new building on University Avenue, it showed figures which gave promise of a very satisfactory future.

	1909	*1914*
Surgical Diagnosis	734	1811
Autopsies	118	216 (45%)
Bacterial Examinations	360	1153
Wassermann Tests	—	1159

J. J. Mackenzie had a great attraction for young men to whom his great knowledge extended with effortless grace. H. W. Caulfield, D. A.

L. Graham, O. R. Maybee, G. W. Lougheed, W. L. Robinson and H. K. Detweiler, his junior associates, were all to provide valuable service to the hospital in the years to come.

When it was decided to organize a new emergency department in 1908 the recommendation of the heads of the surgical service that Dr. N. A. Powell should be in charge, with the rank of Senior Assistant Surgeon, was a natural choice. It had been as a personal tribute to him that the generous bequests of Miss Jane and Miss Agnes Shields had been made to the hospital. The former in her will of 1898 had left money to "purchase a site near the business centre of the city and to erect and maintain a building costing no less than $30,000 in memory of her brother, John Shields, providing the choice of the site and every detail of the building, equipment and management should be submitted to and approved by Dr. N. A. Powell." On the death of the last sister, Miss Agnes Shields, in April 1912, another $95,000 was left to complete the building and provide motor ambulances, as well as an endowment to ensure a degree of independence to the activities of the emergency hospital. This provided for a second storey to be built and in May 1913, Dr. Powell ordered the first motor ambulance for use at the new hospital at a cost of $4,586.10. In addition to special features adding to the comfort of the patient, it was claimed that this vehicle could develop a speed of 35 miles per hour when required. Although Dr. Powell had a long association with teaching and the practice of medicine in Toronto, the outstanding memory he left was the integral part he played in the development of the emergency hospital. None who saw him in his chosen environment will forget the tall, straight figure with the grey pointed beard watching over the care of those who came to his department. He had received his medical education at Victoria and Trinity medical schools with postgraduate training at Bellevue Hospital in New York, where he received the degree of M.D. from the University of New York in 1875. He was one of the faculty members of Trinity University who joined the service of the Gerrard Street Hospital and the emergency hospital on Bay Street, and his appreciation of the immediate needs of the sick and injured made him a valuable teacher of the practical principles of medicine.

The new emergency hospital soon became a hospital within a hospital. The only operating room available at night in the General Hospital was the larger of two in the emergency section and in time of stress the smaller was used as well. At times the demand for patient accommodation over-taxed its facilities for thirty patients on the ground and second floors. The practical experience available to the resident house staff on duty cannot be over-estimated, and they came to appreciate the strong support they received at all hours from Dr. Roy Thomas when he was appointed in 1912 to be assistant to Dr. Powell.

When Dr. George Armstrong Peters died of coronary thrombosis on March 13, 1907, at the age of forty-seven, the General Hospital lost one of the most distinguished surgeons who had served during its long history. He had graduated from the University of Toronto in 1886 with the Gold Medal, and after serving as a house surgeon at the Toronto General Hospital he taught in the Department of Anatomy and was appointed a surgeon to the Out-Patient Department of the hospital. On leave from the hospital he went to England in 1890 where he took the examinations for the Fellowship of the Royal College of Surgeons within six months. He was one of the first Canadians to attain the Fellowship by examination. He served in the Department of Surgery from 1892 until the time of his death, and in the last four years he was the University Professor of Surgery. Dr. W. E. Gallie said he was the best surgeon and surgical teacher he had ever known. He was an advocate of asepsis, with full appreciation of the value of avoiding unnecessary tissue trauma. Working both at the General Hospital and at the Hospital for Sick Children, where he was the Surgeon-in-Chief, he developed original methods of treating malformations of the bladder, extraperitoneal transplantation of the ureters in ectopia vesicae, hyatid cyst of the pancreas, fusiform dilatation of the oesophagus, and club feet. He wrote authoritatively for several surgical textbooks.

His two great interests, apart from his profession, were closely related: horsemanship and the cavalry. This prompted him to organize a mounted rifle regiment, the Toronto Light Horse, of which he became the commanding officer, and when the time came the regiment paraded in his honour to his graveside. He was active almost to the end of his life, reading a paper on the "Choice of Operation in the Surgery of the Gall Bladder" a month before his death and dictating to his secretary a description of his angina pectoris just before the end. His great contribution to the standard of surgery at the General Hospital was appreciated fully by all who knew him.

Another untimely death occurred on November 17, 1911, when Dr. J. F. W. Ross died as a result of a motor accident near Richmond Hill, just north of Toronto. The son of Dr. James W. Ross, who in his day had had an extensive practice in Toronto with a particular interest in midwifery, he received his undergraduate training at the Toronto School of Medicine and obtained his degree from the University of Toronto in 1879. After a year as house surgeon at the Toronto General Hospital, he went to England to train under Jonathan Hutchison in London and also Lawson Tait of Birmingham, at that time the most active and progressive abdomino-pelvic surgeon in Britain. He then went to Berlin and to Vienna, receiving further instruction under Virchow, Schroeder, Braun and Bilroth. On his return he received an appointment to the surgical staff of the General Hospital and a short time later to the newly organized department of gynaecology. In 1897 he was appointed Associate Professor of Gynaecology and in 1903, on the retirement of Dr. Uzziel Ogden, he became Professor of Gynaecology and head of the gynaecological service at the hospital.

He was a man of great energy and leadership. It was largely due to his influence that the special pavilion for women was erected in 1882, and in March 1908 he persuaded the trustees of the value of a special out-patient clinic that he organized in a house on Christopher and Chestnut streets, in what was then known as the new hospital area. Finally, he was responsible for planning the accommodation of the Department of Gynaecology at the new College Street Hospital.

His ability in his special field received international recognition, and his surgical competence within the abdomen went beyond the strict confines of gynaecology. He was President of the American Association of Obstetricians and Gynecologists and Abdominal Surgeons in 1908, and his presentations before this Society showed sound reasoning and confidence in his ability to discard the outworn and to develop techniques and procedures made possible by improved facilities. A leader in organizing the Academy of Medicine in Toronto, he served as its first president. He appreciated clearly the value of an institution's uniting the whole profession in the community, and was constant in his demands for a liberal support of its library. At a meeting in the academy on December 5, 1911, his colleagues united to pay tribute to one who had given liberally of himself to his profession, the university and the General Hospital.

IX

The University and the General Hospital

WHEN THE FACULTY OF MEDICINE OF THE UNIVERSITY OF Toronto was re-established in 1887, the anomaly of the University's granting degrees to graduating students over whose clinical training it had no control came to an end. The re-organization was based on an agreement with the Toronto School of Medicine, whose staff became the Faculty of Medicine at the University. The departments of Biology, Physiology, Chemistry and Physics, already maintained by the University, now became available to the enrolled students so that they might acquire an acceptable knowledge of the basic sciences essential to the modern study of disease.

During the period from 1853 to 1887, which is generally referred to as the period of the proprietary medical schools, both Trinity and Victoria universities had faculties of medicine. Under John Rolph the Toronto School of Medicine, incorporated in 1851, had become the Medical Faculty of Victoria in 1855 and although the dean was deserted by the faculty members a year later when they re-established the Toronto School, teaching had continued under Rolph with a freshly recruited staff, on Asquith Avenue. On Rolph's death William Canniff became dean and the faculty moved to a new building close to the General Hospital on the corner of Gerrard and Sackville streets. Even the new environment did not delay the inevitable, and in 1875 Victoria students as a body joined the Toronto School of Medicine, which had grown to increasing importance under W. T. Aikens, and with the collapse of the Victoria faculty the Gerrard Street building came under its jurisdiction.

The history of the Faculty of Medicine of Trinity University was no less involved. The Upper Canada School, founded by Edward Hodder and James Bovell in 1850, became the Medical Faculty of Trinity University the next year, but after five years this association came to an end because of the dictatorial attitude of the university hierarchy. The Trinity school was re-established in 1871 with Hodder as Dean and Walter Geikie as Registrar and Secretary-Treasurer. With a good staff it soon became an outstanding school of medicine. For a few years the association with Trinity University was largely nominal as the students were free to obtain their degrees from other universities, but as the need for greater knowledge of the basic sciences became obvious a closer affiliation developed, and the school once again became the Medical Faculty of Trinity University.

Walter Geikie, who had followed the tortuous academic path of many others, became dean of the faculty and carried on an aggressive program so that in 1879 the building which the school occupied on Gerrard Street was enlarged to provide "two large Lecture Rooms, a new Chemical Laboratory, a new Dissecting Room (lighted from the ceiling), a Museum and a Reading Room for Students."[1]

At the inaugural meeting of the Board of Management of the Medical Faculty of the University of Toronto in 1887, W. T. Aikens was elected Dean and Dr. Adam Wright Secretary of the faculty. From this time there was close collaboration between the faculty and the university, and the following year it was announced that a new Science Hall was to be built on the site of Moss Hall, the original building of the Medical Faculty of 1843. The new building, which came to be known as the Biology Building, provided laboratory and teaching facilities far beyond the means of Trinity University. At the same time a feeling was growing that the General Hospital on Gerrard Street was becoming inadequate to meet the needs of a growing community and also the increasing demands for medical education. It was also felt that the location of the hospital was unsatisfactory, and so a new site in the Queen's Park was considered by the faculty, the trustees of the University and the board of the hospital. The Vice-Chancellor of the University, William Mulock, Professor Ramsey Wright, the Hon. John Macdonald, and Dr. Charles O'Reilly visited hospitals in Boston, Baltimore, Philadelphia and New York to see the desirable features of a new hospital, and shortly before he died John Macdonald offered to

[1] *The Canadian Practitioner*, XIII (1888).

provide $40,000 towards the new project. Naturally there were many obstacles to overcome, but these two developments presaged the ultimate amalgamation of the Trinity and Toronto medical faculties.

In the meantime high hopes developed that the "Park Hospital" would soon be established, and at a meeting of the faculty Dr. George Peters and Dr. A. B. Macallum expressed the hope that the hospital would be under the control of the Senate of the University, pledging the support of the faculty to bring about this proposition. At the same time, to meet the immediate necessity of providing accommodation for final year students, the university leased the old building from the Toronto School of Medicine at Gerrard and Sackville streets for $1,000 per annum for the next five years, despite the necessity for making extensive repairs.

Very shortly after the inauguration of the School for Nurses at the Toronto General Hospital, the demand that women should be given the right to a medical education could no longer be denied, and in 1883 the Ontario Women's Medical College was organized. Dr. Michael Barrett, a Professor of Physiology at the University of Toronto and a strong advocate of medical education for women, announced names of the faculty of the new college, of which he was to be the President and Lecturer on Institutes of Medicine. Nearly all the faculty members were physicians and surgeons already engaged in teaching at the established schools, namely George Wright, Practice of Medicine; I. H. Cameron, Surgery; A. H. Wright, Obstetrics; Alexander McPhedran, Materia Medica; S. T. Duncan, Anatomy; R. A. Reeve, Diseases of Eye and Ear; R. B. Nevitt, Sanitary Science; F. Kraus, Medical Jurisprudence; A. R. Pine, Chemistry; and Augusta Stowe-Gullen, Demonstrator in Anatomy. It was also announced that nearly fifty applicants had applied for admission and had been informed that they would be required to attend the General Hospital for a period of twenty-four months which might be distributed over four winter sessions. Bedside instruction would be given and the trustees of the hospital had proposed to erect a special gallery to allow women students to view operations and clinical demonstrations.

Dr. Augusta Stowe-Gullen was the first woman to receive a medical degree from a Canadian university. She was an undergraduate student at the Toronto School of Medicine, obtaining her M.D., C.M. from Victoria University in 1883. Although she was never on the staff of the Toronto General Hospital it was in this hospital that she received the clinical education which was the basis for her professional career.

Her special interest was paediatrics and in later years she became a member of the Senate of the University of Toronto. Throughout her life she was a vigorous proponent of equal rights for women.

In 1897, 1898 and again in 1899 the trustees of the General Hospital were unable to grant the request of R. B. Nevitt and D. J. Gibb Wishart for the appointment of a graduate of the Women's College as a resident assistant physician. Finally, however, in May 1901, Dr. Helen McMurchy was appointed and the following year it was decided to appoint a female intern each year. At the same time two women graduates were to become registrars, the first two appointees being Dr. Jenny Gray and Dr. Jean Williams. In 1902, although the Toronto Faculty of Medicine still did not accept women as students, Dr. Alexander Primrose, the Secretary of the Faculty, requested the hospital to appoint one of the teaching staff of the Women's College to act with representatives from the Trinity and Toronto faculties in advising on the appointment of house surgeons and in considering any improvements which might be made in the clinical facilities of the hospital.

By 1906 the testing time was over, and the Faculty of Medicine of Toronto University agreed to accept female medical students. The Women's Medical College thus ended the performance of its primary function. During twenty-three years the average total yearly attendance had been thirty students whose fees were only sufficient to pay the running expenses of the college, leaving the gratitude of the students as the only reward of their teachers. Although its history was short, the college left a tradition which has been fostered for a much longer period by the Women's College Hospital, which since 1958 has been a teaching hospital of the University of Toronto.

By the end of 1902, the amalgamation of the medical faculties of Trinity and Toronto universities was under serious consideration. In its final phases this was part of the federation which constitutes the University of Toronto as it is today. Although most of the Trinity faculty were convinced that this progressive action should not be delayed, there was a "die-hard" faction under Dean Geikie who fought to the last to maintain a separate tradition. Even in the final calendar for 1902–03 the statement was made "that the Corporation of Trinity Medical College has finally and definitely decided against amalgamation" and "students will pursue their studies and go on to graduation precisely as successive classes have done for the past 30 years."[2]

[2]George W. Spragge, *Trinity Medical School*, p. 92.

Although Walter Geikie now retired at seventy years of age, a distinguished group of teachers holding appointments on the staff of the Toronto General Hospital joined the new united faculty, including Frederick Grasett, Charles Sheard, Sterling Ryerson, Luke Teskey, John L. Davidson, George Bingham, Allan Baines, D. J. Gibb Wishart, H. B. Anderson, J. T. Fotheringham, H. C. Parsons, C. B. Shuttleworth, Newton Powell and B. Z. Milner.

The union of the faculties was sealed by the opening of the new Medical Building on October 1, 1903. Situated on the university campus just south of the Library and built at a cost of $170,000, it provided the best laboratory and teaching facilities of its time. Charles Sherrington, Professor of Physiology at the University of Liverpool, gave the inaugural address before a distinguished audience with representatives from Johns Hopkins, Philadelphia, Harvard, Yale, McGill, Chicago and Michigan. In the evening, William Osler, returning "as an old student of this School," addressed the students of the Faculty on "The Master Word in Medicine." It was one of his greatest addresses, for the occasion was close to his heart, and he led his listeners from a tale of Rudyard Kipling down through the ages of medicine to his final eloquent conclusion.

> It seems a bounden duty on such an occasion to be honest and frank, so I propose to tell you the secret of life as I have seen the game played and as I have tried to play it myself. You remember in one of the "Jungle Stories" that when Mowgli wished to be avenged on the villagers he could only get the help of Hathi and his sons by sending the master word. This I propose to give you in the hope, yes, the full assurance, that some of you at least will lay hold upon it to your profit. Though a little one, the master word looms large in meaning. It is the open sesame to every portal, the great equalizer in the world, the true philosopher's stone which transmutes all the base metal of humanity into gold. The stupid man among you it will make bright, the bright man brilliant and the brilliant student steady. With the magic word in your heart all things are possible, and without it all study is vanity and vexation. The miracles of life are with it; the blind see by touch, the deaf hear with eyes, the dumb speak with fingers. To the youth it brings hope, to the middle aged confidence, to the aged repose. True balm of hurt minds, in its presence the heart of the sorrowful is lightened and consoled. It is directly responsible for all advances in medicine during the past twenty-five centuries. Laying hold upon it Hippocrates made observation and science the warp and woof of our art. Galen so read its meaning that fifteen centuries stopped thinking and slept until awakened by the *De Fabrica* of Vesalius, which is the very incarnation of the master word. With its

inspiration Harvey gave an impulse to a larger circulation than he wot of, an impulse which we feel today. Hunter sounded all its heights and depths, and stands out in our history as one of the great exemplars of its virtues. With it Virchow smote the rock and the waters of progress gushed out; while in the hands of Pasteur it proved a very talisman to open to us a new heaven in medicine and a new earth in surgery. Not only has it been the touchstone of progress, but it is the measure of success of every-day life. Not a man before you but is beholden to it for his position here, while he who addresses has that honour directly in consequence of having had it graven on his heart when he was as you are today. And the Master Word is WORK, a little one, as I have said, but fraught with momentous consequences if you can but write it on the tables of your heart and bind it upon your forehead. . . . A conscientious pursuit of Plato's ideal creation may teach you the three great lessons of life. You may learn to consume your own smoke. The atmosphere of life is deafened by the murmurings and whimperings of men and women over the non-essentials, the trifles, that are inevitably incident to the hurly-burly of the day's routine. Things cannot always go your way. Learn to accept in silence the minor aggravations, cultivate the gift of taciturnity and consume your own smoke with an extra draught of hard work, so that those about you may not be annoyed with the dust and soot of your complaints. More than any other, the practitioner of medicine may illustrate the second great lesson that we are here not to get all we can out of life for ourselves, but to try to make the lives of others happier. This is the essence of the oft-repeated admonition of Christ: "he that findeth his life shall lose it and he that loses his life for My sake shall find it"; on which hard saying if the children of this generation would lay hold, there would be less misery and discontent in the world. It is not possible for anyone to have better opportunities to live this lesson than you will enjoy. The practice of medicine is an art, not a trade; a calling, not a business; a calling in which your heart will be exercised equally with your head. Often the best part of your work will have nothing to do with potions and powders, but with the exercise of an influence of the strong upon the weak, the righteous upon the wicked, the wise upon the foolish. To you as a trusted family counsellor the father will come with his anxieties, the mother with her hidden griefs, the daughter with her trials and the son with his follies. Fully one-third of the work you do will be entered in other books than yours. Courage and cheerfulness will not always carry you over the rough places of life, but will enable you to bring comfort and help to the weak hearted, and will console you in sad hours when, like Uncle Toby, you have "to whistle that you may not weep."[3]

[3]William Osler, *Equanimitas and Other Addresses* (London: H. K. Lewis, 1914).

Harvey Cushing, as he described the occasion, said that any student incapable of being uplifted by an exhortation of this kind is beyond the pale.[4]

With the appointment of Joseph Flavelle as Chairman of the Board in 1904 the future of the hospital was under constant consideration. An Advisory Medical Board, made up largely of the Committee on Hospital Facilities of the University and consisting of Doctors R. A. Reeve, George Bingham, J. F. W. Ross, Bruce Riordan, Alexander McPhedran, I. H. Cameron and N. A. Powell, discussed with the board the need for reorganization of the staff to improve the care of the patients, and the great need to improve the facilities for clinical teaching. It was clearly evident that neither the buildings nor the staff organization were meeting standards required of a first-class institution.

The reaction of the provincial government to this situation was presented in an Act "to enable the Trustees of the University of Toronto to assist in the reorganization of the Toronto General Hospital to provide means by which the students of the Faculty of Medicine should be instructed for the betterment of public health and the prevention of disease." A sum not exceeding $250,000 was to be provided for this purpose, and if a proper agreement with the trustees of the hospital could be reached a further sum of $50,000 was to be advanced to pay for the site of a new hospital.

In May 1906 the basis of the agreement with the university was laid before the board which consisted of Joseph Flavelle, representing the hospital subscribers; P. C. Larkin, Cawthra Mulock and M. J. Haney, appointed by the government; and Thomas Urquhart, the mayor of Toronto. It was stipulated that a sum of $400,000 would be paid by the University of Toronto to acquire the block of land bordered by College Street, Elizabeth Street, Hayter and Christopher streets and University Avenue, except that part owned by the Royal College of Dental Surgeons, and that a new hospital building costing not less than $900,000 should be erected. The hospital was also to agree to the payment of reasonable fees by students for the medical instruction they were entitled to receive. After due consideration, the agreement sponsored by Sir William Meredith for the university and Mr. Flavelle for the hospital received the approval of the board. At the same time the Toronto General Hospital Act of 1906 established a new hospital Trust consisting of Professor A. B. Macallum, Cawthra Mulock, William

[4]Cushing, *Life of Sir William Osler*, vol. I, p. 619.

McKenzie, William J. Douglas, Charles Cockshutt and Dr. Joseph O. Orr, appointed by the government of Ontario; the Chairman of the Board of Governors; the President of the University of Toronto; Byron E. Walker, Rev. J. A. MacDonald and W. T. White appointed by the University of Toronto; the Mayor, Dr. John Noble, Mr. Alfred Jones and James McGhie, appointed by the city of Toronto; and J. W. Flavelle, W. E. Rundle, C. D. Massey, H. C. Cox, H. H. Fudger, P. C. Larkin and M. J. Haney elected by the hospital subscribers. From this board the Chairman, Joseph Flavelle, appointed various standing committees—an executive committee under himself, a house committee for the old hospital under P. C. Larkin, a finance committee for the new hospital under H. H. Fudger and a building committee for the new hospital under M. J. Haney.

The hospital was empowered to expropriate lands for the new site and the National Trust Company became the official agent for the purchase and subsequent rental of the properties so obtained. As a beginning in May 1906, 109 College Street was purchased for $4,128 and 111 College Street for $13,875, and by January 1907, over $240,000 had been expended on properties in the area.

Although the provincial government acting through the university was obviously going to provide liberally for the new hospital, and the city of Toronto was giving $200,000, it was evident that the benevolence of good citizens would be a major factor in meeting the financial demands of the building committee. The initial stimulus had come in a letter which Mr. Flavelle received from Cawthra Mulock in September 1904. This emphasized the urgent need for an Out-Patient Department to provide services to the needy poor as well as clinical instruction for medical students. He offered to give $100,000 to build, equip and furnish a separate building or wing for this purpose. Anticipating the future, it was thought for a while that this building might be constructed on the Gerrard Street site, but already progressive minds among the board of trustees were planning the move to College Street, and so this gift became the beginning of the contributions that made the construction of the new hospital possible.

Shortly after this the Mayor made a general appeal to the citizens for financial support for the building of the new hospital, and P. C. Larkin and H. H. Fudger undertook to organize a campaign committee. Through Mr. C. D. Massey the Massey Estate subscribed $100,000 and Senator George Cos and his family gave $100,000 to provide a Nurses' Residence in memory of his wife. John C. Eaton offered to provide a fully equipped surgical wing, including wards and operating theatres in memory of his father, the late Timothy Eaton. The bequests of Agnes and Jane Shields, estimated at between \$100,000 and \$140,000, went to erect and maintain the emergency hospital and ambulance as described in the preceding chapter. Several benefactors provided sums of from \$25,000 to \$50,000, and by October 1911, when the cornerstone had been laid and the hospital was under construction, the total public subscriptions had amounted to \$866,000. None the less, considerable problems remained for the Citizens' Committee, working at that time under W. E. Rundle and Mark Irish.

Darling and Pearson were appointed architects in 1906, and after considerable study and discussion it was decided that the new hospital should be built on the block system; that is, a group of buildings consisting of wards, administration building, laboratories and other structures being of three or more storeys and only situated far enough apart to provide good light and air. In addition separate buildings would be required for the Burnside Lying-In Department, the Nurses' Residence and the Out-Patient Department. To these were added, a little later, separate buildings for private and semi-private patients, an emergency department, a laundry, a power house and also accommodation for the hospital help. An early estimate in 1908 anticipated that these buildings would cost \$1,388,000, and by the end of that year the purchase of a site of approximately ten acres was completed at a cost of \$586,830, including the property of the Royal College of Dental Surgeons. But even in those days the penalty for delay was constantly rising costs. Originally it had been planned to erect a modern fire-proof 400-bed hospital. By 1910 this had become a 550-bed hospital at an estimated cost of \$2,900 per bed, and a year later when another fifty beds were added the cost had risen to \$3,700 per bed.

In his formal address at the opening of the hospital on June 18, 1913, Mr. Flavelle presented the financial situation very succinctly. He traced the development of the hospital from its modest beginning in 1819 to the institution of his own day, a hospital of 670 beds representing an expenditure of \$3,450,000. To this the City Council had voted grants now totalling over \$600,000, and he challenged the citizens to contribute another \$500,000 so that their hospital should have its beginning free from debt. He prompted their generosity by recalling the obligations which had been met by generations of trustees and the gratuitous services rendered the sick and suffering by the physicians and surgeons of the hospital staff:

> We know of no parallel in any field of activity for the work performed in the public wards of hospitals the world over by professional men who, by day and night, have ungrudgingly served suffering men and women without monetary return. The Trustees wish to express their deep sense of appreciation for the unassuming, sincere and efficient daily attention by the men of the profession who minister to the needs of the sick in the Wards of the Toronto General Hospital.

He concluded by referring to a quarter-century of service from Dr. Charles O'Reilly and Miss Mary Snively, and the continuing faithful work of A. F. Miller, now Secretary-Treasurer of the Trust, for over thirty-five years. He drew attention also to the group of fifty gentlemen designated as "honorary governors" who had for some years subscribed $100 annually toward the maintenance of hospital services.

The main building facing College Street had a frontage of 620 feet and consisted of a central administrative area extending on either side to three-storey medical and surgical wings. These contained large wards of twenty-four and sixteen beds on each floor, with laboratories and central nursing stations. On the ground floor, extending back from either side of the central entrance hall, were wards available for semi-public patients and above these on the second floor were located the Eye, and the Ear, Nose and Throat departments and similarly, on the third floor, the Department of Gynaecology. Fully staffed operating rooms and special examining rooms were available on both floors.

A large lecture theatre had a central location in the basement, in which also were located the Department of Radiology and Hydrotherapy and, among many other services, the sterilizing rooms and surgical supply room. Built separately from the main hospital but in close proximity to the east end was the hospital kitchen.

The Shields Emergency Hospital and the Cawthra Mulock Out-Patient Building faced University Avenue. The former had conveniently located ambulances in service and the latter many examining rooms, with the hospital dispensary surrounding a large central hall for the waiting patients. The Admitting Department was located to the south of the Medical Wing, where it was approached from the Out-Patient and Emergency departments. Here, in addition to examining rooms, were special rooms set apart by a long covered wall, for the temporary accommodation of infectious diseases and obstreperous patients.

Facing Elizabeth Street on the east were a building for servants' accommodation and the Burnside Lying-In Department, which was a complete unit with accommodation for eighty patients in small four-bed rooms and arrangements for out-patient clinics and special laboratories. To the south of this were located the power house and the laundry. Approached from the south and centrally located and facing one another were the Private Patients' Pavilion, and the Nurses' Residence which had accommodation for 180 nurses, with teaching facilities and the amenities so essential to a residence of this type.

On the fourth floor of the central area of the College Street building, accommodation was provided for the Assistant Medical Superintendent, Dr. A. K. Haywood, and twenty-six house physicians and surgeons.

One source of controversy was the separate operating rooms on each floor of the surgical wing and in the special departments. While the surgical staff felt that they provided a sense of unit organization, those responsible for their maintenance criticized the greater demand which was made for the services involved.

Apart from its strictly utilitarian aspects the hospital presented some outstanding features giving it a character of its own. Considerable thought had been given to the bricks with which the buildings were faced. It was thought that red brick would have a factory-like appearance, and white would appear too cold, so a special beige-coloured brick was prepared and exhibited by the architects to the Board to justify an additional expense of from $45,000 to $50,000. There is no doubt that the balconied building of modest height connected by covered passageways and set on spacious grounds benefited greatly from the trees and greenery and well-kept gardens that gave an air of restfulness, to the benefit of not only the patients but also those who worked for them.

Shortly before the hospital was opened Sir Edmund Osler, one of the honorary governors, informed the building committee that their efforts had received the hallmark of approval, as his brother, Sir William Osler, in visiting the new buildings, had been delighted with them and felt they could not have been improved.

The new building was clearly the basis for a strong interlocking of the interests of the hospital trustees and the governors of the University of Toronto. As the plans for the new hospital had developed, the financial problems of the trustees were unrelenting. In addition to requiring extra grants from the city of Toronto, the trustees were forced to approach the University for a further major contribution. When the University agreed to contribute a further $300,000 to the hospital, it stipulated that this was to be in the form of debentures to be retired over a period of forty years, and in return the hospital trustees were asked to convey a block of land to the University upon which it would erect a building for the use of the departments of Pathology, Bacteriology and Pathological Chemistry, or any other department of the Medical Faculty. This building was to cost between $100,000 and $130,000, the money to be provided by the trustees who agreed to purchase the land and building for $38,500 if it was not to be used by the University for its original purpose. The new Pathological Building was erected just south of the Out-Patient building on University Avenue and was attached to it by a covered way, and it was to serve its dual purpose to the students and the patients of the hospital for many years to come.

Considerable groundwork had been accomplished by the advisory committee of the medical staff and the hospital trustees between 1906 and 1920 in regard to the reorganization of the medical services. In 1907 coordinated services were established: three in medicine, including dermatology and neurology, three in surgery, one each in obstetrics, gynaecology, ophthalmology, and ear, nose and throat, as well as a department of anaesthesia. Each of the services was to consist of a head, with his associates and assistants, and was to be responsible for indoor and outdoor patients. Appointments were to be made on an annual basis, and appointees were forbidden the right to serve on the staff of another general hospital. The heads of services were appointed for a period of ten years but the heads of the surgical services, including the specialties, were to retire at fifty-five years of age and the medical heads at sixty years of age. It was ruled, however, that after special consideration, another five years might be added to this length of service. The trustees also undertook to limit the type of practice of the heads of services. No general practice was to be permitted; only consulting practice for the physicians, surgical practice for the surgeons, obstetrics and paediatrics for the head obstetrician. The chief of gynaecology was permitted to do general surgery, while the ophthalmologist and the head of the nose and throat service could engage in reciprocal practice. All public ward patients would come under the heads of services and would be available for clinical teaching. Finally, senior members of the staff who, through age or length of service, had reached the time of retirement might be appointed to the consulting staff, along with professors of medicine and of surgery at the University of Toronto, as ex-officio members of the active staff of the hospital. Medical practitioners not on the hospital staff were to be permitted to attend private, semi-private or semi-public patients.

There was considerable controversy over the arrangements governing staff appointments, which to date had been the responsibility of the Board of Trustees. The designation "ex officio" as applied to the senior professor of medicine and the senior professor of surgery was evidence of this authority. However, when the agreement between the hospital and the university was sealed by the formal signatures of Joseph Flavelle and Byron E. Walker on December 1, 1910, it established the Joint Hospitals Relations Committee which from this time on was to have the primary consideration of all medical staff appointments. The members of the committee were Joseph Flavelle, P. C. Larkin, D. A. Wilkie and Alderman McCarthy representing the hospital, and the Chancellor, Sir William Meredith, President Robert Falconer, Sir Charles Moss and the Rev. Dr. D. Bruce MacDonald representing the university. One of the first actions of this committee was to authorize a fourth service under I. H. Cameron, with C. L. Starr as his senior assistant, and Doctors Norman Shenstone and W. E. Gallie as junior assistants. At the same time, since the university was responsible for all students' fees, it began to pay twenty-five dollars per annum for the hospital privileges each received.

June 13, 1913, was a gala day. Two thousand guests were invited to attend the official opening. It had been expected that the Governor General of Canada, H.R.H. the Duke of Connaught, would perform the act of opening the door with a gold key. But the serious illness of the Duchess of Connaught prevented his attendance and Sir John Gibson, the Lieutenant-Governor of Ontario, acted in his place. Church and state combined in the ceremonies and Sir John Gibson, the Hon. James Whitney, the Prime Minister of Ontario, and Mayor H. C. Hocken all paid tribute to those who had worked so hard to make the new hospital possible. Above all they praised Joseph Flavelle, whose unfailing energy had stimulated others in their outstanding efforts.

According to the press, the opening of the hospital was appreciated by large numbers of the citizens as an event in the history of Toronto. While other general hospitals were now in service, some working in close association with the university, the very name of the General Hospital stirred a feeling of civic pride, for it was now the largest and best equipped of Canadian hospitals, comparing with the best in the world.

Spontaneous applause from a crowd of several thousand gathered in front of the hospital greeted the opening of the doors, and that evening, while the bands of the Queen's Own Rifles and the 48th Highlanders played on the balconies, over 30,000 people went the rounds of the buildings, while half as many more asked in vain to be admitted. There was something highly significant for the future in the new location next to the Hospital for Sick Children on College Street, for it was visible evidence of the enduring partnership between two great teaching hospitals of the University of Toronto.

On July 3 the board of trustees passed another milestone when it held its first meeting in the new board room on College Street. The membership at the time is worth recording. Appointed by the government of Ontario were Professor A. B. Macallum, Cawthra Mulock, Sir William Mackenzie, Eugene O'Keefe and J. C. Eaton. Appointed by the University of Toronto were Dr. John Hoskin, K.C., President R. A. Falconer, C.V.O., Sir Edmund Walker, Z. A. Lash, K.C., and Sir Edmund Osler. Appointed by the city of Toronto were Mayor H. C. Hocken, Alderman A. E. Burgess, Alderman J. W. Meredith, Alderman J. Wanless and Alderman S. M. Wickett. Elected by the subscribers were J. W. Flavelle, Chairman, H. H. Fudger, P. C. Larkin, D. A. Dunlap, W. E. Rundle, C. D. Massey and H. C. Cox.

When the first patients were admitted to the new hospital on June 10 and the transfer of 275 patients from Gerrard Street took place a few days later, the Burnside Lying-In Hospital had not been completed, and for another year the obstetrical patients were cared for in the old Burnside Hospital on Gerrard Street. The Private Patients' Pavilion was also still under construction and the house surgeons' quarters were arranged to provide accommodation for a very limited number of patients. F. W. Marlow performed the first major operation in the new hospital on July 15, 1913.

X

The War Years: 1914-1918

WHEN DR. J. F. W. ROSS DIED, THE UNIVERSITY OF TORONTO decided to combine the departments of Gynaecology and Obstetrics. In November 1912 the Joint Committee on University and Hospital Relations appointed Dr. B. P. Watson to the chair of the new combined department. Dr. Watson, a Scotsman, had graduated from Edinburgh in 1902 and had already proved his ability as a teacher and clinical investigator. With this appointment Dr. K. C. McIlwraith, who had been in charge of the Department of Obstetrics since the retirement of Dr. Adam Wright in 1907, along with Dr. F. W. Marlow, who had served similarly in Gynaecology after Dr. Ross's death, became the Senior Assistant. Certain other appointments were continued in the separate departments, but from this time on all new appointments recognized the combined department under Professor Watson, and his two house surgeons alternated between Obstetrics and Gynaecology on a six-month basis.

B. P. Watson lost no time in introducing new services to increase the efficiency of his department. A pathological laboratory was equipped in the Burnside Building where his technician prepared material and he himself was responsible for the surgical pathology. In the next room he developed a pathological museum for students working in his department. Here they could study the correlation between case histories and the gross and microscopic pathological material which was available to them.

An out-patient maternity service had been developed in 1908 by Dr. K. C. McIlwraith which, in cooperation with the Victorian Order of Nurses, assisted in the home confinements of a considerable number of women. At a time when the large majority of women were delivered at home the value of this experiencc to house surgeons, senior students and pupil nurses was very great.

On the other hand, however, the necessity for antenatal care had not been appreciated by more than a few physicians. An obstetrical textbook used in the department at the time stated that the mortality for eclampsia was twenty-five per cent, and that "the accoucheur will generally have seen the patient before labour."[1] Dr. Watson's appointment of Dr. J. G. Gallie in 1913 changed this situation completely, for he applied the routine that he had learned at the New York Lying-In Hospital and the Manhattan Maternity, and regular antenatal clinics were organized in the Burnside department under his supervision, with a social service nurse in attendance. Although his service was interrupted during the war by his appointment to No. 4 General Hospital, the antenatal clinic he had organized carried on. Dr. J. W. S. McCullough, reporting on progress in public health in Ontario between 1910 and 1920, presented figures from the Burnside showing that the maternal death rate in supervised public ward patients was less than one-quarter of that which occurred in semi-private patients admitted to that hospital, and this he attributed to the clinic that Dr. Gallie had developed.

Another major development in the General Hospital was the appointment of Miss Jean Gunn in September 1913 to succeed Miss Robina Stewart as Superintendent of Nurses. Born in Belleville, Ontario, Miss Gunn had graduated from the Presbyterian Hospital of New York in 1905. She had been a supervisor on the hospital staff and later was engaged in social service work in New York City. Prior to her appointment in Toronto she was Superintendent of Nurses at the Memorial Hospital in Morristown, New Jersey. On Miss Gunn's recommendation, Miss Helen Locke, a fellow graduate of the Presbyterian Hospital, was appointed as Assistant Superintendent of Nurses. Thus Miss Gunn acquired the services of an effective right arm, and for some years to come these two ladies seemed inseparable as they directed the care of the patients and the instruction of the nurses.

The Training School was facing a great increase in the number of pupil nurses and a constantly broadening field of instruction. In her annual report in September 1914 Miss Gunn stated that 1,694 applica-

[1]Adam H. Wright, *A Textbook of Obstetrics* (Toronto: Moran, 1905).

tions had been received for probationary instruction and that the nursing staff now included 32 supervisors and head nurses and 207 pupil nurses, including probationers. As a result the Nurses' Residence was full to capacity and an annex had to be opened on Queen's Park. Pupil nurses were now receiving instruction in home obstetrical care through the Out-Door Department of the Burnside Hospital and in public health services through the Social Service Department.

Almost before the trustees and medical staff had settled down to face their new duties and responsibilities, war was declared between Britain and Germany, and Canada's response was that of British people throughout the Empire. The tradition of the General Hospital had always been one of unquestioning service to the country in time of war. J. D. Thorburn had been the first Regimental Surgeon to the Queen's Own Rifles when that regiment was raised to meet the threat of the Fenian Raid in 1866. Sterling Ryerson was the Regimental Surgeon of the Royal Grenadiers at Batoche when that victory put an end to the Northwest Rebellion, and E. E. King also served in the campaign. Dr. Ryerson and Dr. James Roberts served during the South African War in 1901–1902, and now this example was to be followed by a great number of surgeons and physicians, while medical students were to break their studies by service in the Army, the Navy and the Air Force.

Among the first to go was Dr. Alfred Haywood, the Assistant Medical Superintendent, who went as Medical Officer of the Third Canadian Battalion and won the Military Cross at the Second Battle of Ypres. Others on the medical staff, holding commissions in the Army Medical Corps, volunteered promptly: C. E. Cooper Cole and R. D. Rudolph left from Valcartier with the first Canadians to go overseas, and John T. Fotheringham became the Senior Medical Officer for the Toronto area. So, as the hospital prepared for the fall term of 1914, there was an air of uncertainty as to the future of teachers and students alike.

The first impact of the tragedy of the war was the outbreak of cerebrospinal meningitis in the late fall of 1914. Although the epidemic that developed among the Canadian soldiers on Salisbury Plain in England received greater publicity, many cases developed among the troops in winter quarters in Canada. In Toronto thousands of soldiers were quartered in the buildings of the Toronto Exhibition, and in the first winter 32 cases of meningitis, of whom 18 died, were accommodated in the Shields Emergency Hospital. In addition, 29 meningococcic carriers were admitted so that this hospital proved, as it would again in years to come, an isolation centre where epidemic patients could receive the best treatment available.

Although the members of the medical staff served with many units from front line battalions and field ambulances to clearing stations and base hospitals, it was the mobilization of No. 4 Canadian General Hospital early in 1915 that had the closest association with the Toronto General Hospital. This came as a result of a meeting of members of the medical faculty who were already associated with the militia, convened by the President of the University, Robert Falconer. The establishment of a hospital of 1,040 beds was shortly authorized by the British War Office.

Lt.-Col. J. A. Roberts was appointed as Commanding Officer with Lt.-Col. W. B. Hendry as Second-in-Command. Physicians and surgeons from many hospitals and others with only university affiliations volunteered for service, but there was a great preponderance from the General Hospital, many of whom held senior appointments. The list included Graham Chambers, Andrew R. Gordon, Alexander Primrose, W. J. O. Malloch, Stanley McVicar, Harold Parsons, Stanley Ryerson, D. King-Smith, Robert Armour, George Boyer, A. H. Caulfield, Robert Gaby, J. G. Gallie, D. A. L. Graham, S. R. D. Hewitt, W. H. Lowry, J. J. Mackenzie, Gilbert Royce, H. J. Shields, B. P. Watson, George Wilson, Harold Wookey, A. Almon Fletcher, N. C. Sharpe and Norman Yellowlees. In addition fifty-three of the nursing sisters were graduates of the Nurses' Training School, including Miss Annie Hartley who was matron of the hospital. There were also among the NCOs and privates some students who would come to appointments in the General Hospital in the years after the war, as well as one who would in later years become the Prime Minister of Canada and who appeared on a nominal roll as "Private—Pearson, Lester Bowles." In his case service brought its reward as later on, before the hospital left Salonika, he was wearing the stripes of a corporal on the sleeves of his tunic.

The hospital sailed for overseas on May 15, 1915, and in July took over Moore Barracks Hospital in Shorncliffe. At this time Britain and her allies were engaged in the Dardanelles campaign and, on a smaller scale, fighting a rearguard action in the Balkans. It was decided to send No. 4 General Hospital out to the base in Salonika, where it arrived after a protracted voyage on November 10, 1915. The nursing sisters, sailing on hospital ships, did not arrive until November 17 and by that time, with the aid of officer fatigues, the men had already erected the tents and the hospital was caring for the first convoy of patients with frost-bite and wounds, from the 10th British Division which had been driven back to the Serbian border. With no beds but blankets covering straw on the ground, the conditions were harsh indeed.

Malaria, dysentery and jaundice accounted for most of the patients received at the hospital, and sanitation became an important feature of the work of both the surgeons and the physicians. Early in 1916 the hospital moved to accommodation in huts on a new site; as a result weather conditions were no longer so disturbing and the efficiency of the hospital was greatly increased. It now had a capacity of 2,000 beds and the average daily number of patients was 1,000. By the time the hospital left Salonika in June 1917, nearly 18,000 patients had been cared for in its wards. The laboratory services made No. 4 the scientific centre for the Salonika area and an X-ray service was developed under Sgt. H. A. McTaggart, who had been a professor in the Department of Physics of the University of Toronto. Two activities developed that were unique in the service: a course of lectures was given to the twenty-one medical students serving with the hospital, and a medico-scientific society was organized in cooperation with the staffs of the other base hospitals in the area. Many interesting meetings were held, the hospitals vying with one another in the quality of the papers that were presented.

The one tragedy suffered by the unit was the death of the Adjutant, Captain Norman Yellowlees, who drowned while trying to swim his horse across the Vardar River on his way to see the remains of a Zeppelin that had been shot down some miles away the previous night. He was a very popular young man, and had served as physician to the Nurses' Training School at the Toronto General Hospital prior to the war. Although a number of officers and nurses contracted contagious diseases from the patients, it was remarkable that only one nursing sister died after her return to England from blackwater fever.

Col. W. B. Hendry took over command at the end of 1916 and the hospital was re-established in England in August 1917. Here it was located in the Basingstoke Asylum, a modern well-equipped building. The hospital remained in this location for nearly two years. The daily number of patients was about 1,200 and a large number of wounded Canadian soldiers came to the Canadian Military Hospital at Basingstoke. A chief interest was the treatment of comminuted fractures by the Carrel-Dakin method. The principle of this was the continuous irrigation of widely open wounds with a solution of sodium hyperchlorite modified with boric acid, after the removal of foreign material and bone fragments. Amputations were obviated, and the healing process initiated before many of the patients were evacuated further on their way home to Canada.

Duncan Graham, who originally had been the bacteriologist to the hospital in Salonika, became the senior physician in Basingstoke and many new officers came as replacements for some of the original staff which had included "those gallant middle-aged men who left with No. 4."[2] William Goldie, R. R. Graham, W. R. Campbell, A. H. Rolph, W. A. Scott and W. L. Robinson were all members of the Toronto General Hospital staff coming to No. 4 on this basis.

John T. Fotheringham was a physician in charge of one of the medical services at the General Hospital when the war broke out. He had come to his appointment of Assistant Professor of Clinical Medicine at the University of Toronto by way of the Trinity College Medical School. He had graduated with honours in Classics from the University of Toronto in 1883 before becoming a medical student, and this background was always evident in his teaching. He had a long association with the volunteer militia, having been a private in the Queen's Own Rifles in 1879, and after being assistant surgeon to this regiment for a number of years he became one of the original commissioned officers of the Army Medical Corps when it was organized in 1900. He was appointed Assistant Director of Medical Services of the 2nd Canadian Division and proceeded overseas when he was fifty-seven years of age to direct the medical services of the Division all through the heavy fighting at St. Eloi, Mt. Sorrel and on the Somme during 1916, for which service he received the C.M.G. He returned to Canada early in 1917 and became Director General of Medical Services in Ottawa, with the rank of Major General, serving in this capacity until 1922. He was appointed honorary physician to the Governor General of Canada, and following the war he received honorary degrees from Queen's and Toronto universities. No one surpassed his patriotic spirit nor the service that he gave.

Another physician whose service was outstanding was Dr. George Strathy. After serving as a registrar of the Toronto General Hospital, he was appointed to Dr. Fotheringham's service and on the outbreak of war he joined No. 2 Casualty Clearing Station, going to France in September 1915. After two years' service, during which he was in charge of the medical patients coming to the unit, he overcame the

[2]J. J. Mackenzie, *No. 4 General Hospital: The Letters of J. J. Mackenzie* (Toronto: Macmillan, 1933).

restrictions of red tape to serve as a battalion medical officer in the severe fighting of the Battle of Passchendaele, enduring the appalling conditions which existed during those months in Flanders. He developed trench fever and after evacuation to England served as a Lieutenant-Colonel in charge of medicine with No. 16 Canadian General Hospital at Orpington.

Many house surgeons went directly into the army to serve at the front, and Dr. C. K. Clarke in his report of September 1917 stated that two assistant superintendents and seven housemen had won the Military Cross and one the Distinguished Service Order, and that Dr. Cooper Cole had been severely wounded serving in the front line as medical officer to the Princess Patricia's Canadian Light Infantry.

It is not possible to recount all the services which were rendered by so many. Mr. I. H. Cameron, Professor of Surgery, C. L. Starr, F. N. G. Starr and Norman Shenstone all gave their best at various hospitals in England and France and at times there was plenty for them to do. H. A. Bruce went overseas in 1914 as consulting surgeon to a number of British hospitals in France, and for some time held a senior staff appointment in the Canadian Army Medical Corps. Dr. Rudolph, overseas from the first, served during the latter part of the war as Chief Medical Consultant to the Canadian hospital on the Western Front.

The war years threw a great strain on the depleted staff of the Toronto General Hospital. Not only had many of the senior staff members gone on active service, but appointments to the house staff suffered from the departure of graduating students, and in 1915 this also applied to a considerable number even before their final year was completed. Twenty-eight students from the graduating class left to serve in the ranks with the locally recruited No. 2 Casualty Clearing Station only to be commissioned by the Royal Army Medical Corps after arrival in England, for even at this early phase of the war the number of casualties in the Medical Corps was beginning to threaten seriously the number of young British doctors available for service in the front line. Those representatives of Toronto who received their degrees in absentia served with British regiments and field ambulances at Gallipoli and on the Western Front. Several received awards for gallantry and two were killed in action.

There was also an unrelenting desire to press on constantly with the teaching of medical students, many of whom were returning from war service to complete their training. Others continued their clinical instruction without the usual vacation breaks of peacetime, so that each year graduated months ahead of what it ordinarily would have done.

By 1915 the volume of work in the hospital had increased steadily, especially in the Out-Patient Department where Dr. William Goldie, in charge of the Medical Service, had twelve assistant physicians and B. Z. Milner in Surgery had ten assistant surgeons. By 1918 over 46,000 patients were attending the Out-Patient Department annually. In addition to the general clinics in medicine and surgery, there were now special clinics for tuberculosis, neurology, dermatology and venereal disease, gastrointestinal disease, psychiatry, obstetrics, gynaecology, otolaryngology, ophthalmology and male genito-urinary conditions. By this time the out-patient staff numbered eighty and it required the services of three dental surgeons to do the work in that clinic.

The increasing incidence of venereal disease required a special treatment clinic for syphilis. Ever since the introduction of Salvarsan, a considerable number of patients had been admitted to the hospital while receiving treatment, but gradually, with refinements in the treatment, this became almost completely an out-patient department service. In 1917, 557 patients attended this clinic under the direction of Dr. C. H. Hair. Routine Wassermann reactions were begun in the hospital in 1912, and by 1918 9,500 were being done annually.

Dr. William Warner Jones was the first specially trained urologist on the staff of the General Hospital. After graduating from the University of Toronto in 1896 he had trained in St. Peter's Hospital for Stone, London, England, and on returning home he was appointed junior surgeon on Dr. Bruce's service in 1907. In those days and for some time after, lithopexy, lithotomy, prostatectomy and the treatment of urethral stricture were considered to be within the scope of the general surgeon, and it was not until the new hospital was opened that Warner Jones was recognized as having any special status, when he was put in charge of the male genito-urinary out-patient clinic where many cases of gonorrhoea were treated. Under wartime conditions he acquired the service of two assistants, and in 1920 the Department of Urology acquired in-patient status under his direction, with a definite number of beds available on the surgical wards.

With all this activity the Social Service established itself as the linchpin of the Out-Patients Department. A good example of the need for such service was seen in the problem presented by the considerable number of unmarried mothers now being admitted to the Burnside. In 1917, on investigation, it was found that only 14 of 138 patients were of normal mentality and many of them only applied for help when labour was imminent.

In the spring of 1916 the Department of Militia and Defence undertook to rent the old buildings on Gerrard Street from the trustees for use as a base hospital. With the erection of tents this provided accommodation for 1,000 patients and based on the assessed value of the property the rental was $10,000 per annum. This hospital was under military jurisdiction and continued in service until February 1920.

In 1916 the trustees agreed to provide accommodation in the College Street building for acutely ill military patients. The demand for this accommodation increased so that eventually it involved the whole second floor with a per diem occupancy of 190 to 200 patients. The patients were under the care of a visiting and resident staff, all holding military rank, many of whom had returned from overseas service. In the later years of the war an increasing number of wounded came for surgical treatment, and eventually this centre in the General Hospital became recognized particularly for the treatment of chest and head wounds. The total number of military patients admitted to the General from October 1916 to July 1919 was 6,100.

In 1917 the Bureau of Municipal Research made an administrative survey of the General Hospital, for the war was accentuating the problems, and it was obvious that on a day-to-day basis recurring deficits could not possibly be overcome. Dr. C. K. Clarke had resigned in 1916, but agreed to remain as superintendent on a temporary basis until reorganization could be effected. When Mr. Horace L. Brittain, who had been responsible for the survey, was appointed Hospital Superintendent he undertook to serve under him as medical director. At the same time Mr. Allan Miller retired, terminating his long service wth the hospital, and it was recognized that from now on there would be only one executive head.

Mr. Brittain's reports for the years ending September 1917 and September 1918 presented very clearly the financial problems as he saw them:

> While it had been accepted that the hospital would run behind in its current expenses in the first few years, it had been hoped that by 1917 or 1918 it would be on a self-supporting basis. This bade fair to be realized but war-time conditions altered this completely.
>
> No institutions had felt more keenly the effects of the war than the public hospitals. The chief elements of cost were food, fuel, medical supplies, salaries and wages. In every one of these classes there had been a large increase in cost. All citizens understood how food prices

> had gone by leaps and bounds but few realized that this affected hospitals more seriously than private homes. It was impossible to economize by using substitutes in any institution which cared for the sick, because the sick must have the best. High fuel prices were even more serious for the hospital than the high food prices. The General Hospital used about 8,000 tons of coal a year and within a year the cost had risen from $3.65 to $7.50 a ton. Most drugs had doubled in price while the prices of others had gone up 1,000 per cent or more.
>
> Public hospitals were limited by law in their charge for the maintenance of patients in the public wards. The government grant for ward patients was also a fixed sum per patient day. It was true that hospitals had recently been authorized to charge $1.25 instead of $1.00 per day as formerly and that the Province had increased its payments from .20¢ to .30¢ per day. But these rates had to remain fixed until changed by the legislature, while no law had been passed or could be passed to prevent the cost of operation from going up. Commerce and industry would be impossible if purveyors of food were compelled to sell for less than cost. The relations between the Government and municipalities on the one hand and the hospitals on the other made it necessary at the end of the year for hospital authorities to go before governing bodies hat in hand, asking for a lump sum of appropriation to meet unavoidable deficits. This was neither dignified nor financially sound for either party. Hospital endowment funds and annual private subscriptions to the hospital enabled the Board to supply the citizens with care for the city's poor at a price less than cost, but it was impossible for hospital authorities to continue to supply essential services at a cost greater than the total income from private gifts plus the regular grants from the Province and Municipality.

The deficit for the years 1917–1918 was over $60,000, including depreciation and interest on the building fund loan.

The hospital was also facing a large deficit from the out-patient department, where there had been great increases in the number of patients under treatment. In 1914 there were 25,000 out-patients while in 1917 there were 40,000. The greatest increases had taken place in the dental clinic, which had risen from 18 to 3,513 patients, and in the psychiatric clinic, from 319 to 1,345. The venereal disease clinic, which was started in 1915, was attended by 6,473 patients in 1917 and, in addition, there were 2,299 patients who had attended the male genito-urinary clinic.

Thus it was seen that the long-range financial problems were to a very large extent a legacy from the war. After a thorough study by the Finance Committee—at this time consisting of George H. Gooderham, Mayor T. L. Church, H. H. Fudger, Sir John Eaton, Alderman

F. G. Whetter, Vincent Massey, Sir Edmund Walker, W. T. Kernahan and the Chairman and Vice-Chairman, Sir Joseph Flavelle and P. C. Larkin—a report was presented to the trustees by the Committee Chairman, W. E. Rundle. The existing debt of $835,600 was largely due to uncollected subscriptions and increased carrying charges, in all amounting to $548,000. It was proposed that if the Gerrard Street property could be sold for $125,000 the city and the university could be approached once again for contributions of $125,000, and another appeal would be made to the public to raise the remaining $500,000.

The trustees were well aware of the effort that would be required to accomplish this plan, because they realized that they themselves had contributed over sixty per cent of the original subscriptions that had come in the first campaign. The hospital had reached the limit of its capacity on a number of previous occasions, and they felt that the citizens must be made to understand that the facilities had to be maintained to meet any emergency which might develop in the future. The statement was made that "no community on this continent contributes less for the care of its sick poor, either for capital or maintenance expenditure, and if the accommodation of the General Hospital had to be provided today the cost would be twice what it had been." This was the swan song of Horace Brittain, who retired as Superintendent after three great years of service, to be succeeded by his nominee, Mr. Chester Decker, who had been associated with him as an assistant for a number of years.

The success that attended the efforts of the board was such that a year later, in December 1920, Mr. Rundle was able to report that the debt had been reduced to $184,000, which he felt would be largely covered by the sale of the Gerrard Street property. Once again the trustees and their friends shouldered the chief burden and dug deeply into their own pockets. At the same time the thanks of the board were tendered to the chartered banks of the city, who had formed a syndicate in 1912 and arranged the debentures which were now redeemed. It was emphasized that it was the action of the banks that had made the completion of the College Street enterprise possible.

The months of victory in 1918 saw the spread of epidemic influenza across Western Europe and the British Isles, which, with ominous similarity to the cholera epidemics of years ago, came with the soldiers returning by ship to Canada. Beginning early in October the newspapers reporting the great battles around Arras and Cambrai and on the road to Mons, with the toll of mounting battle casualties, began to express concern over the rapidly increasing occurrence of influenza and pneumonia. The severity of the infection was seen first of all as it affected the troops. Between mid-September and mid-December there were 11,496 cases of influenza among 61,000 soldiers and airmen in Canada, with 716 deaths, as well as 1,160 patients in the base hospital on Gerrard Street, with a five per cent mortality rate.

The epidemic soon involved the cities, towns and villages across the whole countryside. Hospital accommodation everywhere was inadequate to meet the flood of patients, and general practitioners were working around the clock to attend the multitude who were sick at home. Public gatherings were forbidden, schools were closed and churches were holding only one service on Sunday.

At the General Hospital, Wards C and I and half of F, H and E became isolation accommodation, as well as the better part of two floors in the Private Patients' Pavilion, and a separate area served the same purpose in the Burnside Lying-In Department. Fortunately, Dr. E. A. Gray had been appointed as Assistant Superintendent at this time and he organized the services in the hospital. There were 657 patients with influenza admitted in October, many of whom were moribund and survived only a few hours after admission. At the height of the epidemic there were eight to ten deaths a day. The strain on the nursing staff was terrible. In October eight head nurses, seventy student nurses and twenty probationers were off duty, of whom thirteen developed pneumonia, and Miss Gunn reported the death of three nurses, Hope Aylesworth, Bessie Barr and Jean Thistlewaite.

Dr. J. C. Hastings, the Medical Officer of Health for Toronto, opened emergency accommodation in the Arlington Hotel, which received 155 patients in October. Miss Helen Locke, the Assistant Superintendent of Nurses, contracted the disease while supervising the arrangements and became seriously ill with pneumonia. Even at the end of the month, when the epidemic was much less severe, one-quarter of the nurses were off duty. Throughout the whole critical period volunteers from the V.A.D. and the Neighbourhood Workers and other ladies' auxiliaries worked night and day on the wards of the hospital, at one time providing forty volunteer nurses in the daytime and ten on night duty. Volunteers were also organized to provide home nursing services, and by the time the epidemic was over it was estimated that there had been 150,000 cases in the city, with 1,750 deaths.

There was a recurrence of the epidemic in January and February 1920, but it was much less severe and the death rate was only half that of the first epidemic. Once again the public was warned against crowded gatherings, and for a few weeks there was no clinical teaching in the hospital. Although specific sera were developed, the experience did not show any particular benefit. An evening paper suggested, as a prophylactic measure, that kissing should be avoided and onions should be eaten.

A death that occurred in Toronto in February 1919, ended the distinguished career of Lt.-Col. W. J. O. Malloch. Prior to the war he had been the Senior Assistant Surgeon on Dr. Herbert Bruce's service at the General Hospital,and he was an original officer with No. 4 Canadian General Hospital and senior surgeon to that unit at Basingstoke. After graduating in Medicine from Toronto in 1898 he had obtained his F.R.C.S., England, in 1905 and received his appointment to the hospital and Medical Faculty in 1907. His graphic and anecdotal manner of teaching was a delight to his students, and his kindly and sympathetic interest in those who worked under him was the basis for his exceptional popularity. He contracted an infection on his voyage home and died of pneumonia a few days later. He left the memory with those who knew him of a good surgeon and a patriotic citizen.

The war years and their disastrous aftermath came to an end in 1920. Although the pattern differed from that of a hundred years before, the same two apocalyptic horsemen had taken their toll—war and pestilence. This time 60,000 young Canadians marched outward and died for their ideals and the old loyalties, and John McCrae, an ex-houseman of the General Hospital, voiced their requiem:

> If ye break faith with us who die
> We shall not sleep, though poppies grow
> In Flanders Fields.

The temporary migration of a large percentage of Canadian doctors, young and old, brought about a massive sophistication in Canadian medicine and the alteration of the professional viewpoint. Changes that would inevitably have occurred came much sooner because of the maturing ideas of leaders whose influence was to shape Canadian medicine in years to come.

XI

Reform

THE GRADUAL DEVELOPMENT OF CLOSE BONDS BETWEEN THE University and the Hospital reflected an experience which was repeated all over the continent. As might be expected, the rate of evolution varied considerably and often progressed by slow stages. In many schools demands for proper pre-medical education were entirely lacking, and the accepted students received clinical instruction inferior to even the earliest efforts of our own proprietary medical schools. Where university affiliation existed it was often in name only, and the finished product could hardly have been worse.

Concern over these conditions resulted in the investigation sponsored by the Carnegie Foundation and carried out by Abraham Flexner in the first decade of this century. Flexner's approach was that of an experienced educationist. A graduate of Johns Hopkins University, he was inspired in his undertaking by the enthusiasm of William Welch. It was natural, therefore, that he came to apply the standard presented by the Johns Hopkins Medical School, built as it was on the firm foundation of Osler, Halstead, Kelly and Welch, as the yardstick by which to measure shortcomings prior to correcting many intolerable situations.

Based on his observation of 155 medical schools in the United States and Canada, a report was published in 1910 on medical education in America. Later Flexner visited Great Britain and Germany, an experience which allowed him to compare the great Practitioner-Teacher with the scientifically orientated "Herr Professor." He saw the former on his rounds of the wards or, with his masterful technique in the operating room, developing an almost hypnotic effect upon his enthralled students. Through brilliance and experience he transferred knowledge, and by his presence he offered a model to maintain an ideal. In contrast to this was the scientist-turned-clinician, completely dominant in his university and hospital appointment. Characteristically he sought a scientifically based answer to the problems of disease and was rarely satisfied with evidence from bedside observation which lacked laboratory confirmation. His area was the control and cure of disease rather than the care of the individual patient. Naturally the truth in both cases lay well within the limits of two extremes, and it could be realized that with the passage of time they would merge ever closer to one another.

Flexner saw the solution in the development of clinical departments under full-time professors within the organization of a university. He felt that on this basis medicine would become more of a science and less of an art. Thus in close association with the scientific departments of the medical faculties, teaching would be established on a standard hitherto impossible to attain. Coming from the mind of an educationist this presented a radical change which was open to question even in the minds of the most sympathetic of established teachers of clinical medicine.

William Osler, at this time Regius Professor of Medicine at Oxford University, was well aware of the need for change. In 1911, speaking before the Northumberland and Durham Medical Society, he suggested the value of developing hospital units in the teaching hospitals. On this basis sufficient laboratory services would be readily available to the clinical professor so that in addition to the care of the sick the problems of disease could be investigated. As a result both students and nurses would receive much better instruction. Osler's opinion had developed as a result of his experience at Johns Hopkins. Here, for fifteen years, he had been Professor of Medicine and Physician-in-Chief to the hospital, introducing to American medicine the British practice of bedside teaching under conditions that were the nearest approach to a full-time professorship existing in that country. It stopped short of this ideal only because the excellence of its staff made Johns Hopkins a Mecca for patients and troubled physicians alike; as a result, private practice forced its way into the busy life of the physician, the surgeon and the gynaecologist who made this school famous.

Osler felt that the professor should enter his career through a previous scientific interest, or as he put it, "through one of three doors —physiology, chemistry or bacteriology and pathology. He should live in his wards like his faculty colleagues lived in their laboratories." Although he feared the possibility of a man with an overwhelming scientific interest, he felt that the daily contact with students on the wards would prevent the staleness of a pure researcher. Osler had an inherent fear that Flexner's advice might endanger the type of school a hospital should be:

> a place of refuge for the sick poor of the city—a place where the best that is known is taught to a group of the best students—a place where new thought is materialized in research—a school where men are encouraged to base the art upon the science of medicine—a fountain to which teachers in every subject would come for inspiration—a place with a hearty welcome to every practitioner who seeks help—a consulting centre for the whole country in cases of obscurity. . . .[1]

This appraisal emphasized the great importance of the chosen professor, whose personality and wisdom could decide the success or failure of his position.

Llewellys Barker succeeded Osler at Johns Hopkins in 1905. A graduate of Toronto who had won the Gold Medal in 1890, he had been Resident Physician at the Toronto General Hospital in 1890–1891. He was willing to take his appointment on an entirely full-time basis, but the lack of sufficient endowment would not permit it.

In June 1911, speaking at Convocation at McGill University on "Some Tendencies in Medical Education in the United States," Barker foretold the future very clearly. Proper endowment was necessary for progress, affecting the departments of anatomy, physiology and pathology as much as the clinical departments. The major problem was the rising cost of living. Honour and respect were good rewards, but the pecuniary weakness of the university chairs often demanded the supplementary finance met only in part by the writing of textbooks. He welcomed the period of reform in which universities were entering into arrangements with the hospitals, as well as the corollary development by which their professors were coming to control the hospital staff through their skill in diagnosis and treatment, their ability as teachers and their power to guide original investigation. He looked forward to the time when special wards would be set aside for clinical investigation, and he stressed the importance of good out-patient departments where all the activities of the clinic would have full play.

In such an organization practical work by senior students under

[1]Cushing, *Life of Sir William Osler*, vol. II, p. 292.

supervision would replace didactic teaching. Postgraduate students would find full value for the years spent in such an environment, and if university salaries could not satisfy the needs of the professor and his staff some modification might permit limited full-time service.

Finally, he warned that there is always the danger of confusing alteration with progress, reminding his audience that attempts at betterment invariably excite some animosities and antagonisms. The truth of this latter statement has stood the test of time.[2]

Flexner had reported favourably on conditions in Toronto, referring to "splendid provision which has been made for laboratories of ideal construction and admirable equipment . . . that are amongst the best on the continent." He was probably aware of the plans for the new buildings on College Street, and must have appreciated the growing co-operation of the university and the hospital. In 1908 the medical course had been extended to five years, two years of basic science followed by three spent on the wards of the teaching hospitals, and the quality of the graduates of Toronto was becoming well known in the United States.

Teaching in the pre-clinical years was extending into widening fields of physiology. Professor Ramsey Wright and his pupil J. M. MacCallum were unceasing in their efforts to keep abreast of scientific advances. MacCallum, a graduate in Arts from Toronto in 1880, received his medical degree in 1899, becoming in 1891 Professor of Physiology in the Faculty of Medicine and University professor in 1901. His reputation was international, and he was responsible for the appointment of T. G. Brodie, who came out from London, England, to be Professor of Physiology in 1908 when MacCallum transferred his interest to the Chair of Biochemistry, a post that he held for the next ten years.

In 1909 J. B. Leathes, another distinguished English scientist, was appointed to a new Chair of Pathological Chemistry, and from this time on medical students learned the importance of chemical methods of investigation in the study and diagnosis of disease. When the new hospital was opened, a clinical chemical laboratory under the direction of a member of his staff was available for students to examine material from patients on the wards who had been under their observation. A considerable number of the junior members of the medical and surgical

[2]Llewellys F. Barker, "Some Tendencies in Medical Education," *JAMA*, LVII (1911).

staffs of the hospital held part-time appointments in these departments, and an increasing number of medical students were entering the clinical years after completing honours courses in the basic sciences.

Professor MacCallum served for twelve years as a trustee of the hospital. Another faithful member of this board was Robert Falconer, the President of the University. Their close relationship with the heads of the clinical departments made all aware that the problems of the immediate future would be shared by both institutions.

The time had also come when Alexander McPhedran was to retire from his positions as Professor of Medicine and as Senior Physician to the General Hospital, for he had passed threescore years and ten and his association with the faculty and the hospital had spanned the full period from Professor H. H. Wright to the postwar years.

Born on a farm in Halton County, he had begun his teaching career in the Normal School when he was a student of medicine at the Toronto School before the re-establishment of the Medical Faculty of Toronto University. He graduated at the head of his class and was appointed as a demonstrator in medicine by Professor Wright in 1885. After a long association with James E. Graham, he succeeded him as Professor of Medicine and Senior Physician to the hospital when Graham died in 1903.

In tribute to McPhedran, Thomas McCrae, Professor of Medicine at Jefferson Medical School, Philadelphia, said "he was a skilled diagnostician and his treatment was simple and based on common sense. Therapeutic vagaries did not meet with approval. I look back on the period spent as his house officer as most profitable—for he was the best teacher of medicine for undergraduates with whom I ever came in contact. I doubt that if in the early '90's medicine was better taught anywhere on the continent."[3] Llewellys Barker, another of his students and house physicians, said "his teaching was of outstanding excellence for these reasons—that he brought his students into direct personal contact with the object studied—to use their powers of observation and each to think for himself in all his clinical work. Although of a conservative nature he was progressive in action and quick to sense the advantage of new ideas. He was one of the first to establish himself as a specialist consultant in internal medicine."[4] William Goldie, his associate for years, recalled "the clear piercing eye intent on the patient

[3]D. K. Foerster, *U. of T. Medical Journal*, XXVIII (1953).
[4]*CMAJ*, XXXII (1953).

and the reacting or unreacting student . . . the concise wording of logical sequence, dramatic gestures, and the insistent questions 'Why? How? Where?' were impressive and never-to-be-forgotten." It was no wonder that his abilities received international recognition. He was a Fellow of the Royal Society of Canada, a rare distinction for a practising physician, but through it all he sought no other degree than his M.B., Toronto.

On April 28, 1919, Sir Robert Falconer announced that after careful consideration the full-time appointment of Professor of Medicine had been offered to Dr. Duncan Graham, and the trustees of the General Hospital had agreed to the proviso that he should have a free hand to allow him to reorganize the medical services of the hospital. As a matter of fact the trustees had anticipated the situation by passing a by-law the previous March, stating that there was to be only one service in Medicine (including dermatology and neurology) and one service in Surgery. The by-laws respecting the medical staff of the hospital were to be amended accordingly.

It might well be said that the new Professor of Medicine, who had graduated from Toronto in 1905, had spent the intervening years in good preparation for his appointment. Graham had held junior appointments in physiology and pharmacy before spending two years in London, various German centres and Vienna. When he returned to Toronto in 1911 he became Lecturer in Bacteriology and profited greatly from a close association with Dr. John Amyot of the Provincial Department of Health. His studies of the bacteriology of cerebrospinal meningitis and the efficient laboratory service which he organized in Salonika established his reputation beyond question. During the busy years at Basingstoke, where he was in charge of the Medical Service, he came to know and to be known by the men who would be his colleagues in the future, and the experience fostered the qualities of leadership which were to prove his strongest asset in the years to come.

In all progressive communities there are certain individuals who, although they do not sit in the seats of the mighty, show their larger vision and enduring influence. Of such was William Goldie, who brought to the wards of the hospital and the out-patient department, its patients and his students, the same sound appraisal that was characteristic of his private practice. When he spoke all listened, and it was he more than anyone else who had made it possible to establish the full-time Chair of Medicine, for it was through the generosity of his patients, Sir John and Lady Eaton, that the chair was endowed—the first to be established in the British Empire. The Eaton bequest of $25,000 annually was sufficient not only to pay a salary of $10,000 to the full-time professor, but it provided for the appointment of W. R. Campbell, H. K. Detweiler, A. A. Fletcher and N. M. Keith as full-time members of his staff.

William Osler had watched the development with interest, and although he still reserved his final approval of a full-time appointment he had no hesitation in endorsing the appointee. He wrote to Sir Robert Falconer that "Graham's appointment has been very well received over here and I am asking the Professors of Medicine in the United Kingdom to meet him next week at dinner at the Atheneum."[5] And in a more personal way he paid his tribute to Duncan Graham:

Oxford,
March 31st.

Dear Graham:
Delighted and hearty congratulations! Do come down and spend a night with us and before you go I should like to have a few friends meet you at dinner in London.

Yours sincerely,
WILLIAM OSLER

The reorganization of the medical service of the hospital became a reality when at a meeting in September the board approved the nominations of the Joint Hospitals Relations Committee. Besides confirming Duncan Graham's appointment as Physician-in-Chief, they also designated the following as Clinicians to the Hospital:

Robert G. Armour
W. R. Campbell
A. H. W. Caulfield—T.B. Clinic, Out-Patient
H. K. Detweiler
A. A. Fletcher
William Goldie—Supervisor, Ward H
Norman Gwynne
H. S. Hutchison
Goldwin Howland—Supervisor, Ward I
Ross Jamieson
N. M. Keith
F. S. Minns—T.B. Clinic, Out-Patient
Donald McGillivray
A. G. McPhedran
Fletcher McPhedran

[5]Cushing, *Life of William Osler*, vol. II, p. 646.

Leonard Murray
John Oille—Supervisor Ward G
H. C. Parsons—T.B. Clinic, Out-Patient
F. W. Rolph
David King-Smith
G. S. Strathy—Clinician in Charge of General Medicine Clinic, Out-Patient
Emerson J. Trow
G. S. Young

By the fall of 1921 the staff was fully organized with the addition of E. E. Cleaver, H. A. Dixon and W. R. Hodge and the university and hospital appointments to the Sub-Department of Therapeutics of Professor R. D. Rudolph and Drs. C. E. C. Cole and W. V. Watson. At this time, voluntary assistants to the Medical Out-Patient Department included G. H. Armstrong, C. M. Black, R. J. Brook, H. M. Harrison, E. G. Hodgson, F. W. Hipwell, G. W. Lougheed, J. W. Reddick, V. F. Stock, C. H. Warner, F. W. Weston, John Maynard, W. E. Sparks, T. H. McKillop, W. H. Holmes, F. L. Thompson, R. S. Richardson and R. Barraclough.

At a meeting of the Council of the Medical Faculty in December 1919, a letter was presented which had been received from Dr. George E. Vincent, President of the Rockefeller Foundation in New York, announcing a large grant "for the promotion of medical education and public health in different parts of the world." Mr. Rockefeller himself was quoted as expressing an interest in Canadian medical education.

> My attention has been called to the needs of the medical schools in Canada, but as the activities of the General Education Board are by its charter limited to the United States, I understand that the gift may not be used for Canadian medical schools. The Canadian people are our near neighbours; they are closely bound to us by the ties of race, language and international friendship, and they have without stint sacrificed themselves, their youth and their resources to the end that democracy might be saved and extended. For these reasons, if your Board should see fit to use any part of this new gift in promoting medical education in Canada, such action would meet with my cordial approval.

The result was that approximately $5,000,000 would be made available by the Rockefeller Trustees for use in Canada.

On the suggestion of the President, Sir Robert Falconer, a committee was appointed to clarify the position of the faculty in regard to the proposed gift. On March 1, 1920, it presented a long and exhaustive report to the council which, as it affected the Toronto General Hospital, recommended that "all matters affecting directly or indirectly professional care of the sick, including nursing, should be under the direct control of the professional staff of the hospital."

The committee also recommended complete reorganization of the Department of Surgery. The Professor of Surgery at the University of Toronto was to be Surgeon-in-Chief to the Toronto General Hospital and in charge of the surgical wards, as well as the outdoor and emergency departments of the hospital. This would do away with separate surgical services, as all patients admitted to the public ward beds would be under his control. After consultation with the hospital authorities, he would recommend to the President of the University the members of the staff to be appointed as university teachers or to the Out-Patient Department. He was to have similar control of the university appointments to the staffs of all hospitals having a university affiliation. It was recommended that he should receive a salary of at least $10,000 a year, and while he was allowed three hours daily for private work, his mornings from 9.00 a.m. to 1.00 p.m. must be devoted to his duties as Head of the Department. He was not to go out of Toronto on professional work and was to confine his surgical practice to the Toronto General Hospital. A salary of $1,000 a year would be paid to his resident surgeon, who must have spent a year as a senior house physician or surgeon and a year in an approved laboratory.

The committee also advised that hospitals other than the Toronto General Hospital which granted facilities for university teaching should establish a service of surgery with control of an adequate number of beds, organized and staffed along the lines proposed for the General Hospital. Finally, the committee recognized an urgent need in recommending that a new building should be erected on the General Hospital grounds for the accommodation of the Department of Pathology and Pathological Chemistry, with equipment for research, accommodation for animals, animal operating rooms, and other amenities.

Plans for reorganization of the Departments of Obstetrics and Gynaecology, and Otolaryngology and Ophthalmology did not proceed to the same extent as in Surgery at this time, but the committee's recommendations were similar, defining clearly that the heads of these university departments would have control over the teaching in the hospitals granting university facilities.

The time was opportune for the reorganization of the Surgical Services at the hospital, for Mr. I. H. Cameron had resigned as Professor of Surgery and Surgeon-in-Chief of the hospital in 1920, bringing to an end a long association with the Toronto General Hospital. Born in 1855, he was the son of Sir Matthew Crooks Cameron, Chief Justice of the Court of Common Pleas in Ontario, and had been educated at his father's old school, Upper Canada College. After briefly considering a legal career, he entered the Toronto School of Medicine in 1871 and graduated three years later with his M.B., Toronto. When the Medical Faculty was re-established in 1887, he was appointed Professor of the Principles of Surgery and Surgical Pathology, succeeding his old teacher Aikens on his retirement from the Chair of Surgery at the University in 1897. He became an Honorary Fellow of the Royal Colleges of England, Edinburgh, Ireland and Canada, and of the American College of Surgeons.

An early advocate of Lister's teaching, he governed his practice by unchanging principles, and even in the final years he operated wearing a short-sleeved gown, with hands and arms prepared by scrupulous washing, but without gloves, to allow, he claimed, a better tactile sense. His lectures, interlaced with classical references, both in Latin and Greek, were a bridge with the past and to his students he personified the courtesy and bearing of a true gentleman.

His retirement resulted in a series of changes in the staff of the hospital. Dr. Alexander Primrose became Acting Head of the University Department of Surgery and took over the Cameron Service at the General Hospital. As a result, Dr. F. N. G. Starr culminated his long career by becoming Chief of the Primrose Service. When Dr. Primrose retired the following year, Dr. N. S. Shenstone assumed his duties at the hospital, and when Dr. George Bingham died in 1922, Dr. Charles Shuttleworth, his senior assistant, became the Senior Surgeon on Ward A.

Both George Bingham and Alexander Primrose had had long and distinguished service in the General Hospital. Dr. Bingham was born in Durham County, Ontario, in 1860 and in his early years was a public school principal. He received his medical education at Trinity Medical College and on graduation in 1884 received both an M.D., C.M. from Trinity and an M.B. from Toronto. He taught at the Trinity Medical School, becoming Professor of Anatomy in 1890 and later Professor of Clinical Surgery. He was on the surgical staffs of the General, St. Michael's and the Hospital for Sick Children and on the amalgamation of the faculties of Trinity and Toronto universities in 1903 he became Professor of Clinical Surgery at the University of

Toronto and Chief of one of the services in the General Hospital. His sound surgical judgment and abilities as a clinical teacher combined with immense personal dignity, an impressive appearance, and a clearness of expression left a lasting memory with his students.

Alexander Primrose was another outstanding personality in Canadian medicine. Born in Nova Scotia in 1861, it was through the influence of Dr. John Stewart of Halifax, one of Lister's favourite assistants, that he sought his surgical career. He received his medical education in Edinburgh, earning his M.D., C M. in 1886, and after two years spent at the Middlesex Hospital and the Great Ormond Street Hospital for Children in London he came to Toronto in 1888. Two of his outstanding characteristics were a graphic ability to present his knowledge of anatomy and the meticulous records of his patients, which he maintained for a period of fifty-five years. He was Professor of Anatomy at the University of Toronto School of Medicine from 1896 to 1907, and from 1918 to 1931 Professor of Clinical Surgery. He was interested in the whole broad field of surgery and was ever ready to apply new procedures as they developed.

During the war he was the Senior Surgeon with No. 4 General Hospital at Salonika, returning to Canada on leave when his only son was killed in action in Flanders in 1916. He continued on active service as Consulting Surgeon to the Canadian Army Medical Corps in England in 1917, and was awarded a C.B. for his war services.

He became Dean of the Medical Faculty in 1920, retiring in 1932. An outstanding administrator, he held many offices including that of President of the Academy of Medicine, Toronto, President of the Canadian Medical Association and President of the American Surgical Association in 1931.

The hospital lost the services of another distinguished surgeon when Dr. D. J. Gibb Wishart reached the age of retirement in 1922. He was not only the progressive hard-working Chief of the Department of Otolaryngology, but over the years he approached the problems of the faculty with wise judgment. A son of the manse, he was born in Madoc, Ontario, in 1859, graduating in Arts from Toronto in 1882 and in Medicine from McGill University in 1885. He confined his practice to Otolaryngology, and in addition to the General Hospital he held appointments to the Hospital for Sick Children and St. Michael's Hospital. As a teacher he was on the original staff of the Women's College Hospital from 1886 to 1905 and also taught at Trinity Medical College from 1889 to 1903, in which year, with the amalgamation of

Trinity Medical College and the University of Toronto, he became Professor of Otolaryngology, continuing this post until 1922. He served for thirty-two years on the General Hospital staff, being Chief of the Department of Otolaryngology from 1914 to 1922. He also organized the well integrated out-patient and in-patient services at the new hospital. In those days, before the advent of antibiotics, the vast majority of operations performed in his department were for diseases of the tonsils and mastoid, and for nasal septal deviation. But Dr. Wishart with clear foresight established an increasingly broad basis of investigation which was of great value to his successors.

In June 1921 the University and the General Hospital agreed that Dr. C. L. Starr should be appointed as Professor of Surgery and Surgeon-in-Chief to the Toronto General Hospital. Dr. Starr had already established an outstanding reputation. The son of Dr. Milton H. Starr of Georgetown, who had been a graduate of Bellevue Medical School in New York, he received his undergraduate education at the Toronto School of Medicine, and his M.B. from the University in 1890. Following this he undertook postgraduate training in Corning, New York, later serving as house surgeon in the Hospital for the Ruptured and Crippled in New York City under Dr. William T. Bull and Dr. Virgil T. Gibney and receiving his M.D. from Bellevue Hospital Medical School. He then spent a year in England and in Germany before returning to Toronto to commence his practice in 1894. His special training in orthopaedic surgery resulted in his appointment as junior surgeon to the Hospital for Sick Children in 1895. He was a registrar to the General Hospital in 1899 and was appointed to the Out-Patient Department in 1902. From this he came to serve under Dr. Alexander Primrose on the In-Patient Service and finally became Senior Assistant Surgeon to Mr. I. H. Cameron in 1909. In 1911 he became Surgeon-in-Chief to the Hospital for Sick Children. Here his staff appointments showed his sound judgment: W. E. Gallie, D. E. Robertson, Bruce Robertson and Arthur LeMesurier, under his guidance, soon established the international reputation of the surgical service of that hospital.

During the war he served as Senior Surgeon in the Granville Canadian Special Hospital in Ramsgate from 1915 to 1917. Returning to Canada, he was appointed consultant in orthopaedic surgery and organized this service in the military hospitals across the country, developing a reputation second to none. In 1920 he resumed his duties at the Children's Hospital, and now that the Rockefeller Foundation had made it possible to establish a full-time Chair of Surgery his appointment was received with great satisfaction.

His appointment as Surgeon-in-Chief was confirmed by the Board of Trustees in September 1921.

Professor Starr did not re-appoint any members of the service who had been under the direction of Dr. Herbert A. Bruce, and as an immediate consequence Dr. Bruce tendered his resignation as a surgeon on the active staff of the hospital, though he continued to act as a consulting surgeon. This, as well as the fact that some of the older members of the medical staff had not been re-appointed, was responsible for an outburst of criticism in both the medical and the lay press, in which the deposed were presented as victims of a lack of appreciation for years of service.

Influence was brought to bear on the provincial government which set up a committee, under the chairmanship of Prime Minister E. C. Drury, to inquire into the matter as it affected both the University and the General Hospital. Some of the physicians and surgeons who appeared before the committee expressed the fear that the status of the "family doctor" was endangered by the training of too many specialists, the new system of medical education being concerned with the "ultra-scientific" rather than with the practical.[6] To a protest directed by some against a "closed hospital," the committee responded by suggesting that the university and the hospital should devise means to enable practitioners who were not on the hospital staff to attend their patients in the public wards. With reference to the Eaton endowment and the Rockefeller Foundation's gifts, it was suggested that in a publicly owned university private endowments should not be accepted if they presented conditions binding the university governors to a particular course of action.

In response to a request from the special committee, the Board of Trustees submitted a memorandum presenting their reactions to the controversy, reading in part:

> . . . As the single service system has been more or less criticized in this investigation, as a hospital board, we would like to express our opinion on our experience in the single service as introduced into our hospital against the duplicated heads of service system as previously carried on.
>
> So far as our experience has gone, we unhesitatingly state that we believe the single service is much preferable from the patient's stand-

[6]Bruce, *Varied Operations.*

> point, and the student body, as well as more efficient and smoother operation of our hospital work, and the great majority of our doctors, as well as our superintendent and nursing staff, speak most highly of the improvement in our service, we desire to emphasize this, as a change of organization has caused some dissatisfaction and criticism that to our mind is uncalled for and not in accordance with the facts.
>
> We exceedingly regret, in connection with this change of service, that there apparently has been some irregularity or technical mistake occasioned by a misunderstanding between the Secretary of our Board and the Provincial Secretary's Department at this time. . . .

Shortly after this, and before any further action was taken, a provincial election resulted in the defeat of the Drury government. As is invariably the case, the newly elected government found many other matters of immediate importance to deal with, and the controversy died away. Moreover, the benefits of the transformation in hospital authority and organization, not possible before, were soon obvious. Just as the appointment of Mr. Horace Brittain had resulted in unified control of the internal economy of the hospital, so now Duncan Graham and C. L. Starr unified the medical and surgical services, inaugurated the residency system, and established modern postgraduate training in the hospital.

Although there was no change in the status of Professor B. P. Watson, funds were made available from the Rockefeller Grant to allow for the appointment of a full-time Fellow as a junior member of his staff and also to provide a salary for a resident in Obstetrics and Gynaecology. By this time Dr. Watson had become a most influential member of the staff of the General Hospital, and it was with great regret that the university and the hospital learned that he had accepted the invitation to return to Edinburgh as Professor of Obstetrics and Gynaecology at his alma mater. Without doubt this came as a result of his work in Toronto. Although he was only here for ten years, broken by his service in Salonika with No. 4 General Hospital, he established an unrivalled reputation as a teacher and left a legacy which was to influence his staff for many years to come. At all levels they learned the fundamentals of the physiology and pathology of women, and his museum in the basement of the Burnside was a classroom and study for the undergraduates, where they saw visual evidence, both through the microscope and with the naked eye, of the facts which he presented so clearly in his lectures. Watson also set aside living-in accommodation for senior students so that they would be immediately available for obstetrical cases.

Dr. Watson was very fortunate to have two outstanding assistants at the Burnside Hospital. Dr. Alan Brown, the young Physician-in-Chief of the Hospital for Sick Children, accepted his appointment as a Clinical Assistant in 1914 so that he might apply to the newborn in the Burnside nursery his diets which were influencing young mothers from near and far who sought his advice. His nurse/disciplinarian was ready at hand. Miss Helen Kelly, the Supervisor at the Burnside, was a graduate of the Presbyterian Hospital in New York, and from the time of her appointment her pupil nurses maintained a service in keeping with the white-starched primness of their director. A pinnacle was reached in 1919 when a premature nursery, provided through the generosity of Alan Brown, was opened, and this nursery became a model of efficiency. Here, with conveniently located sterilizing facilities and a meticulous routine, near-miracles of infant survival became possible and liaison between the Burnside and the Hospital for Sick Children was firmly established.

The postwar years presented an immediate problem with the great increase in the number of medical students. In 1924, 234 students, including the last of the veteran airmen and soldiers, crowded the wards of the hospital, but this only presaged the great number of students who would demand a medical education in the following years. The Medical Advisory Board realized that this would overtax the facilities for clinical instruction in the wards of the hospital and welcomed the changes which had been made by the University. In 1919 a sixth year had been added to the course under the Medical Faculty. Higher entrance requirements were demanded, and further organization of the clinical teaching departments of St. Michael's and the Toronto Western Hospital, under the control of the University professors, helped to meet this problem for the time being at least.

It seemed almost a fitting climax to these momentous changes that Sir Joseph Flavelle retired as Chairman of the Board of Trustees of the hospital in May 1921. For seventeen years he had given unrelenting service and leadership to the hospital: not only had he overseen the move from the antiquated and picturesque hospital on Gerrard Street to the great buildings on College Street, but by his reputation and personality he had attracted a generation of notables to the Board of Trustees. Together they maintained an indissoluble association with the University of Toronto and presented to the government of the province and the citizens of Toronto a veritable "Who's Who" of the leaders of trade and finance in the community.

It was undoubtedly through his influence that W. E. Rundle, the General Manager of the National Trust, became a member of the Board of Trustees. Rundle's great contributions were the detailed review of the financial state of the hospital in 1919 and the campaign which re-established its solvency, to which Sir Joseph made his personal contribution of $25,000. Another of his associates on the Board of Trustees, and certainly the closest to him, was Mr. P. C. Larkin. For eighteen years he served on the board and for most of this time acted as vice-chairman. He retired in February 1921, and the following year was appointed Canadian High Commissioner to London, a fitting honour to climax a life of generous service to Toronto and to Canada.

During the war years Flavelle had been Chairman of the Imperial Munitions Board in Canada, and as such his service was of inestimable value in the war effort of the Empire. It was particularly in recognition of this service that he was made a baronet. But his work for the General Hospital might well have earned him the same reward. In the rotunda of the College Street building of the General Hospital is a great bronze tablet set in a dark oak frame, erected as a tribute by his fellow trustees to commemorate the man through whose energy, foresight and perseverance these buildings were erected.

XII

Years of Progress

In MARCH 1921 THE BOARD OF TRUSTEES ELECTED MR. C. S. Blackwell to succeed Sir Joseph Flavelle as chairman. He had been appointed as trustee the previous year, representing the Ontario government, and it was significant and of good promise that his career, like that of the retiring chairman, combined industry and finance. His primary interest was in the packing industry (he eventually became Chairman of Canada Packers Limited), but in addition he was Vice-President of the Toronto General Trust and Chairman of the Board of the Dominion Bank. It was soon evident that he brought to his work in the hospital not only a trained business mind but also deep human sympathy.

When the new hospital was opened in 1913 no one thought that within twelve years it would prove to be inadequate. Yet by 1925 the public wards, private patient accommodation, out-door department and nurses' residence were all found lacking and the facilities of the power house and the laundry were incapable of providing for the extension which could no longer be delayed.

In those twelve years the population of Toronto had increased from 375,000 to over 556,000. At the same time the reputation of the hospital had grown considerably and many patients were being referred to it for investigation and treatment not available in community hospitals across the province. It was also true that when the university had accepted the grant of $1,000,000 from the Rockefeller Foundation it had undertaken to erect a new anatomy building, to establish a psychiatric institute, to provide increased laboratory facilities in connection with the pathology building, and to limit the number of medical students.

The new Anatomy Building was built in 1922, and Dr. C. K. Clarke realized his most cherished ambition when he took part in laying the cornerstone of the Toronto Psychiatric Hospital near the General Hospital on November 12, 1923. In addition to 85 beds, this hospital contained an out-patient department with social service workers, laboratories for research in metabolism and pathology, and psychiatric facilities for treatment by physical and occupational means.

In the latter part of 1926 it was decided to invite a hospital consultant, Dr. S. S. Goldwater of New York, to meet with the board to review their plans for extension and to advise them as to how they should proceed. Realizing the difficulty of planning additions to an established hospital, he found himself in general agreement with the situation as it was presented to him, thus concluding his report: "there are many fine hospitals in America but the Toronto General is one of the few which might be called beautiful; upon completion of the projected buildings the General Hospital will more than ever rank as one of the beauty spots in the hospital world."

Following this a building committee was appointed consisting of C. S. Blackwell, G. A. Morrow, Mark Irish, Frank P. Wood, T. A. Russell, Dr. Bruce D. Macdonald, Alderman T. M. Macdonnell, Frank Y. McEachern and E. H. Gurney. After due consideration they recommend that Darling and Pearson should be appointed architects for the new building and expansion program.

The over-all plan was to extend the east and west wings and the south medical wing of the College Street building to provide accommodation for more public ward patients, expropriating a block of land extending from University Avenue to Elizabeth Street for 286 feet south of the present hospital property. This would necessitate closing the west end of Christopher Street and the northern ends of Centre and Chestnut streets. Gerrard Street would then be extended to University Avenue and would provide the southern boundary of the new hospital property.

A new Private Patients' Pavilion to accommodate 280 patients would be erected facing University Avenue south of the present Pathology Building. The original Pavilion would be converted into a second Nurses' Residence, which was badly needed as there were already 130 nurses requiring accommodation not available in the present residence and living in the basement of the Pavilion, the old servants' quarters, and in houses on College Street and University Crescent. The Department of Radiology, which had completely outgrown its quarters, was to be moved to the present Pathology Building and the Out-Patient Department, also working to the limit of its capacity, would extend into an addition to the Pathology Building which was to be built for this purpose.

As the university and the hospital were both involved in the anticipated change in the Pathology Building, the Faculty Council joined with the Medical Advisory Board and the trustees in considering various possible sites and types of building. One of the first demands of Professor Duncan Graham on his appointment as Physician-in-Chief had been that the hospital should provide clinical laboratories conveniently located as to the medical wards. But it was not until Mrs. A. R. Clarke, through the influence of Dr. John Oille, made a donation of $20,000 in May 1921 that he was able to have a properly equipped laboratory developed in one of the small rooms on Ward H. This set an example that emphasized the great importance of the close association of a new pathological and clinical laboratory building with the hospital. After various alternatives had been considered, it was finally decided that a building should be built by the university on the north side of College Street and connected with the hospital by a tunnel under College Street. The old Pathology Building and the land on which it stood was to become the property of the hospital, which would then free the university from a promised subscription of $500,000 towards the hospital building program.

There was little delay in expropriating the land to the south of the hospital. At this time the narrow streets were lined with old dilapidated little houses, and the whole area had an assessed value of only $197,000. At the same time, work on the extensions to the wings of the College Street building went on to completion by May 1928, and provided accommodation for 185 more public ward patients.

Construction of the new Private Patients' building commenced in midsummer 1928 and was finished by April 1930. The nine-storey building presented the latest features of hospital construction, providing accommodation for 320 patients, and as it reached completion the daily papers vied with one another in presenting to the public the new services that would be available. There would be fifteen operating rooms on the ninth floor, two floors for obstetrical patients, with nurseries of the latest design, accommodation for relatives and a private dining-room and kitchen designed for an efficiency previously unknown. There were comfortably furnished lounges available on the operating room floor for surgeons and physicians, and the one available to the obstetricians was particularly welcome during their frequent nocturnal vigils.

The trustees viewed the result of their labours and were well pleased. In a brochure commemorating the opening of the Pavilion, Mr. Blackwell paid tribute to the practical sympathy of the generous public, saying "a modern hospital second to none marking the very latest advances in medical and surgical eqiupment, this is their achievement. To the inspiration of their example may we confidently leave the future of this great enterprise."

It was remarkable how the trustees, and especially the building committee, had planned to meet their financial obligations. In preparation for the building program the trustees had passed a by-law in October 1929 empowering them to borrow from time to time up to $1,500,000. Starting with grants totalling $1,400,000 from the city of Toronto and from the province of Ontario through the university, they were able to raise another $1,100,000 within two months from private donors and corporations. The total expenditure was $4,500,000, major items being $2,500,000 for the Pavilion and $450,000 for the new power house and laundry. But in succeeding months donations both large and small continued to come in—the trustees themselves, as in the past, being an unfailing source of support to the institution.

In all the long association of the University of Toronto and the General Hospital there was never a more memorable occasion than the opening of the Banting Institute on September 18, 1930. It was the Chancellor of the University, the Rt. Hon. Sir William Mulock, who led a group of citizens in raising a fund for medical research and obtained further financial support from the provincial government for the new building which was to contain the pathological chemistry departments, clinical laboratories and laboratories for medical research under Dr. Frederick Banting's direction. As this building developed it became necessary and expedient to provide the heads of the clinical departments with facilities for the administration of the work of their departments. Badly needed student laboratories, rooms for an ever-growing pathological museum, laboratories for the hospital pathologist and bacteriologist, a post-mortem room and a large lecture theatre were features of the new building. For the first time, operating rooms and animal quarters were available to clinical investigators as well as for the scientists attracted to the Institute.

The ceremony marked the decade since the great discovery of insulin by Banting and his close associate Charles Best, and in his introductory remarks the Chairman of the Board of Governors of the University, the Rev. Dr. John Cody, emphasized that the name chosen was one that brought honour to all. There were representatives from thirty medical schools and greetings were sent from many others. Lord Moynihan of Leeds, President of the Royal College of Surgeons of England, formally opened the Institute, and the conclusion of his great address is worth quoting:

> The inauguration of the Banting Institute of the University of Toronto is for me one of the happiest duties of my whole life. This is a moment of high romance in a "Land of Dreams Come True." Dr. F. G. Banting, reading for the Primary Examination for the Fellowship of my College and still keeping his mind on problems of general medicine, became possessed of the idea of extracting the hidden virtues of the Islets of Langerhans, and of using them in the treatment of diabetes. As often will happen with the dreamer of dreams he surrendered every other object to this quest. He came to Toronto, was allowed the use of the physiological laboratories, and the help of an assistant, Best, whose name is forever linked with his own. The result of his labours announced ten years ago is now the common possession and the equal pride of the Nations of the World.
>
> One man with a dream at pleasure
> Shall go forth and conquer a crown.
>
> Banting has conquered, and to-day, as a gift from all mankind he wears with so becoming humility the crown of immortality. In his honour we raise to-day this Temple of Science.
>
> Memorials are of many kinds. Some are graven in stone, some are cast in bronze, some are written in letters of gold upon the scroll of honour which enshrines the names of the saviours of their Country. There is yet another memorial, born in the hearts of those from whom a heavy load of suffering and of sorrow has been lifted, and dedicated by them as an act of homage to a great deliverer. Take the journey of Autolycus and gaze down into the multitude of homes in which live the men and women and children of every nation, of every race, of every creed, from whom the cold hand of death has been turned aside by the skill of him whose services to humanity we commemorate to-day. Consider too that this is not the work of a moment nor even of an age but that it will continue forever. In the grateful hearts of those rescued from death and from those who spend their lives in the sacred ministry of healing the true memorial to Banting will be found. Is not his indeed a crown of immortality?

A special convocation was held for the conferring of honorary degrees, and among a distinguished company C. S. Blackwell was presented to the Chancellor by Sir Joseph Flavelle to receive the degree of Doctor of Laws, *honoris causa.* Sir Joseph traced the long association of the Toronto General Hospital with medical education and the University of Toronto. Referring to the constant responsibilities of the Board of Trustees in administering the affairs of the hospital, he emphasized the unselfish devotion of the present Chairman to his self-imposed daily duties, which had won for him the respect, affection and confidence of his associates as well as the esteem and support of the members of the medical faculty.

The Banting Institute will always recall those hot summer months in 1921 when Banting toiled with Best in the cramped quarters of Professor J. J. R. Macleod's laboratory. With the enthusiasm of youth, the young surgeon-turned-physiologist and the young scientist with the analytical mind formed a perfect team. As has so often been the case in the great discoveries of medicine, though the facilities were meagre the minds were great and, by November, literally living on the job, and financed largely by the sale of a Model T Ford, they reached their goal—their insulin controlled diabetes. J. B. Collip, Professor Macleod and others contributed to the production of a purified insulin, and when animal experimentation proved its efficacy the final test of treating diabetic patients was then undertaken.

There is no doubt that it was the authoritative position of Duncan Graham that prevented any delay in the treatment of diabetic patients at the General Hospital. He already had physicians on his staff who were well trained in the field of metabolic disturbances and experienced in the dietary control of diabetes. W. R. Campbell and A. A. Fletcher were responsible for the treatment of seven patients in 1922. The first to receive insulin, on January 11, 1922, was a fourteen-year-old boy, Leonard Thompson. He was suffering from severe diabetes with ketosis and was unresponsive to dietary control. But after a course of insulin he was discharged six weeks later and survived with controlled diabetes to die thirteen years later from bronchopneumonia. The great problem was the production of sufficient insulin, and Collip worked all day and sometimes all night to meet the constant demands of an increasing number of patients. In June, Duncan Graham organized a diabetic clinic on the second floor of the Pavilion, with a well equipped laboratory for private and semi-private patients. The public ward patients were treated on Ward H. In addition to Duncan Graham and his two associates, Frederick Banting was appointed to the staff of the hospital and William Goldie served as supervisor for those patients who were treated on Ward H. The staff of the clinic included a dietician and graduate nurses specially trained to take care of the patients under this treatment. Dr. E. S. Jeffrey became an important member of the team, as he was the Senior Intern constantly on duty.

By the end of the year, all the complications of the disease and sometimes the effects of over-treatment had been studied in fifty patients. Many came to visit the new Mecca and classes of instruction were organized. Instruction was given by Doctors Banting, Campbell and Fletcher to weekly classes of forty physicians, followed by laboratory demonstrations and dietary exhibits so that family physicians might be capable of supervising their own patients. An invariably fatal disease was now controlled and long life became the expected result. In 1962 Almon Fletcher received a Christmas note from one who said "1922, remember." The original clinic was discontinued at the end of May 1923, and the Departments of Physiology, Medicine and Pharmacology and the newly established Connaught Laboratories cooperated in the preparation of insulin under the direction of Dr. R. D. Defries. The little old building (1888) of the University Y.M.C.A. became the production centre so that insulin could be available for wide distribution. Frederick Banting became an Honorary Consulting Physician to the hospital and John D. Rockefeller, as his tribute, gave $10,000 to the hospital to support the treatment of indigent diabetics in the community.

When the hospital purchased its first X-ray equipment in July 1900, a major consideration in its use was as a means of physiotherapy. And while two of Dr. C. R. Dickson's assistants at different times were designated as being in charge of the X-ray Department, it was not until a technician, B. J. Fenner, was employed in 1910 that any real service developed. A stereoscopic X-ray unit was purchased that year for $10,040, and in 1911 the Superintendent reported to the board that 1,439 radiographs had been taken and 1,134 electrotherapy and radiotherapy treatments had been given. Fenner's salary was $500 a year with a right to fifty per cent of the net profits of the department. At this time Dr. Dickson's eyesight was failing rapidly, and after twenty years' service in charge of the electrotherapy department he continued his service in a consulting capacity only. Fenner produced radiographs of fractures, arthritic changes and a few abdominal and chest X-rays on glass plates that were then interpreted by physicians and surgeons. But as his knowledge grew through experience his interpretations of the X-ray findings were usually accepted. Percy Ghent, who was later to serve with Dr. Gordon Richards for many years, was first interested in radiology through association with Fenner. He recalled that Fenner transported a small X-ray unit in a home-made Ford truck in order to take radiographs at the Wellesley and St. Michael's hospitals.[1]

The volume of work increased rapidly at the General, and in 1914 the report showed 4,201 radiographs, 1,446 screenings and 1,476 treatments. The Medical Advisory Board, however, recommended that the time had come for the hospital to appoint a qualified physician to direct the radiological services. Wartime conditions caused delay and it was not until January 1917 that Dr. Gordon Richards was appointed as radiologist and hydrotherapist to the Toronto General Hospital.

Gordon Richards had graduated from the University of Toronto in 1908 with the Gold Medal, and his career was characterized by his ability to steer an undeviating course towards the goal that he had set for himself. After graduation he went to British Columbia as physician to a mining camp. His interest in radiology developed through association with Dr. C. W. Proud of Vancouver, who later became radiologist to St. Paul's Hospital in that city. Richards joined the Royal Army Medical Corps early in the war and became radiologist to a British General Hospital in the Mediterranean zone. It was with this experience that he came to the Toronto General Hospital to organize diagnostic radiology on a professional basis. The service had already become a source of revenue to the hospital and in a formal agreement it was decided that he and Fenner should have a share in the net profits in addition to their salaries. By March 1919, the volume of diagnostic work had increased to such an extent that Dr. W. H. Dixon, an experienced gastrointestinal X-ray diagnostician, joined Dr. Richards and in February 1921 a new agreement was arranged by the hospital with Doctors Richards and Dixon which established the diagnostic services on a very satisfactory basis. At this time, as far as the hospital was concerned, X-ray therapy was still to all intents and purposes largely another agent of physiotherapy. Other forms of electrotherapy were falling into disuse. Although diathermy was accepted as of benefit, the indications for its use were not clearly defined. It is interesting that in collaboration with the Department of Medicine Richards undertook the treatment of pneumonia by this means, but without any appreciable effect on the course of the disease.

[1]*Telegram*, May 15, 1951.

At the time Dr. Richards took on his duties at the hospital minor forms of physiotherapy services, such as they were, were carried on by a self-taught technician. In the latter years of the war, however, with the return of large numbers of wounded soldiers, the importance of remedial gymnastics and massage resulted in organized training for professional physiotherapists. In Toronto this developed from the efforts of Professor Edward Bott and Dr. William Blatz, and through the generosity of Vincent Massey accommodation was provided in Hart House, then under construction. Later the school was moved to the Christie Street Hospital of the Department of Soldiers Civil Re-establishment.

Application of this service to civilian patients had its beginning at the General Hospital in 1920 when Miss Ruth Green, who had been trained in Montreal and afterwards at Christie Street, was employed by Dr. Richards. As the work increased, other therapists trained at Christie Street were employed in the department. When Miss Green retired she was followed by Miss Jean Masten, who later had a distinguished career as Director of Nurses in the Sick Children's Hospital.

The value of physiotherapy as a means of rehabilitation was soon appreciated by the Medical Advisory Board. As a result, prompted by Mrs. Bruce Robertson, a course of instruction was given on the wards of the hospital in September and October 1920. This established a readily available special service which, a short time later, came to include instruction in occupational therapy. Gradually the status of the physiotherapists became more widely recognized and in 1929 the first fully organized course was established by the University of Toronto, making use of instructional facilities at the General Hospital.

The first physician to practise radiotherapy in Toronto was Dr. W. H. B. Aikens. He had a long association with the General Hospital as a physician and as a pathologist and finally was appointed to the consulting staff of the hospital. He was one of the founders of the American Radium Society and its first President in 1910. His many publications showed the wide range of conditions he undertook to treat by radium therapy in those early years, including rodent ulcer, skin cancer, sarcoma, keloid, naevis, cancer of the lip, benign and malignant gynaecological conditions, exophthalmic goitre and hyperthyroidism, and finally leukemia and Hodgkin's disease. In 1914 Aikens published a study of the histological and clinical changes induced by radium in carcinoma and sarcoma. Although it was admitted that this was purely empiric therapy, it was already presenting a reasonable alternative to the surgical treatment of malignant disease. One thing is certain, that Aikens' practice, conducted from his office on Bloor Street, was a challenge both to the General Hospital and to Gordon Richards.

Richards, through his efforts to treat superficial lesions with the X-ray equipment available, was convinced that the hospital must acquire some radium to justify continuance of radiotherapy. In February 1921 he complained to the trustees that he was forced to refer many patients to clinics in American cities, and asked that the hospital consider the purchase of 250 mgm of radium which, with the necessary appliances, would cost between $27,000 and $30,000. The board responded favourably, and in May of that year it was decided to make use of a gift of $20,000 from Mr. William Addie, along with the final payment from the Department of Militia and Defence for the Gerrard Street property, to purchase radium—which would be known as the William Addie gift to the hospital. In September, 150 mgm of radium in various forms of containers was received by the hospital and Dr. Richards was permitted to purchase a new X-ray unit for therapy purposes.

Richards' case book shows the promptness with which he undertook to use the new equipment. In the last two weeks of September 1921, he treated fifteen patients for various lesions, including the first patient to receive radiotherapy for cancer of the cervix. This did not effect a cure but in 1922, combining external X-ray therapy with local radium, the first patient was cured of cancer of the cervix and survived for sixteen years.

Early in 1922 Richards spent two months visiting various German clinics, an experience which enlightened him as to the type of radiotherapy department he should develop. As the new building plans developed on College Street and it was decided that the Pathology Building would not be required for its original purpose, the trustees undertook to carry out renovations to make it suitable to accommodate both the Departments of Radiology and Urology. In 1925 the hospital received a legacy of $250,000 from the estate of D. A. Dunlap. Mr. Dunlap had served on the board for eleven years, and it was decided as a tribute to his memory to name the building the Dunlap Building. Co-incident with this, the Medical Advisory Board recommended to the trustees that a radium institute should be established at the hospital under a committee chosen by the staff of the hospital.

In June 1930 Dr. Richards, who was now designated as the Director of the Department of Radiology, requested one gram of radium and the installation of an emanation plant at the hospital. The board agreed to purchase the radium at a cost of not more than $12,000. However, by this time the provincial government was facing demands for support for radiotherapy from a number of hospitals across the province and it decided that the situation required thorough investigation.

The following year a Royal Commission was established to report on "The Use of Radium and X-ray in the Treatment of the Sick." This commission consisted of the Hon. and Rev. John Cody, Chairman, J. C. McLennan, Professor of Physics at the University of Toronto, W. T. Connell, Professor of Medicine, Queen's University, Kingston, and Arthur Ford of London, Ontario. It first held meetings in Ontario, then proceeded to visit the leading cancer radiotherapy centres in the U.S.A., Great Britain, Germany, Sweden, France, Belgium and Denmark, accompanied by the Minister of Health, Dr. J. M. Robb, and Dr. J. W. S. McCullough, Chief Inspector of Health for Ontario. The comprehensive report which the commission presented to the legislature in 1932 has since been the basis for government support of radiotherapy in the province. It emphasized the importance of public and professional education, research, radiation physics, centralization of treatment in hospitals associated with medical schools and close cooperation with surgeons, physicians, and pathologists in the diagnosis, study and treatment of cancer. The principles that it emphasized still apply today. The Commission noted very favourably the extensive service that had already developed in the General Hospital, and as a consequence decided that the major cancer institute would be established in Toronto.

The Hon. Dr. J. M. Robb, Provincial Minister of Health, and Mr. Mark Irish signed an agreement on November 24, 1932. The result was that the department in the hospital became designated as the Ontario Institute of Radiotherapy, and while the government undertook to supply radium and radium emanations the hospital agreed to provide a building with fifty beds and facilities for the scientific study and applications of treatment by X-rays, radium and radioactive substances.

An administrative committee appointed to supervise the activities of the institute consisted of three members, including the Minister of Health, representing the government, three (including the chairman) representing the trustees of the hospital, and two representing the University of Toronto through its representatives on the Board of Trustees of the hospital. The Chairman of the Board of Trustees of the Toronto General Hospital was to be chairman of this board. The Head of Radiology at the General Hospital was to be the Director of the

Institute, and the heads of all the clinical departments of the hospital were to form the consulting staff and nominate representatives to constitute the active staff of the institute. Patients were to be accepted on referral by any practitioner, and referred back to him should they require operative treatment. It was proposed that the active staff at the institute should cooperate fully in both the investigation and the treatment of all patients referred to the institute, and that the institute should be under the direction of the hospital and controlled by the Board of Trustees.

The Supervising Committee of the Ontario Institute of Radiotherapy held its first meeting on February 26, 1934. Present were H. H. Williams, J. Stanley McLean and Thomas E. McDonnell on behalf of the government of Ontario; the Rev. Dr. H. J. Cody and T. A. Russell on behalf of the university; and Mark H. Irish (Chairman), G. A. Morrow and Frank P. Wood on behalf of the hospital trustees. The first patients were admitted to the institute located in the Dunlap Building on April 3, 1934, and on April 20 the Lieutenant-Governor of Ontario, the Hon. Dr. Herbert A. Bruce, the Prime Minister, the Hon. George S. Henry, the Minister of Health, and the Board of Trustees made a formal inspection of the building which now provided forty-nine beds for the Department of Urology and fifty beds for the Radiotherapy Institute.

Even before the Dunlap Building was opened, follow-up clinics were organized in special fields of surgery and gynaecology and all the patients were seen on admission and for follow-up by Richards and the departmental representatives. Radiotherapy equipment, much of it designed locally, brought treatment standards to a high level unsurpassed elsewhere. Richards and T. B. Hurst designed a 400 KV high-voltage unit produced by Picker X-Ray Engineering, which was capable of treating four patients at one time. They also devised a rotational feature containing four grams of radium as a modification of a Seivert teleradium unit. This unit was designed for the treatment of neck and breast areas. Another original development was specially designed radium applicators for the treatment of cervical cancer. Made from nylon, they prevented the harmful effect of secondary irradiation from the metallic applicators in rubber sheaths which were used at that time. It is of interest that Richards anticipated the value of hypothermia in controlling tissue metabolism when, following the work of Temple Fay of Philadelphia, he built a refrigerating unit as a means of delaying the progress of extensive lesions. It was a time of trial and error, and careful physical examination was the only means to determine the course of treatment in anticipation of more precise biophysical services.

At this time the institute had just under six grams of radium: 1½ grams belonging to the hospital and the remainder being provided by the Ontario government. Two years later, in March 1936, the first Canadian radium produced by Eldorado Gold Mines from the Bear Lake deposit came into use and 3½ grams of Belgian radium were replaced by the Canadian product in the head of the so-called radium bomb.

Although the government was generous in supplying radium to the Radiotherapy Institute at the General Hospital, the radium emanation plant was assembled in the Department of Physics at the University of Toronto and was under the control of the Department of Health. From this source radium emanations in the form of gold seeds were supplied not only to the Radiotherapy Institute and the clinics but also, on application, to a considerable number of private doctors in the province.

Richards' colleague, W. H. Dixon, died in October 1932. Under his supervision improvements in the diagnostic radiological service at the General had kept pace with Richards' own work in therapy. Dixon had received wide recognition as an outstanding authority on the diagnosis of gastro-intestinal conditions and it might well be said that he not only established the quality of the work in the Department but also prepared for his successors by training the young men who were to follow him, A. C. Singleton and Malcolm Hall.

In 1919 the University had appointed Richards Lecturer in Radiology, and the next year he became an Associate and Head of the Department with W. H. Dixon and A. H. Rolph as his assistants. In 1923, cooperating with Professor J. C. McLennan of the Department of Physics at the University, the first postgraduate course in radiology was organized. The first two graduate students to receive the Diploma of Radiology from the University of Toronto were E. H. Shannon and Omar Hague, who was also Richards' first resident in radiology. By 1932 the department was firmly established and Richards had become an Associate Professor and Chief of the Hospital Department of Radiology, with W. H. Dixon, A. C. Singleton and M. R. Hall as Assistant Radiologists.

Towards the end of these eventful years two unexpected deaths occurred which profoundly affected the Toronto General Hospital. Dr. C. L. Starr died on Christmas night in 1928. He had not been in good health for some time, but he was not one to lay down a burden because it was becoming heavy. In his own quiet way in the short period of seven years he had moulded his Department of Surgery and set a firm foundation for his successors. His ideals determined the nature of his service. It was Starr who, before Banting went to London, Ontario, trained him at the Sick Children's Hospital, and the list of his residents at the General formed an honour role of which the hospital was very proud. Dr. Shenstone voiced the feeling of his staff in his final tribute:

> Dr. C. L. Starr, by his courageous organization of the Department, his great executive capacity, his surgical skill, his innate honesty and unusual aptitude as a teacher had earned the admiration and respect of all his associates. His personal interest, his sympathy and the kindness of his criticism won their wholehearted affection and appreciation. As Chief of the Department he has been an inspiration to his fellows and his influence will be a lasting force.

C. S. Blackwell died in London, England, on June 12, 1932. His sudden death came as a profound shock to all his friends and associates, as he had been in good health and had only arrived in London on a well-earned vacation two days previously. It was a rare day when he did not visit the hospital, and in the eleven years he had served as chairman of the board there had been tremendous developments. The minutes of the Board of Trustees repeatedly pronounced admiration for his leadership and self-sacrifice. At the annual meeting in 1930 Dr. Bruce Macdonald, the Vice-Chairman of the Board, had moved that

> at this Annual Meeting the Trustees of the Toronto General Hospital desire to place on record their deep appreciation of the untiring and unselfish interest shown by the Chairman of the Board in all the activities of the hospital. The excellent position occupied by the hospital to-day is largely due to his daily attention to the arduous duties of an honorary position of high public trust and a readiness to give of his judgment and experience without stint or thought of self.

The eulogy pronounced by his close associate, the Rev. H. J. Cody, at his funeral service in Convocation Hall at the University ended with these words: "He was a gallant gentleman, who did justly, loved mercy and walked humbly with God." The trustees had a marble arch erected in his memory as an entrance to the east wing of the Private Patients' Pavilion.

XIII

Post-War Renaissance

AMONG THE SENIOR OFFICERS OF NO. 4 GENERAL HOSPITAL when it went overseas in 1915 was Lt.-Col. Andrew R. Gordon. At this time he was the senior member of the service of Alexander McPhedran at the General Hospital, having been Associate Professor of Medicine at the University since 1903. His success in practice had resulted in his limiting his work to a consulting practice and as he had spent considerable time in London, England, working with Sir James MacKenzie, he came to be one of the first physicians in Toronto to be recognized as an authority on cardiac disease.

About this time the advent of electrocardiography was providing a new approach to the study of the physiology and pathology of the heart. In 1912 Professor T. G. Brodie installed an electrocardiograph in the Department of Physiology, and early in 1914 Dr. Gordon gave the General Hospital $1,500 so that this instrument could be moved to the hospital and become available for the clinical investigation of cardiac patients. Unfortunately, both Dr. Gordon and Professor Brodie died in 1916, and it was not until Dr. Ross Jamieson returned from his overseas service at the end of the war that any cardiography was carried out at the General Hospital, the cardiograph having been stored in the basement of the hospital in the custody of Dr. Gordon Richards.

Dr. Jamieson's experience had made him very familiar with the use of the new diagnostic procedure. He had graduated from Toronto in 1910, spending the next two years at the Bellevue Hospital in New York working under Dr. Van Horn Norrie, who was one of the leading cardiologists in the United States. This was followed by a year at the

Rockefeller Institute under Dr. G. E. Cohen, one of the pioneers of electrocardiology in America. During the war Jamieson went overseas with No. 16 Canadian General Hospital and was seconded to the Royal Army Medical Corps, serving first at the special heart hospital at Hampstead and then at Colchester. As a result he had a long and invaluable association with Sir Thomas Lewis and other leading British cardiologists.

By the time Dr. Jamieson returned to Toronto and was appointed to the staff of the General Hospital, Dr. John Oille had already established a growing reputation as a cardiac specialist. Graduating in 1903 with the Gold Medal, he was awarded the George Brown Scholarship in Medical Science. He was a house physician at the Toronto General Hospital in 1904–1905 and then practised at Byng Inlet on Georgian Bay. After a year spent in London, England, under Sir James MacKenzie at a time when Sir Thomas Lewis was beginning his study of the significance of abnormal electrocardiograms, he returned to start practice in Toronto, having a special interest in heart disease. He was given a junior appointment in the Department of Medicine and in the service of Alexander McPhedran in the General Hospital in 1912.

For a period of ten years Oille and Jamieson formed a perfect team, and Ward G at the General Hospital became an investigative, treatment and teaching unit outstanding in Canadian medicine. John Oille had a logical and methodical mind. He solved the problems of diagnosis on a broad basis to which cardiography made a large contribution but his students also learned from his intensive teaching that signs and symptoms were still of great significance in establishing a diagnosis and prognosis, and both house physicians and postgraduates profited by the atmosphere he engendered. As a result the cardiovascular unit under his supervision came to produce such men as John Hepburn, Harold Rykert and Carl Burton.

William Edward Gallie became Professor of Surgery and Surgeon-in-Chief to the Toronto General Hospital in July 1929. In the interregnum following Dr. C. L. Starr's death, at the request of the university and of the trustees of the hospital, Dr. Norman Shenstone had carried the dual responsibility. Gallie had graduated from Toronto in 1903, and after serving as house surgeon at both the Hospital for Sick Children and the Toronto General Hospital he spent another year as house surgeon to Royal Whitman at the Hospital for the Ruptured and Crippled in New York. From this training he came back to spend fifteen years in the closest association with C. L. Starr and eventually to become his senior assistant surgeon at the Children's Hospital. Under this leadership the Department of Surgery was never complacent and attracted such outstanding young men as D. E. Robertson, A. B. LeMesurier, and Bruce Robertson. The result was a standard of investigative surgery unsurpassed in Canada. Here W. E. Gallie established his reputation and found the answers to three great problems, namely tendon fixation, the repair of bone and the fate of bone grafts, and the transplantation of fibrous tissue, especially fascia lata, in the form of living suture to control inguinal and other hernias. His original work received worldwide recognition. When Dr. Starr became Professor of Surgery and Surgeon-in-Chief to the General Hospital, W. E. Gallie succeeded him as the Chief Surgeon at the Children's Hospital. During the eight years in which he held this post he chose his staff with care, and stimulated its enthusiasm with his personality. His numerous publications, produced with the cooperation of his associates in Canadian, American and British journals, showed the result of the teamwork that he engendered. A great honour came to him when he delivered the Hunterian Lecture before the Royal College of Surgeons of England in 1924 on the "Transplantation of Fibrous Tissues."

Shortly after his appointment Dr. Gallie approached Charles Best, at that time the Professor of Physiology, to see whether it would be possible to undertake joint research in a problem of interest to their two departments. As a result, Dr. Gordon Murray began investigation of the use of heparin in the prevention of thrombosis, leading eventually to his great contributions to cardiovascular surgery. Following his graduation from Toronto in 1921, and after a year spent in general practice near Stratford, Murray had had an exceptional training under many outstanding surgeons in London and New York over a period of six years. He obtained his Fellowship in the Royal College of Surgeons of England and on returning to Toronto became resident surgeon under Dr. C. L. Starr. The following year he was appointed a junior surgeon to the Toronto General Hospital. From this broad experience he launched into an almost endless career in investigative surgery.

A preliminary study was carried out in the laboratories of the Department of Physiology and the Connaught Laboratories by Arthur Charles and E. A. Scott resulting in the isolation of a purified form of heparin that animal experimentation proved to be non-toxic. In May 1935 Murray gave the first intravenous heparin to a patient at the General Hospital and it proved its value in the case of post-partum pulmonary embolus with literally a life-saving result. Further clinical experience led, four years later, to an invitation to Murray to give the Hunterian Lecture before the Royal College of Surgeons of England on "Heparin in Thrombosis and Embolism." He referred to the seven years he had spent on this research, which included the treatment of over four hundred patients at the Toronto General Hospital. For Murray there were always more worlds to conquer, and as early as 1939 he was involved in studies on the reconstruction of the valves of the heart, the first step towards his knowledge of cardiac surgery that gained him worldwide recognition.

The postwar years saw another outstanding development at the General Hospital in the Department of Surgery. Dr. Norman Shenstone had been appointed to the service of the University Professor I. H. Cameron in 1909. After receiving a B.A. from the University of Toronto he had taken his medical training at Columbia University, New York, afterwards serving as house surgeon at the New York Hospital and at St. Mary's Hospital for Children. On his return to Toronto he proved himself a most capable general surgeon, able to contribute something of the progressive nature of American surgery to the hospital and to the Medical Faculty.

During the war he served overseas with No. 16 Canadian General Hospital, and when Professor C. L. Starr nominated the surgical staff of the General Hospital in 1921 he became the senior surgeon and supervisor of the service on Ward C. As a result of his wartime experience with chest wounds and the numerous cases of persistent empyema that were seen in the General Hospital as a complication of influenza, he devised improved and less traumatic methods of treating infective thoracic lesions. This led eventually to his increasing interest in the field of chest surgery, to which he was to make such valuable contributions.

He was soon joined by a very able assistant. Dr. Robert Janes was the first resident surgeon appointed by Professor C. L. Starr, to whom he had been house surgeon in the Children's Hospital. In 1922 he was appointed as a junior surgeon under Dr. Norman Shenstone, and a close relationship developed between two progressive minds. Together they studied the problems associated with the removal of lobes of the lung involved with otherwise incurable bronchiectasis. Following a successful one-stage lobectomy performed at the General Hospital on May 4, 1929, they devised the Shenstone-Janes tourniquet that became a feature of successive operations. This allowed closure of the bronchus by a continuous catgut suture, which proved to be a very effective feature for obviating bronchial fistula. With increasing experience multiple lobectomies were undertaken and in January 1943 they performed their first pneumonectomy for cancer of the lung. In 1938 they had undertaken their first lobectomy for tuberculosis, and with much-improved techniques between 1940 and 1944 they performed seventeen partial and fifteen total pneumonectomies for pulmonary tuberculosis. Never was teamwork more unselfish or the results more gratifying: their collaboration provided the basis of training for a group of thoracic surgeons such as F. G. Kergin, Robert Laird and Norman Delarue, who always attributed their success to the principles they had learned from the teaching of Norman Shenstone and Robert Janes.

In 1922 the Faculty of Medicine awarded the Charles Mickle Fellowship to Harvey Cushing of Boston in recognition of his outstanding contribution to the advance of medical science. Cushing was then at the height of his career as a neurosurgeon, and as a consequence of his high regard for Professor C. L. Starr he offered to accept his nominee Dr. K. G. McKenzie on his house staff and to contribute the prize of $1,000 that he had received towards his maintenance during his year in training. It was a happy coincidence that the grant to the University of Toronto by Charles Mickle, whose lifetime career was involved in neurology, should prove to be the basis for the beginning of neurosurgery in Canada.

Kenneth G. McKenzie graduated from Toronto with the Silver Medal in 1914. His war service with the Royal Army Medical Corps took him to Mesopotamia and on his return he commenced general practice in downtown Toronto. He always had ambition for greater things, but a wife and young family made prior demands. However, when the opportunity for a surgical career became possible he did not hesitate: hearing of the extraordinary opportunity that was available he was so persistent with his application that finally C. L. Starr recommended that he should go to Boston. Here he spent a thrilling year of hard work under an exacting master, learning the routine investigation of neurological patients and the meticulous technique of a great pioneer in neurosurgery. He returned in 1923 to succeed Robert Janes as C. L. Starr's resident surgeon. After a year's service that great moulder of men gave him his desire when he was appointed as a junior surgeon on Ward A under C. B. Shuttleworth.

These were the days of trial for McKenzie. As he recalled in later years, there was no competition with others as to the treatment of the patients whom he felt were his prerogative. Prolonged operations were not usual in those days, and only afternoon hours were available to him. When he was in trouble he was dependent on his own resources, as there was no one else to turn to.

Fifth nerve section for tic douloureux was accomplished with the patient sitting upright on a kitchen chair, and painstaking clinical examination generally located the site of central nervous system and spinal cord tumours. Similarly, brain abscess was treated successfully in many cases with a proper diagnostic and surgical approach. In the early years he faced a mortality rate that would have defeated a less courageous surgeon. Yet those who watched realized the progress that was being made and the techniques that were being evolved. In 1926 a specially equipped operating room was organized for him, and in 1930 he became an associate surgeon in charge of neurosurgery. At the same time his first house surgeon was appointed to work with him in this sub-division of the Department of Surgery.

The impact of McKenzie's work started a chain reaction at the General Hospital. The first to be involved was Professor Eric Linell, who had come out from Manchester in 1921 at the request of Professor J. P. McMurrich to be an assistant professor in charge of neuro-anatomy. Stimulated by a constant association with an enthusiastic student, K. G. McKenzie, he accepted the invitation of Professor Oskar Klotz to establish a new department of neuropathology at the Banting Institute in 1932. Here Linell and McKenzie studied fresh surgical material and Linell organized a bi-weekly conference for the surgeons and physicians of the General Hospital, which was to become the basis for ever-increasing knowledge and for many valuable scientific reports.

Of equal importance was the fact that the new neurosurgical service was responsible for a renewed interest in neurology in the Department of Medicine. Up to this time Dr. Goldwin Howland and Dr. Robert G. Armour, both very capable neurologists, had established a good service on Ward G. But now Professor Duncan Graham, well aware of the potentialities of cooperation between the physician and the surgeon, appointed Dr. H. H. Hyland in 1930 to the position of full-time junior neurologist. Hyland had just completed eight months of postgraduate training under Gordon Holmes, George Riddock and Sir Charles Symonds in the National Hospital, Queen Square, London, and he brought as his contribution a knowledge of neurology that could not have been obtained elsewhere.

As yet there were no radiologists with special training in neuro-radiology. Opaque contrast media were not as yet acceptable. Therefore, it was on the initiative of McKenzie and Hyland that air encephalograms and ventriculograms were done and both the radiologists, Gordon Richards, W. H. Dixon and Arthur Singleton, and the clinicians learned to interpret the pictures which were produced. Fortunately it was a progressive science and its value increased with the growing experience of all who were involved.

Having in mind W. E. Gallie's surgical background, it was natural that he would appreciate the great need to develop orthopaedic surgery beyond the capabilities of general surgery at the General Hospital. He did not have far to look for his choice of someone to establish such a service, for he had worked long enough with R. I. Harris to realize his ability not only as a surgeon but also as an investigator.

Robert I. Harris had stood at the top of his graduating class in 1915. He went overseas and served with a field ambulance and as a battalion medical officer with the R.A.M.C., winning a bar to the Military Cross for his service in the holocausts of the Somme and Passchendaele. After being wounded in 1917 he was invalided home to Canada, and his appointment to the staff of the Davisville Military Hospital in Toronto in January 1918 was the beginning of his interest in orthopaedic surgery. Here and at the Christie Street Hospital he was responsible for the care of patients suffering from nerve injuries and the treatment of surgical tuberculosis. His success with heliotherapy won the gratitude of his patients and the approval of his peers.

His appointment to the staff of the Hospital for Sick Children in 1919 brought him under the influence of C. L. Starr and W. E. Gallie, and gave his career a clear direction. Here he spent ten valuable years perfecting his knowledge of orthopaedic surgery and developing his appetite for clinical investigation. His appointment to the General Hospital in 1929 recognized the status he had gained at the Children's Hospital, as he was appointed an associate surgeon. With Dr. Gallie's wide responsibilities as Surgeon-in-Chief, Harris found himself from the start accepted as the authority in his own particular field, in addition to his duties on a general surgical service. For the General Hospital it was the beginning of this special field of surgery which was to expand with his guidance, so that scientific methods would completely alter the treatment of fractures and painstaking effort would overcome the problems of deformity and of chronic bone and joint disease.

When F. N. G. Starr retired as Professor of Clinical Surgery and Senior Surgeon on Ward B in May 1928, the hospital lost one of the most distinguished members of its staff. In those days of the burgeoning

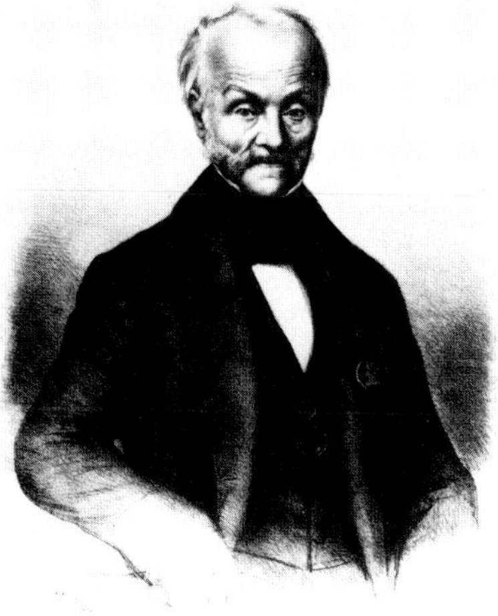

Christopher Widmer
1780–1858

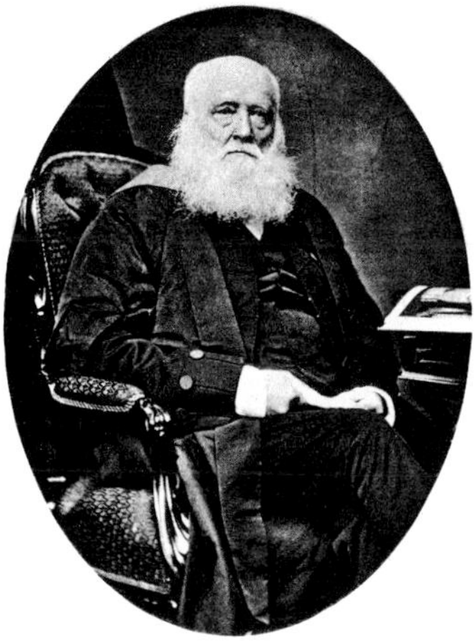

John Rolph
1792–1870

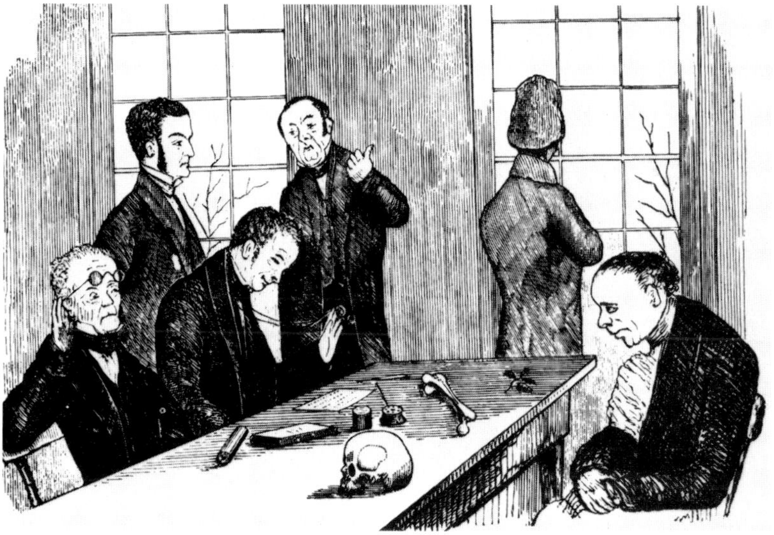

THE STUDENT EXAMINED
The Medical Board of the College of Physicians and Surgeons of Upper Canada

From left to right: Christopher Widmer, James Bovell, John King, George Herrick, Joseph Workman, John Gamble, the candidate.

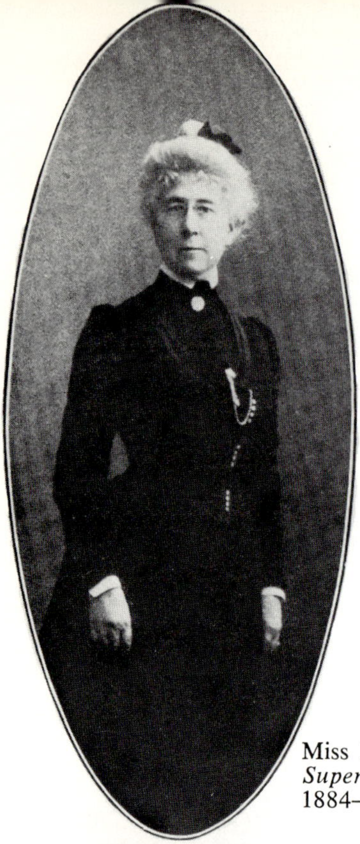

Miss Mary Agnes Snively
Superintendent of Nurses
1884–1910

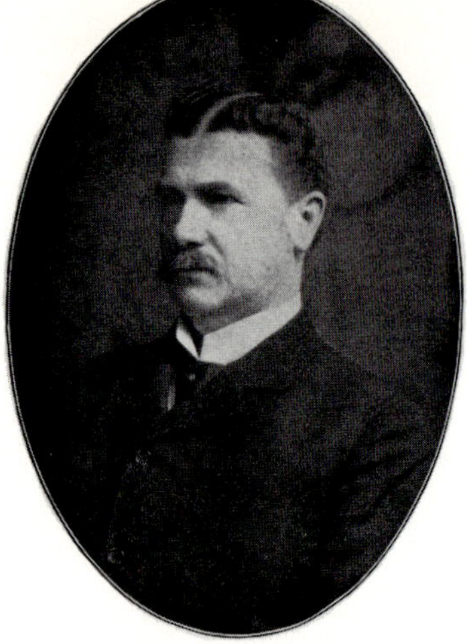

Dr. Charles O'Reilly
Superintendent
1876–1905

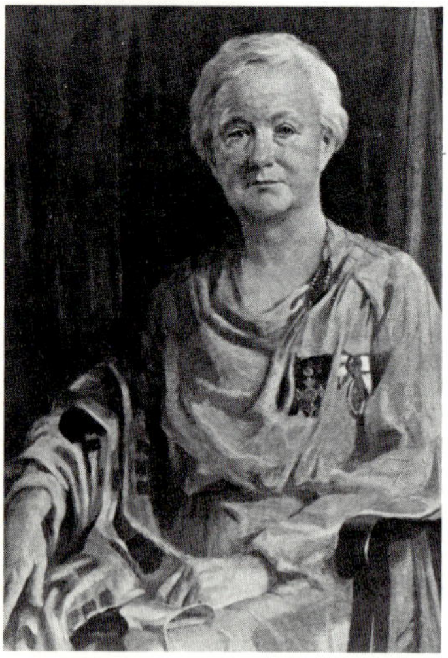

Miss Jean I. Gunn
Superintendent of Nurses
1913–1941

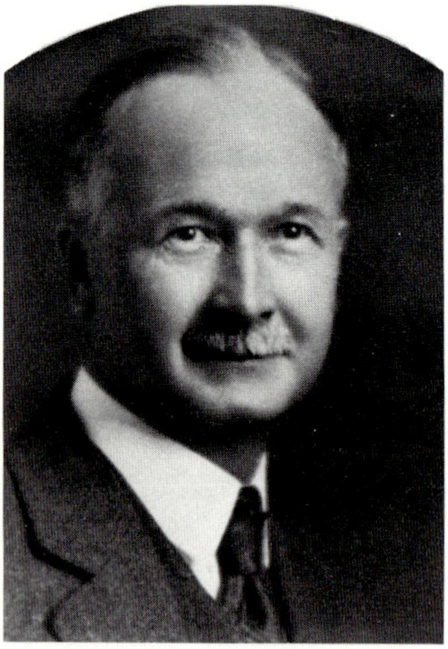

Dr. C. L. Starr
Surgeon-in-Chief
1921–1928

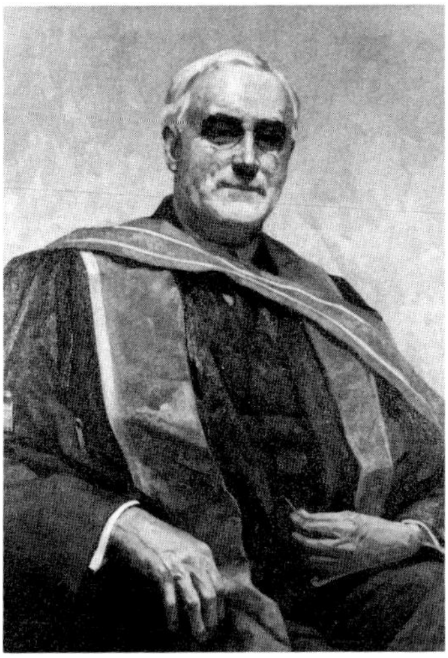

Dr. W. E. Gallie
Surgeon-in-Chief
1929–1945

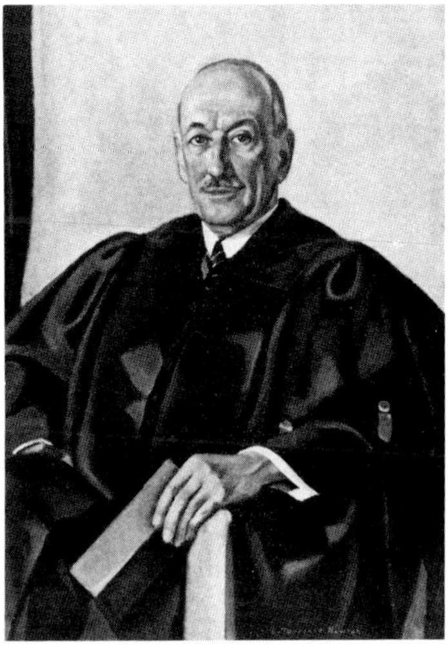

Dr. Duncan Graham
Physician-in-Chief
1919–1947

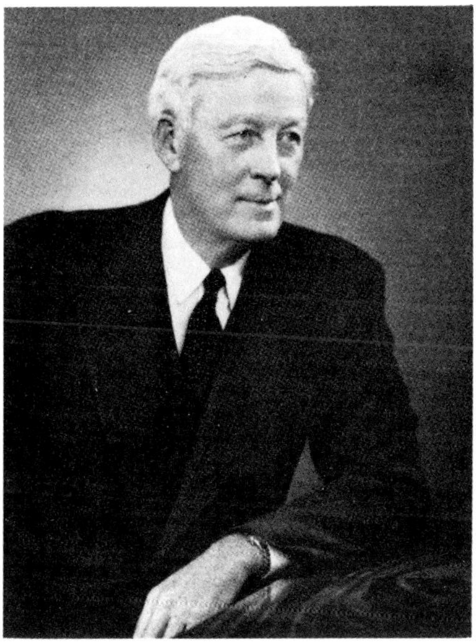

Dr. R. M. Janes
Surgeon-in-Chief
1947–1957

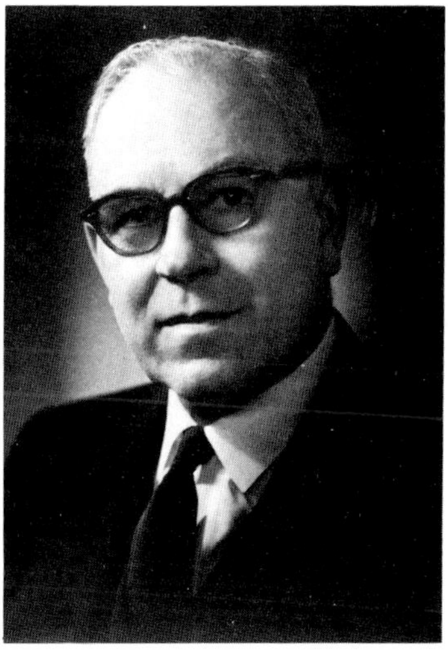

Dr. R. F. Farquharson
Physician-in-Chief
1947–1960

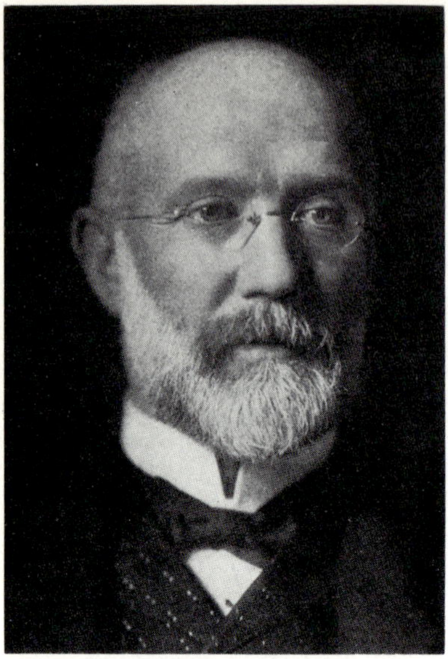

J. W. Flavelle, LL.D.
Chairman, Board of Trustees
1904–1921

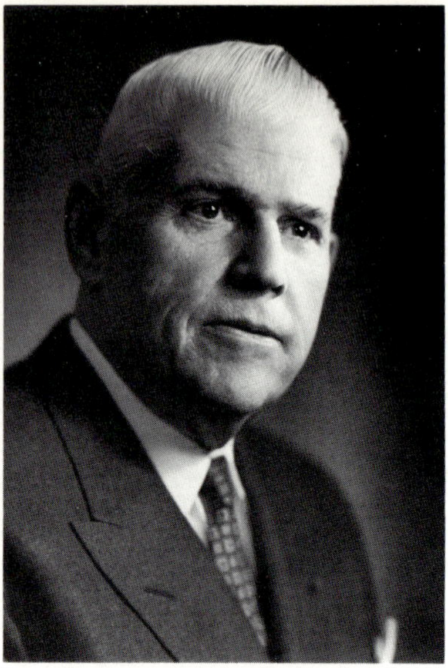

Norman C. Urquhart
Chairman, Board of Trustees
1946–1966

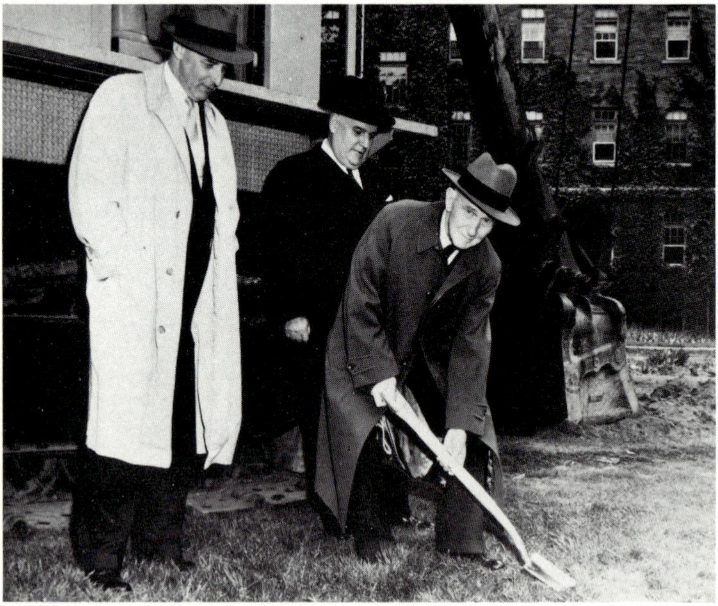

Turning of the Sod for the New Central Building, June 2, 1954.
From left to right: Mr. H. M. Turner, Vice-Chairman of the Board and Chairman of the Building Committee; Mr. Norman C. Urquhart; and Mr. Walter C. Laidlaw, Senior Trustee.

of surgical specialties, he personified the all-competent general surgeon in whose hands abdominal surgical techniques had developed to a very high level. At the same time he emphasized the post-operative care of the patient as the main factor in deciding success or failure. His name became almost a household word in Toronto, and at a time when the north side of College Street was the Harley Street of Toronto, his tall erect figure almost wore a pathway to the entrance of the hospital. He was born the son of a Methodist minister in Thorold, Ontario, in August 1867. He decided early on a medical career, and graduated in 1889 with an M.D., C.M. from Victoria University and an M.B. from Toronto. He was proud to refer to the influence which W. T. Aikens had on him and he always insisted that a good surgeon should have the background of general practice. His first appointment at the General Hospital was to the staff of the old Emergency Hospital on Bay Street. He then became a junior surgeon at the Toronto General Hospital, joining a distinguished group which included George Bingham, Alexander Primrose, N. A. Powell and Herbert A. Bruce. In 1906 he decided to confine his practice to general surgery, and served as a senior assistant surgeon under Alexander Primrose until the reorganization of the staff in 1921. Besides the demands of a large practice and the routine of his hospital and teaching responsibilities, he took a prominent part in medical organization on an international, national and provincial basis. During the war he served on the staff of a base hospital in France and became a consulting surgeon in the Royal Army Medical Corps, for which service he was awarded the C.B.E. in 1919.

He was President of the Canadian Medical Association in 1927, taking a prominent part in the campaign that resulted in the founding of the Royal College of Physicians and Surgeons of Canada as well as serving as chairman of the committee responsible for the incorporation of the college. With Duncan Graham he shared the first vice-presidency, which was divided into medical and surgical divisions, and two years later he became the first surgeon to be President of the Royal College.

Two names were inseparable at this time: F. N. G. Starr and Roscoe R. Graham. Graham had graduated from Toronto in 1910, and after an early appointment at St. Michael's Hospital was appointed in 1915 to Dr. Alexander Primrose's service when Dr. Starr was the senior assistant surgeon. His rise to prominence as surgeon and teacher was meteoric. He developed a manual dexterity that made him an abdominal surgeon without peer. He combined a charm of manner with unrelenting industry and enthusiasm, to win the admiration of house surgeons and students alike. So, in the depth of their friendship and understanding F. N. G. Starr saw with great satisfaction his natural successor come into a dominant place in the Department of Surgery.

The close cooperation which developed between medical and surgical staffs of the hospital was clearly evident in the first clinically diagnosed case of islet cell tumour of the pancreas. The patient presented a history of six years' duration of convulsions and coma which, after laboratory investigation by Dr. W. R. Campbell, was shown to be associated with low blood sugar levels. After prolonged clinical observation that eliminated other possibilities, Dr. Goldwin Howland and a newly appointed assistant physician, Dr. Ray Farquharson, diagnosed a pancreatic tumour. This was successfully removed on March 15, 1929, by Dr. Roscoe Graham, and Dr. W. L. Robinson, the hospital pathologist, found that the well circumscribed lesion was a slow-growing carcinoma of the island tissue. Twenty-three years later the patient was alive and in good health with no recurrence of her hypoglycaemic symptoms. A few years later Dr. Graham reported a series of eleven cases of a similar nature.

Dr. Robin Pearse succeeded Dr. W. W. Jones as senior surgeon in Urology in 1933. Warner Jones had recruited him for his service in 1914 from his old hospital, St. Peter's Hospital for Stone in London, England. But Pearse went on active service with No. 4 General Hospital and did not return until after the war. Now, however, when he became Chief in Urology he had the satisfaction of seeing the establishment of his department as a 49-bed unit in the Dunlap Building, profiting greatly from the convenient service of Doctors Singleton and Hall in the Department of Radiology. He also had the good fortune to have Baltimore-trained Robert McComb and J. C. McClelland as members of his staff. With first-class facilities for diagnosis, surgical treatment improved and the general surgeons realized that a new specialty was well established in their hospital. It is also true that the great influx of patients with various pelvic cancers required their services to overcome complications of the urinary tract, with the result that ureterosigmoid transplants and total cystectomy were undertaken with increasingly beneficial results.

The progress in surgery which marked this period could not have occurred without a corresponding improvement in anaesthesia. Specialization in this service only came by slow degrees. During the first year the hospital was on College Street, the staff under Dr. Samuel Johnston consisted of R. J. MacMillan, Thomas Hanley, E. A. Smith and M. D. McKichan, all of whom were engaged in medical practice when not on duty at the hospital. Innovations in methods of anaesthesia were accepted with reservation, the primary consideration with Dr. Johnston always being the safety of the patient. It was not until after the war that the routine of ether and chloroform was altered. Then, with the return of Dr. H. J. Shields from four years' service with No. 4 Canadian General Hospital, a more progressive service developed and intracheal and spinal anaesthesia gradually became routine procedures.

Dr. W. Easson Brown of the Department of Anaesthesia worked with Professor Velyien Henderson and Dr. George Lucas of the Department of Pharmacology, doing considerable original work on the development of new anaesthetic gases. In 1923 they produced ethylene and in 1929 cyclopropane. However, in spite of considerable pressure, Dr. Johnston refused permission for these gases to be used at the General Hospital.

By the time that Norman Shenstone, Robert Janes, and Kenneth McKenzie had established their special fields of surgery, Dr. Harry Shields had become the Senior Assistant Anaesthetist and was one of the first to use spinal anaesthesia for thoracic surgery and rectal anaesthesia for McKenzie's cerebral operations. When Dr. Johnston retired in 1935, a new era of rapidly progressive change began under Dr. Shields, whose staff consisted of S. J. Evelyn, John Chassels, W. E. Brown, S. M. Campbell, M. S. Clark, A. R. Wilkins and G. R. Balfour. Although, as was customary in those days, they received no remuneration for their heavy public-ward duties, they were unfailing in service to the in- and out-patient departments of the hospital in which there were more than one thousand operations and between one hundred and fifty to two hundred obstetrical deliveries every month.

A surgeon of outstanding ability now on the staff of the hospital remembers this period in the history of the General Hospital as "the era of the giants of the surgical department. All these men emphasized the care of the patient and teaching and research concentrated on the problems of practical applicability. It was indeed the golden era of surgical practice in our hospital."

Dr. W. B. Hendry succeeded B. P. Watson as Professor of Obstetrics and Gynaecology and as Obstetrician- and Gynaecologist-in-Chief to the Toronto General Hospital in 1922. He had been on the staff of gynaecology under J. F. W. Ross, and during the war had been in command of No. 4 General Hospital in Salonika and at Basingstoke. He received the D.S.O. for his service, and when he took charge of the

Department of Obstetrics and Gynaecology at the General Hospital he demonstrated his knowledge of the chain of responsibility: members of his staff came to appreciate his over-all guidance and support in their work in the department and the investigations which they might carry out.

While the more recent members of his staff rotated in service between Obstetrics and Gynaecology, Drs. F. W. Marlow and K. C. McIlwraith continued to serve as Senior Assistants in the Departments of Gynaecology and Obstetrics respectively. F. W. Marlow at this time was a dominant figure in Canadian gynaecology. He was a thoroughly capable abdominal surgeon and a master technician in his own field. After postgraduate training at a number of London hospitals he had obtained his F.R.C.S. (Eng.) in 1903. He was the Senior Assistant Gynaecologist under J. F. W. Ross, and Acting Head of that Department when the combined Department of Obstetrics and Gynaecology was established in 1912. He was an outstanding clinical teacher, and his numerous publications presented an originality featured by simplicity and a direct approach. He was President of the Toronto Academy of Medicine and of the O.M.A., and took a very active part in bringing about the establishment of the Royal College of Physicians and Surgeons of Canada. Unfortunately ill-health limited his activities, but younger members of the staff and house surgeons learned the crafts of a good surgeon from their association with him.

Dr. Kennedy McIlwraith was a traditional figure in the Burnside Obstetrical Department. In his extensive practice he had progressed over the years from practical midwifery to scientifically based obstetrics. His presence at all hours of the day and night taught house surgeons and students alike. Over a cup of coffee and a cigarette he drew from his vast experience to provide answers to their problems at a time when manipulative obstetrics was at its zenith. The wide esteem he had gained was evident in his chairmanship of the Maternal Welfare Committee of the Academy of Medicine in 1928 and the following years. Sponsored by the provincial and municipal Boards of Health, this committee sought measures to control maternal mortality which at that time was in excess of five per thousand live births. In addition, the advice of the committee resulted in postgraduate clinics and lectures for physicians and nurses, as well as the provision of sterilized bundles of supplies for home confinements.

Major factors in maternal mortality were the toxaemias of pregnancy, and shortly after Dr. Hendry took over the department a metabolic ward was established in the Burnside building where, with the service of a specially trained nurse-dietician, patients with pernicious vomiting and others with the late toxaemias of pregnancy could be kept under constant supervision. Dr. H. B. Van Wyck cooperated with Victor Harding, the Professor of Pathological Chemistry, in investigative studies that not only resulted in establishing efficient methods of control but included many original observations which received international recognition. Probably the most important result of their work was to prove the value of simple observations: these made it possible for even the busy general practitioner to recognize danger signals in carrying out routine pre-natal care of his patients. At this time maternal care was largely in the hands of the family doctor—even in Toronto 25 to 30 per cent of women were confined at home and the contribution of Van Wyck and Harding was thus of great significance.

The last serious outbreak of puerperal sepsis occurred at the Burnside in January and February, 1924. During those months there were numerous cases elsewhere in the city, and five deaths occurred among fifty-four patients delivered during a six-week period at another hospital. Streptococcal infections of the throat and upper air passages were prevalent that winter, and recognized as the source of the maternal sepsis. Seven deaths occurred at the Burnside, all due to proven haemolytic streptococcal septicemia, and two house surgeons, several nurses and a number of the medical students were found to be streptococcal carriers. Treatment with scarlet fever anti-toxin failed to cure any patient with septicemia. At the height of the Burnside epidemic, four cases occurred within a period of five days. The labour room was thoroughly disinfected and closed for a week, and a rigid isolation routine was established. It speaks well for the prophylactic routine that developed at this time that, while occasional cases of sepsis occurred, no further epidemic ever developed—this being ten years before Leonard Colebrook, working at Queen Charlotte's Hospital, London, established the control of child-bed fever by the use of sulphanilamides.

Two junior members of Dr. Hendry's staff, working in conjunction with Professor G. F. Marrian of the Department of Biochemistry, established the beginning of endocrine therapy at the General Hospital in 1934. J. B. Collip and his co-workers at McGill had isolated two gonadotropic hormones which they had given satisfactory trials in the treatment of dysmenorrhoea and functional uterine bleeding. On the basis of this work Dr. Melville Watson undertook a detailed study of 150 patients suffering from severe menstrual pain, using the preparation

Emmenin. He found that approximately one-half of the patients responded favourably to treatment, and that anatomical and psychic factors were responsible for lack of success in the remainder. Dr. Nelson Henderson made a similar study of patients suffering from excessive or prolonged bleeding. Using the anterior pituitary-like hormone that had been produced by Collip, he found favourable response in all but a very few in the absence of demonstrable lesions in the genital tract.

Up to this time surgical procedures had been the method of controlling both of these frequent conditions, and there was still considerable controversy as to the harmful effects that might follow the use of female sex hormones.

The introduction of pelvic X-ray mensuration by Caldwell and Malloy of New York opened a new approach to the problems of difficult labour. Radiographs not only presented accurate measurements of the pelvic inlet and canal but indicated hitherto-unrecognized changes in the shape of the pelvic canal. Dr. James Goodwin, a contemporary of Henderson and Watson, in conjunction with Professor T. F. McIlwraith of the Department of Anthropology, carried out an extensive study of varieties of foetal, maternal and paternal head and pelvic shapes as they were related to primary racial types, indicating the problems associated with racial admixtures as they might influence difficult labour in a new country such as Canada. Unfortunately, the results of this investigation seem to have been of greater interest to the anthropologist than to the obstetrician, but in its classical form it held a basic interest for all obstetricians who came to know of it.

Dr. John Mann was appointed to the staff of Obstetrics and Gynaecology in June 1931. A graduate of Queen's University with postgraduate training at the Toronto General Hospital, he exhibited from the start a unique ability to analyse a problem and find a sound mechanical answer to it. Among the innovations he developed were his obstetrical forceps and an apparatus for the resuscitation of the newborn. In the former he embodied a completely original concept of a split universal joint that permitted accurate application and guided rotation during the descent of the head through the maternal pelvis in the case of a mal-presentation. Also, recognizing the traumatic effect of excessive oxygen pressure on the neo-natal lung in the resuscitating apparatus then available, he designed a piece of equipment with a simple positive and negative resuscitation valve, which delivered oxygen at a fixed pressure of 12 mm of mercury positive and 8 mm of mercury negative, and removed the danger of irreparable damage to the delicate lung tissue. Brief words cannot pay just tribute to the value of his work. It never received the publicity it deserved, but he had the satisfaction of seeing his younger colleagues learn to use his forceps, and in 1957 he received an award from the Royal College of Obstetricians and Gynaecologists for the essay he had published describing this instrument. John Mann's mastery of gadgetry in his teaching of students made him a much sought after teacher, for he never failed to prove his point by demonstrations that had a visual effect not soon forgotten.

After A. C. Singleton and M. R. Hall assumed responsibility for diagnostic radiology, Gordon Richards was left free to devote practically his whole time to therapy. In so doing he opened a new field for young physicians seeking a career. In 1938 Vera Peters and Clifford L. Ash were appointed to his staff and set the foundations for their long and distinguished service in Toronto. Dr. Allan Blair, whose name became a tradition in Canadian cancer therapy, held an appointment under Gordon Richards for two years before he began the work in Regina and Saskatoon which established Canadian priority in the use of cobalt-beam therapy. In 1939 John Hinds, M.Sc., of Queen's University came to work at the Radiotherapy Institute. His training in radiation and nuclear physics provided Richards for the first time with the service of a knowledgeable scientist able to establish accurate mensurations for radiation therapy. Individual isotope curves became available, haphazard estimations were soon a thing of the past, and the indispensable service of the radiation physicist was established. Although the facilities in the Dunlap Building were completely inadequate, Hinds' successors, John Brown and later John MacDonald, worked very effectively to contribute to the ever-broadening use of radioactive isotopes.

There were two representatives of the Department of Surgery whose work showed very clearly the great value of close cooperation with the radiotherapist in the treatment of cancer. Dr. H. W. Wookey, who had served during the war as a surgeon with No. 4 Canadian General Hospital, gained his F.R.C.S. (Eng.) before returning home and was appointed to the surgical staff of the Toronto General Hospital by Professor C. L. Starr. His special interest became the surgical treatment of cancers of the head and neck and of the oesophagus. The procedures that he perfected established his reputation internationally and later, when he became chief of a surgical service, he trained many young surgeons in this field of surgery, in a manner unknown in Toronto before his time. With Richards he reviewed the results of their experience and established an integrated plan for the treatment of these hitherto almost hopeless lesions. In 1947 Harold Wookey gave a Hunterian Lecture before the Royal College of Surgeons of England and presented his experiences in the treatment of cancer of the hypopharynx and the oesophagus, starting with his first case in 1934. In these early years radiotherapy was not of great enough intensity to have any appreciable effect upon tumours in this location. However, for surface lesions, including the lip and tongue, radiotherapy was accepted as a primary method of treatment, with surgery being performed for lymph node extension. Wookey was the first surgeon in Toronto to undertake those formidable operations required for the removal of the lower jaw when bony involvement had taken place. The number of patients coming to the General Hospital as a result of these combined efforts in treatment was such that after a period of thirty years Dr. Clifford L. Ash, by then Dr. Richards' successor, working with Wookey, Keith Welsh and Robert Mustard, reported on the treatment of nearly two thousand cases of cancer of the oral cavity with an overall five-year survival rate of forty-two per cent.

Robert Janes was particularly interested in the treatment of cancer of the breast. Having in mind not only the length of survival after treatment but also the physical state of the patient during survival, Richards and Janes showed that pre-operative radiotherapy often transformed otherwise inoperable lesions so that many became curable and that local recurrences were much less frequent after such treatment. This was at a time when endocrine therapy had not become a major factor in the control of breast cancer, and the five-year survival rate of forty-five per cent which resulted from their efforts has increased very moderately since that time. They found that radiotherapy was of little avail when surgery had been inadequate and surgery would not achieve very much in an effort to overcome radiation failures.

No other field offered a greater use for radiotherapy than the treatment of malignant disease of the female genital system. Previous experience with the surgical treatment of cancer of the cervix had been so disappointing that all were agreed that radiotherapy should become the routine treatment of this condition. By 1949 Richards and his consulting gynaecologists, W. G. Cosbie and J. R. McArthur, were reporting the treatment of nearly four hundred patients by this means. Methods leading to early diagnosis had not yet become established, and more than sixty per cent of the patients coming to the Institute had advanced lesions, so that a five-year survival rate of thirty-five per cent was accepted as a satisfactory result of treatment. Pre-operative radiation became a feature of the treatment of cancer of the uterine corpus, and post-operative radiation was given with the hope of controlling the intraperitoneal spread of cancer of the ovary. The clinic at the institute attracted a large number of cases of cancer of the vulva, and when radiotherapy proved unsatisfactory a routine of radical surgery was developed which proved to be successful for a satisfactory number of patients.

XIV

The Daily Round

DUNCAN GRAHAM, C. L. STARR AND B. P. WATSON INAUGURATED the residency system at the Toronto General Hospital in 1921 with the appointments of W. P. Warner, Robert Janes and D. M. Low. From the beginning these appointments were a mark of distinction that brought its own reward. These senior intern appointments in Medicine, Surgery, and Gynaecology and Obstetrics represented at least three years of postgraduate training, and along with the supervisory responsibility that the resident assumed came the invaluable close association with the chiefs of the departments.

At this time there was no formal organization of postgraduate training in Canada. The situation was shortly to change, however, as Dr. Duncan Graham planned the future of the Department of Medicine. Realizing the inadequacy of mere clinical training for those who aspired to become members of his staff, he required each after a year as intern at the hospital to spend a year of study in a basic medical science—biochemistry, physiology or pathology—before receiving the appointment as resident physician. Following this he arranged appointments for them in the United States or in Britain, where a number passed the membership examination of the Royal College of Physicians of London before returning home. It was from men with such training that he chose his full-time staff, who were then required to spend three or four years in teaching, research and the care of patients on a full-time basis before they were allowed half-time for practice and eventually to become part-time senior members of the staff.

Dr. Graham modified this postgraduate routine when he undertook to train physicians who would not necessarily have an academic career. A year spent as a senior intern on one of his wards, where they were associated with a staff intent on teaching, was followed by further training in paediatrics and obstetrics that the professor arranged for them. An example of the type of young men who sought his appointments is evident in the three senior interns in 1935—F. H. Brien, Robert C. Dickson and J. C. McCreary, men who in years to come were leaders in Canadian medicine literally from coast to coast.

From the beginning it was intended that degrees awarded by the Royal College of Physicians and Surgeons of Canada would signify not only academic achievement but also that its Fellows had received sound practical training to qualify them for recognition in the special fields of medicine and surgery for which they held this high degree. It was in order to meet this situation that W. E. Gallie, with the collaboration of the Departments of Physiology, Anatomy and Pathology, organized an integrated plan for young surgeons in all the major fields of surgery. In his 1932 Report to the Dean of Medicine he announced:

> This year has seen the establishment in this School of a definite plan of postgraduate training for surgeons. Hitherto it has been impossible for a graduate to receive adequate training here in General Surgery, and he has been forced to seek it in hospitals abroad. Now with the support of the Professors of Medicine and Pathology, a course is available extending over three years which it is hoped will place the teaching of Surgery in this School on a high level. The first year—six months of Medicine and six months of Pathology. Second year—one year as senior house surgeon on one of the general surgical Divisions. Third year—one of the following options—
>
> A) Six months as house surgeon at the Hospital for Sick Children and six months as House Surgeon in the Genito-urinary Department of the Toronto General Hospital.
>
> B) Six months as House Surgeon at the Hospital for Sick Children and six months as House Surgeon in the Neurosurgical Department in the Toronto General Hospital.
>
> C) Six months as House Surgeon in the Neurosurgical Department of the Toronto General Hospital and six months in the Genito-urinary Department of the Toronto General Hospital.
>
> There is also a two year service which is open to applicants who have served what may be considered equivalent to the first year of the three year course in some other manner. In this, the first year—one year as Senior House Surgeon on one of the general surgical divisions. Second year, one of the three options described for the three year course. The plan has been in operation for a full year and has become very popular with our interns, seventeen of whom applied for the first three appointments.

> Two features of the plan should be referred to: first, these House Surgeons are no longer treated as chance wayfarers through the wards of the hospital but are accepted as apprentices to the art of surgery and so treated by the attending staff. Secondly, when they accept their appointments they automatically enter the course for a postgraduate degree of Master of Surgery and they undertook to pursue the course of study in Anatomy and Physiology and in Surgery and Pathology required for that degree. Arrangements have been for the House Surgeons to spend two evenings a week in the dissecting room and one afternoon with an instructor in Physiology so that they will be prepared for the primary examination for the Master's Degree or for the Fellowship of the Royal College of Surgeons of Canada or England as they choose.

This was the first course of its kind in Canada. As the years went by it became extended into the other teaching hospitals of the University and broadened in its scope to include other special fields of surgery as they developed. Further organization of postgraduate training in Toronto did not occur for a few years: prior to 1944, in spite of the desire to encourage postgraduate training, the regulations governing examination for the Fellowship in the Royal College of Canada only required one year of hospital training. In that year the primary examination of the Royal College was discontinued, and in 1947 new regulations were drawn up. These gave in detail the nature of the five years' postgraduate training then required for the Fellowship, which had to be taken in a hospital approved by the College.

The golden anniversary of the Training School for Nurses was celebrated in 1931, and many of its 1,867 graduates gathered together to look back with pride to the school from which they had come. In the eighteen years of Miss Jean Gunn's direction she and her staff had served the hospital with outstanding ability and the school had been in the forefront of establishing a new status for the graduate nurse. Miss Gunn always felt a personal responsibility to protect her pupil nurses from overly prolonged hours of duty on the wards—a critical problem in 1919 when the graduate nurses demanded a ten-hour day instead of the twelve hours for which they had been receiving a daily remuneration of four dollars. The monthly salaries of the senior nursing staff at this time were not much better: the Assistant Superintendent earned $100, the Supervisor of the Private Patients' Pavilion (after fourteen years' service) $90, and the head nurses on various wards, in operating rooms and in various departments, anywhere from $65 to $85—many after years of good service.

Affiliation with training in other hospitals, which had had its beginning in association with the Hospital for Sick Children in 1907, now extended to the accepting of nurses from St. John's Hospital and the Wellesley Hospital for short periods of time so that they might have broader experience in nursing. In 1918 a further bond between the hospitals in Toronto came from the centralized course of lectures leading to standard examinations and in 1921 the curriculum extended over a period of 630 hours to include anatomy, physiology, chemistry, bacteriology and pathology, hygiene, materia medica and massage, as well as lectures on the complete range of diseases that it was necessary for the nurses to understand.

In 1922 the provincial government passed a law to control the registration of nurses. This did not affect the entrance qualifications for the General Hospital, but it recognized the importance of special courses which had been developed by the Toronto Department of Health and the University in Social Service and Public Health Nursing, so that no longer were the trained nurses' interests necessarily confined to the routine care of patients on the wards of the hospital. A final step, in which Miss Gunn gave strong support to one of her graduates, Miss Kathleen Russell, came with the establishment of the University of Toronto School of Nursing in 1933. The new school provided a course in administration and teaching, to which a considerable number of graduates of the Toronto General Hospital have gone on a postgraduate basis to meet the ever-growing demand for well-trained senior appointees to the major hospitals across the country.

In 1924 Miss Gunn received an invitation to be the guest of the Rockefeller Foundation in order to visit hospitals and training schools in Europe. Her pre-eminence in Canadian nursing was recognized when she became the first nurse to be a Doctor of Laws of the University of Toronto, and in January 1935 the trustees tendered their congratulations when she received the Order of the British Empire for her conspicuous contributions to the profession of nursing in Canada while serving as Superintendent of Nurses at the Toronto General Hospital.

It was largely through the efforts of Miss Gunn that the Social Service Association of the Toronto General Hospital was organized in 1921. Prior to this the Ladies Committee and the Golden Rule Guild of the Nurses Alumni had combined to provide financial support for social services at the hospital, and had initiated a volunteer service to augment the work of the professional staff. During the war years the Federation of Community Services in Toronto was organized, and it gradually became the financial support for social services in the hospital.

Both Miss Gunn and Miss Mabel Knisely, the Head of the Social Service Department, appreciated the value of active volunteer workers and under their direction various committees were formed. Since the development of welfare services such as Unemployment Insurance, Mothers' Allowance and Old Age Pensions there has been a marked change in the nature of the demands for material help, but three committees set up in 1921 still provide very necessary services. The Serving Committee, which has been particularly associated with the Burnside, has provided clothing for the newborn. The Library Committee, with its book wagons, provides reading material for patients, including newspapers and magazines in several languages. The Occupational Committee has supported this remedial activity and organized the sale of articles so produced. In the following years the Pre- and Post-Natal Committee was organized to meet the wants of patients attending the obstetrical clinics, and the Motor Committee, starting as a voluntary driving group, finally became responsible for funds to provide taxis for patients leaving the hospital or coming to its clinics.

In all these developments it often looked as though the needs of the Out-Patient Department remained a low priority. But change was imminent. In January 1925, Mr. C. S. Blackwell reported to the trustees that during the past year 11,483 patients had been admitted to the hospital, but reminded them that there were other services not to be forgotten:

> The contribution to the community's health and welfare made by the Out-Patient Department of the Toronto General Hospital cannot be estimated in dollars and cents, but some appreciation of the importance which it plays in the life of the community can be had from the numbers apparently dependent upon its guidance and treatment of disease in the earlier stages, for 58,953 individuals, approximately 5,000 per month, have visited the various clinics of the Out-Patient Department during 1924.
>
> I would again draw the attention of the members of the Board to the splendid work of our special departments. The Pre-Natal Clinic, operated under the supervision of the Burnside staff, records a total attendance of 1,592. Again the importance and value of the supervision given to the expectant mother is reflected in the results as shown by these records. During the year there were 534 confinements in the public wards of this department; of this number 356 were clinic patients and 178 non-clinic patients. The percentage of still births amongst the non-clinic patients was 17.9 per cent as compared with

> 1.9 per cent of the patients attending this clinic. The new premature room, completed in the Burnside with a capacity for 16 babies, is a source of great relief and comfort to the staff of that department. The success which we have enjoyed in the handling of premature infants is deserving of the highest commendation to those immediately in charge. Since the opening of the new room some four months ago there has been but one loss—this is indeed a remarkable record. . . .

In spite of this commendation, however, the trustees informed the Medical Advisory Board that funds were lacking to meet their demands for additions to the Out-Patient Building.

The steady increase in attendance at the Out-Patient Department was accentuated in the depression years following 1929. It was with great satisfaction, therefore, that the trustees received in October 1934 a gift of $100,000 from the Salada Tea Company in memory of its late President, Mr. P. C. Larkin. By this time the monthly attendance was over 12,000 patients, and now the trustees were able to undertake the building of the Peter Larkin Annex which, when it was opened in March 1935, met the long-overdue needs of this active hospital service.

During these years two relatively new clinics had become important features of the Out-Patient Department in addition to those long-established. In 1920 Dr. Gordon Bates became Head of the Venereal Disease Clinics, and with characteristic enthusiasm he and his associates campaigned to increase the flow of patients. Treatment was subsidized by matching grants from the Dominion and provincial governments, though this support was gradually phased out, federal assistance stopping in 1933. In March 1936, 2,289 patients received treatment for which the hospital received only twenty-five cents per treatment. Following the outbreak of the war in 1939, there was a considerable increase in the number of patients and the Deputy Minister of Health wrote to the Superintendent regarding the efficiency of the clinic at the Toronto General Hospital, which at $4.60 per cured patient had shown the lowest cost of any clinic supported by the Department of Health. To centralize the treatment facilities, he asked the General Hospital to consider increasing its staff and including another social service worker, so that patients might be accepted who had previously been treated in three other Toronto hospitals.

Dr. Gordon McLean volunteered to re-organize the Dental Out-Patient Service in 1927. He reported to the Medical Advisory Board that after seeing "the infected, filthy, disease-producing oral conditions of the patients" he was not surprised that the hospital wards were filled.

He nominated a group of dental surgeons who served with him on a rotation basis, using the two chairs then available in the Out-Patient Department and providing the services of their own dental nurses. On Dr. McLean's advice a full-time graduate was appointed at a salary of twenty-five dollars a week to care for in-patients, and dental students were permitted to attend clinics. For the future he asked for five dental chairs and the service of a nurse, and a closer liaison with other hospital services. This, he felt, would establish the fact that major dental conditions required hospitalization; in addition nurses in training would be instructed in the value of oral hygiene. The desired facilities were provided in the newly organized Out-Patient building, and after years of invaluable service as Dental Surgeon-in-Chief Dr. McLean retired in 1935 to be succeeded by one of his associates, Dr. Douglas Tanner.

Professor Duncan Graham was very fortunate in the physicians whom he appointed to the Out-Patient Department when the Medical Department was reorganized in 1919. Dr. George Strathy became an Associate Physician in charge of Medical Service in the Out-Patient Department. His knowledge of medicine was most comprehensive, as his postgraduate training included obstetrics and paediatrics. Prior to the war he had been on the staff of the Children's Hospital and the range of his experience during the war years, from battalion officer to senior physician at a general hospital, demonstrated the fullness of his character and the unselfish nature of his service. He was intensely interested in the problems which the out-patients presented, and became not only an inspiration to his staff but also an ideal to his students. His death in June, 1925, as the result of fulminating streptococcal endocarditis contracted from a patient under his care, removed him at the height of his career when he was only forty-two years of age.

Dr. Strathy was succeeded by his senior assistant, Dr. George Young. Dr. Young had graduated from Toronto in 1895 and practised for some years in Prescott, Ontario. Returning to Toronto, he was appointed to the service of Dr. J. T. Fotheringham, and it was from this association with the hospital that he transferred to the Out-Patient Department. He was not only highly regarded as a consultant in internal medicine, but also served his profession in many high offices, as President of the Ontario Medical Association, as member of the Ontario Cancer Foundation and as Chairman of the Board of Directors of the Canadian Cancer Society. His crowning honour was to be President of the Royal College of Physicians and Surgeons of Canada from 1937 to 1939.

Dr. Young was succeeded by Dr. H. S. Hutchison, who had been another of the original Out-Patient staff when the medical service was reorganized. His characteristic modesty almost obscured his excellence as a physician. By this time the Medical Department had attracted an outstanding group of voluntary assistants who contributed the wisdom of their extensive experience to the care of the patients and the training of the undergraduate students and house physicians. In 1933 this medical Out-Patient staff included

Dr. Charles F. Abbot	Dr. W. R. Little
Dr. Kendal Bates	Dr. Gladstone W. Lougheed
Dr. W. Robertson Caven	Dr. W. A. McTavish
Dr. E. J. Clifford	Dr. Eugene Montgomery
Dr. T. A. Crowther	Dr. Harold Rykert
Dr. H. D. Delamere	Dr. David Selby
Dr. Kenneth E. Ferry	Dr. E. O. Shaver
Dr. F. R. Griffin	Dr. W. E. L. Sparks
Dr. W. H. Holmes	Dr. V. F. Stock
Dr. E. S. Jeffrey	Dr. R. W. I. Urquhart
Dr. Murray Jeffrey	Dr. M. J. Wilson

The medical clinics had become a clearing house for the clinics of all the other services and a means of admission to the hospital wards, and even disruption due to the construction work which was then proceeding was overcome by the staff, having in mind better days to come.

Dr. Hutchison had a long experience in life insurance medicine, being at this time Chief Medical Officer for the Crown Life Insurance Company of Canada. He gave a special course of lectures on this subject, and his students learned to assess the significance of incipient signs of ill health. His sudden death in January 1934 from coronary thrombosis was a great loss to the hospital and to all those who knew him.

Dr. Fletcher McPhedran succeeded Dr. Hutchison as Attending Physician in charge of the Medical Clinic of the Out-Patient Department. The son of Professor Alexander McPhedran, he had received his postgraduate training at Johns Hopkins Hospital, Baltimore. He brought to his appointment not only a sound knowledge of medicine and a long association with the Out-Patient Department but also a magnetic and enthusiastic personality which was a constant stimulus to his associates and to his students. He was fortunate to have under his direction a well established group of senior physicians which included A. G. McPhedran, Trevor Owen and G. W. Lougheed in the General

Medical Clinics; Harold Parsons, A. H. W. Caulfield and W. E. Ogden in the Tuberculosis Clinic; and Dr. Gordon Bates who still presided over the Venereal Disease Clinic.

Although he was only indirectly associated with the Toronto General Hospital, John Gerald Fitzgerald was responsible for a development that brought Toronto once again into the forefront of Canadian medicine and proved of the greatest value to physicians on the staff of the hospital who were involved in clinical investigations of the prevention and control of certain diseases. He had graduated from Toronto in 1903, and after prolonged postgraduate training which took him to Baltimore, Harvard, Freiburg and the Lister Institute in London, he settled into his life's work in 1913 with a full-time appointment in the new Department of Hygiene at the University of Toronto. Here he developed plans for an Institute of Research in Preventive Medicine, and for the preparation of public health biological products. Laboratory facilities such as he envisaged were completely lacking in Toronto, but President Falconer and the Board of Governors of the University were soon convinced of the necessity of meeting his recommendations. As a result, a start was made in very meagre quarters in the basement of the Medical Building. Within a year the demands of wartime brought rapid expansion, and the magnificent gift of Sir Albert Gooderham resulted in the building of the Connaught Anti-toxin Laboratories and the University Farm to the northwest of the city. A few years later, through a grant from the Rockefeller Foundation, a School of Hygiene was established. It was to be closely linked with the Connaught, and its fine new building provided greatly increased laboratory facilities. The Connaught and the School of Hygiene never failed in their dual purposes, and from the beginning they attracted and maintained very productive staffs of research workers.

The value of liver extract as a means of generating haemoglobin was established in 1926 and 1927 by various American investigators, including Minot, Murphy and Cohn. In 1928 Dr. E. W. McHenry, working with Professor Charles Best in the School of Hygiene, undertook the preparation of a liver extract for clinical use in the treatment of anaemia. By gradual steps this resulted in 1931 in the product of a solution suitable for intramuscular injection.

Clinical trials were carried out simultaneously at the Montreal General Hospital and at the Toronto General. Dr. Ray Farquharson, after the treatment of twenty-two patients suffering from pernicious anaemia, found that the intramuscular administration was thirty times more potent than previous oral preparations. By this means it was possible to maintain even seriously ill patients in good health and to prevent nervous lesions. The success of this combined effort embodying the research laboratories, the wards of the General Hospital and the clinics of the Out-Patient Department proved another example of a clinical investigative unit at its very best.

One of the first of the medical staff of the hospital to become involved in clinical investigation was Dr. Almon Fletcher. In his undergraduate days his interest in basic science was stimulated by Professor J. B. Leathes, and his contribution in the original use of insulin to treat diabetes was based on this knowledge. In 1928, with the collaboration of Dr. W. H. Dixon of the Department of Radiology, he undertook the study of a group of patients with chronic arthritis. While recognizing the multiple aetiology factors of the condition, they showed that two-thirds of the patients gave evidence of fenestration of the colon, indicating malnutrition. A program of dietary control and the administration of Vitamin B not only demonstrated favourable change in the radiographs, but was co-incident with improvement in the arthritis. Years later an admirer, reviewing the contributions which he made from this time on towards the control of this disease, said he had earned the right to be considered "The Father of Rheumatism in Canada." Inherently he had a profound influence on many others: it was his leadership which brought about the organization of the Canadian Arthritis and Rheumatism Society, and he received international recognition on being appointed to the first Committee for the Control of Rheumatic Disease in the U.S.A.

A physician whose career followed to a considerable degree the path of Duncan Graham was Dr. Herbert K. Detweiler, who left the staff of the General Hospital in 1936 to become Physician-in-Chief to the Toronto Western Hospital. He had graduated with the Gold Medal in 1914, and was one of the first group of full-time medical research fellows appointed by Duncan Graham when re-organizing the Department of Medicine at the General in 1919. His first interest had been bacteriology, and in 1917 he had organized the Wassermann test service in the Pathology Building of the General Hospital, so that routine tests were done on admission on all public ward patients at a time when it was found that twelve per cent of patients had positive tests for syphilis.

During the influenza epidemic of 1919–20, he conducted research into the aetiology of this highly fatal disease. His knowledge of bacteriology and serology gave him a paramount position on the clinical staff of the General Hospital, and in his practice he was recognized as a leading authority in Toronto on allergies and the seasonable causes of hay fever. From this he developed control therapy to prevent many troublesome and often serious respiratory conditions associated with air contamination. Although these were the highlights of the services that he developed at the General Hospital, he had a broad knowledge which made him an outstanding teacher and practitioner of internal medicine as he moved to his important position in an active teaching hospital of the University of Toronto, and by his leadership he contributed greatly to the growing prestige of the Western Hospital.

During the late summer and autumn of 1937 Canada experienced the worst epidemic of poliomyelitis in its history. In Ontario there were 2,544 cases with a paralysis rate of 56 per cent and a mortality rate of 4.3 per cent. The intensity of the epidemic at first threatened to overwhelm the facilities available for the care of the patients. During the previous ten years, which included one slight epidemic, there had only been twenty-five cases admitted to the General Hospital, but in 1937 alone the number increased to sixty-six.

Once again the Shields Emergency Hospital proved to be an ideal unit for accommodating epidemic patients requiring highly specialized treatment, constant supervision and often emergency care. Professor Graham wasted no time in organizing a group of physicians to meet the critical situation: H. H. Hyland, F. C. Heal, W. A. Oille and O. M. Solandt were constantly on duty. It was fortunate indeed that Dr. W. J. Gardiner had had time since his return from England in 1932 to develop an effective department of physiotherapy in the quarters vacated by the radiologists. The result was that an efficient staff was available to provide services essential to the saving of life and to undertake the skilful treatment necessary to combat paralysis before it caused an irreparable condition.

Specific therapy was of no avail, and there is no doubt that the factor that saved many lives was the manner in which the engineering staffs of the General Hospital and the Children's Hospital cooperated in developing a type of Drinker respirator that was much more efficient than any available before. Albert Derbyshire and William Davidson of the General Hospital, with Harry Banforth of the Children's Hospital, manufactured in their own shops the functioning portion of a model of which fifty units were completed for service in the two hospitals. When the Province of Ontario undertook to supply respirators many were sent to other hospitals in the province. At the beginning of the epidemic there was only one respirator in the General Hospital; later there were fifteen in constant use. To meet the emergency, nurses and physiotherapists were specially trained in the routines of artificial resuscitation and the prompt use of anaesthetic equipment to deliver oxygen. This saved many lives.

The General Hospital became a diagnostic centre for many patients suspected of having polio, and some idea of the volume of work is indicated by the fact that about 100 lumbar punctures were done daily at the Emergency Hospital.

By the end of the epidemic there were forty-seven patients who had developed paralysis, but as the result of the treatment featuring good physiotherapy, over two-thirds of them recovered completely or obtained good use of their limbs. Nine patients died, respiratory failure accounting for all but one fatality. This tragic episode is now only of historic interest: the development of an effective vaccine by Dr. Jonas Salk, to which an essential contribution was made by the Connaught Laboratories, practically put an end to the disease that had hitherto threatened death or deformity to so many children and young adults.

From the time the American College of Surgeons undertook the accreditation of hospitals, two problems confronted the Medical Advisory Board of the General Hospital. The first was the proper maintenance of patients' records and the second was the right of the hospital to refuse operating rights in the Private Patients' Pavilion to incompetent surgeons. There never had been any question with regard to the records of patients treated on the public wards. These were remarkably good and showed the effect of the supervision of many good registrars. This did not apply, however, to private patients, especially those treated by physicians and surgeons who were not on the staff of the hospital. A major factor limiting the authority of the medical staff was that the trustees considered the Private Patients' Pavilion to be a separate institution that provided an important source of revenue when its wards were well filled.

In 1921 the Medical Board organized a committee under Dr. Roscoe Graham to develop an efficient method of maintaining medical records. The result was the decision to adopt the unit system of case histories. As so often happens with any innovation, it took some time to overcome the lack of space and trained personnel. In 1925 Miss A. S. Hall was appointed Records Librarian and sent to the Presbyterian Hospital in New York for training. On her return, with the help of three secretaries, she organized a new service located in the basement of the old Pathology Building. With the opening of the new enlarged Out-Patient Building in 1935, it was possible to provide a conveniently located room on the ground floor with facilities for fifteen clerks to work with the current histories, as well as storage in the basement for the bound records going back in obstetrics to 1878 and for medical and surgical patients to 1905.

Mr. Mark Irish, who had succeeded C. S. Blackwell as Chairman of the Board of Trustees, retired in January 1936 after a very short term in office. He had been a member of the Board for thirty years, during which time he had given outstanding service to the hospital. In his final address he referred to his pride in the establishment of the Radium Institute, new facilities for physiotherapy, and the development of an efficient medical records system, and he claimed that the General Hospital now had the most efficient and modern accommodation on the continent for its Out-Patient Department. He then dealt with the constant problem of hospital finance, which was now further complicated by the Radium Institute's presenting the highest per diem cost the hospital had ever experienced. This situation, affecting particularly patients with malignant disease, would become accentuated in the years to come. Finally, he drew the attention of the medical staff to the financial problem of empty beds in the Private Patients' Pavilion, and suggested that this could force consideration of increasing the staff —taxpayers might resent repeated demands to meet yearly deficits to maintain a "closed hospital" which denied service to the great majority of doctors in the city.

The Depression years had presented a constant financial dilemma for the board under Mr. Irish. An overcrowded Out-Patient Department and constantly filled public wards coincided with a decreasing number of patients in the Private Pavilion. The monthly reports of the hospital Superintendent, Mr. Chester Decker, showed the results of rising costs and falling income. Efficient service depended on a larger staff and resulted in much greater expenditure. The unrelenting strain of this situation on the Superintendent prompted the board at the end of 1932 to appoint Mr. R. W. Longmore, Chief Accountant, to be Assistant Superintendent, Administrative. His service already warranted this promotion, and the coming years would emphasize his value to the hospital in this new position.

Dr. E. A. Gray served the hospital as Assistant Superintendent,

Medical, for nearly twenty years, and his sudden death in October 1937 came as a great shock. With his quiet friendly manner was associated a high degree of efficiency: the house staff went to him with their troubles and returned his kindness with real affection. Miss Gunn and her associates in the nurses's training school appreciated his full understanding of their problems, and the staff physicians and surgeons came to feel that he lived for the welfare of the hospital. The Board of Trustees paid their tribute to the loss of a very valued administrator, who, they had come to feel, was capable of meeting any of the problems during the difficult days of postwar readjustment.

XV

The War Years: 1939-1945

EDWARD CAREY FOX BECAME CHAIRMAN OF THE BOARD OF Trustees in January 1936. His career in industry and finance, along wth his interest in higher education, had contributed to make him well fitted for the responsibility he now assumed. A graduate of McMaster University (then located in Toronto), he always maintained a great interest in his alma mater, becoming Chancellor after he retired from the Board of the Hospital in May 1946. He was Vice-President of Canada Packers Limited during his period on the Board and also Vice-President of the National Trust.

The Chairman's yearly reports presented in detail his appreciation of the problems of the Toronto General Hospital, and he reiterated the great need for support from the provincial government and the City of Toronto, realizing that an institution with the triple function of the care of the sick, the education of medical students both undergraduate and postgraduate, and the constant endeavour of medical research, required support beyond that of a simple community hospital. He foresaw that the inevitable effect of rising taxes and succession duties would result in the increased responsibility of governments, both municipal and provincial, for the maintenance of hospitals. In the case of the General Hospital, the greatly increased budget already had made the income from its endowment less than adequate.

No period in the history of the General Hospital made greater demands on the leadership of the chairman and the resourcefulness of the board than the ten years of Mr. Fox's service. The immediate pre-war years were still affected by the Great Depression, and since both the Ontario government and the city council were loath to increase their grants these failed to cover the maintenance of the public ward patients. At this time only sixteen per cent of the other patients were paying enough to cover the cost of their accommodation. Even the receipts from the Private Pavilion and the Department of Pathology were inconstant, and often failed to meet expenses. Due to falling rents and increasing taxes, the income from the endowment had decreased to half of what it had been, amounting to less than $50,000 a year.

Sir Joseph Flavelle's death in March 1939 ended an association of thirty-seven years with the General Hospital, spanning the years of extraordinary progress from the old Victorian institution on Gerrard Street to the great hospital on College Street. As a Governor of the University of Toronto, as well as in his role as indefatigable Chairman of the hospital Board, he was responsible more than any other for the close relationship which developed during these years between the university and the hospital. It was with great satisfaction that the trustees welcomed his son, Sir Ellsworth Flavelle, as his successor on the board of the hospital.

For nearly six years the war transformed the life of Canada. In addition to the mobilization of vast numbers of young men and women for active service, Canadian industry developed at an unprecedented rate to provide the materials for winning the war; and civilian needs, of necessity, were relegated to a secondary role. In spite of this there was an unrelenting demand for skilled physicians, surgeons and nurses and the teaching hospitals rose to the occasion as the result of the combined efforts of the professional staffs and the lay boards of trustees.

To comply with new regulations the annual report presented in 1940 covered a period of fifteen months to the end of December 1939, and therefore showed the effect of the first four months of the war. Within a week, with the mobilization of No. 15 Canadian General Hospital, forty-two of the medical and nursing staff had gone on active service. Summing up the new challenge facing the Hospital, the Chairman stressed that the main task was

> to try and maintain the current high standards of daily operation regardless of the prior demands that the exigencies of war make upon us. Two chief factors must be considered, the human and the financial. The doctors are the mainspring of the former. The fundamental requisite of a doctor on our hospital staff is that he be not only a good operator, per se, but that he be a good teacher. There are many more doctors possessed of one of these qualities than there are possessed

of both, hence it is not easy to replace doctors who leave for war services, and besides we have promised such doctors the equivalent of their present positions when they return.

The financial factor is clear-cut and simple but in prospect very grave, for in the 6 years ending September 30th last, the average per diem cost of main ward patients was $3.03. We received $2.35 per day for this service. This is a peace-time condition. The war greatly accentuates the problem. I am told that if we pass through this present war without some inflation in costs it will be the first time in history. I think we have to assume we are facing higher costs of operation. Even a 10 per cent increase in all round costs, if there be no offsetting increase in revenues would add approximately $150,-000.00 to the already disturbing annual deficits.

One factor offsetting the financial crisis was a bequest left by Mrs. Margaret Bingham to the General Hospital in memory of her husband, Dr. George Bingham. This amounted to $350,000, and a request was considered that it should be used to build a convalescent hospital under the control of the Toronto General Hospital. Since this was ruled to be beyond the jurisdiction of the Board of Trustees, it was decided to use the bequest to cover the cost of centralizing all the operating rooms in the College Street Building, but wartime conditions made it impossible to dispose of mortgages and real estate which together amounted to $125,000. It was also true that a major building project could not be considered under conditions existing since the outbreak of war.

The Superintendent, Mr. Chester Decker, reported that over 25,000 patients had been admitted to the hospital during the fifteen-month period. The distribution, according to departmental accommodation, was 5,000 medical, 10,000 surgical, 2,600 obstetrical, 2,500 gynaecological, 600 in ophthalmology and 2,200 in otolaryngology. He thought it was of interest to note that the in-patients were 86 per cent of British origin, 65 per cent Canadian, while the 160,000 patients in the out-patient departments represented 58 different nationalities.

Mr. Decker drew the attention of the board to studies which had been going on for a period of five years with regard to schemes for group hospitalization. He dealt particularly with the Associated Medical Services, sponsored and supported by the Toronto Academy of Medicine, which provided professional services within the home and during time of hospitalization. The premiums under this plan, he understood, were to be twenty-four dollars per annum for a married man and twenty-one for his wife. He felt that while the plan was commendable its cost precluded that element of the population with which hospitals were mostly concerned, as 63 per cent of the wage-earners of Ontario earned less than $1,200 per annum and 84 per cent less than $2,000—with 85 per cent of the total number of patients admitted to the Toronto General Hospital coming from these two classes. He also referred to the plan which the Ontario Hospital Association hoped to announce in the near future, and suggested that the rates for membership would be as low as 40¢ per month for ward accommodation and 60¢ to 70¢ per month for semi-private and private accommodation. On this basis the hospital would receive from this fund $2.75 to $3.00 per day for ward accommodation, $5.00 per day for semi-private accommodation, and $6.50 per day for private accommodation.

By the end of 1942, twenty-eight doctors and many nurses from the staff of the Toronto General were on active service. The trustees were constantly faced with the problem of maintaining the non-professional staff, as the demands of industry had resulted in a 100 per cent turnover during the year. The new employees often lacked any sense of responsibility—a serious and continual problem, especially on weekends when there were often as many as 100 absentees. As a result it became necessary to organize a group of teenage boys and girls to provide basic services, and up to the end of the war fifteen to twenty medical students often served on the wards as orderlies.

The year 1942 also saw the termination of the ten-year agreement with the provincial government regarding support for the Cancer Clinic. During this time the hospital had received $450,000, but this had been largely expended on the land, building and equipment. The volume of work had also increased greatly. There had been over 1,100 patients with cancer treated in the previous year, as well as approximately 800 suffering from non-malignant lesions. Dr. Gordon Richards had established his place at the forefront of Canadian radiotherapists, and with the help of his technician, T. B. Hurst, had developed much of the equipment in use at the Institute of Radiotherapy in the Dunlap Building. It was intimated to the Chairman that the Department of Health, looking to the future of radiotherapy in the province, was considering the possibility of organizing a centre independent of the General Hospital. A year later, when the Ontario Cancer Treatment and Research Foundation was incorporated by the government, Mr. Fox and his Radiotherapy Committee began to consider the importance of maintaining a close relationship between the General Hospital and the enlarged Institute of Radiotherapy which might be developed in Toronto. The trustees felt that, as the Radiotherapy Clinic had developed to this point within the General Hospital with the cooperation of its surgeons, it would be a retrograde step to break this association.

In 1944 an amendment to the General Hospitals Act raised the municipal and provincial grants for the first time in seventeen years. The hospital would now receive $2.25 per day from the city and 75¢ per day from the province for indigent patients, though this was still inadequate to cover the public ward expenses, which had risen to $3.98 per day. It did, however, increase the hospital income by $25,000 annually—welcome news for the trustees, as the deficit for the year, after subtracting the income from the endowment, had been $90,000. By this time wages were responsible for over fifty per cent of the running expenses of the hospital, and some employees were demanding a 38-per-cent raise in their wages, for compared with industrial workers they were poorly paid. There was certainly some justification for their demands, as a married man who received forty-two dollars a month in 1938 was only receiving seventy-eight dollars in 1942.

During the war years the hospital first felt the impact of organized labour. The difficulty of facing demands that were reasonably applicable to industry cannot be over-emphasized. In spite of protests submitted by the Board of Trustees and the Ontario Hospitals Association to both the provincial and dominion Labour Relations Boards, the hospital services employees became members of an international union of the American Federation of Labor, and wage increases agreed upon amounted to a total of $204,000 a year.

Despite insufficient government grants the trustees were reluctant to undertake the alternative of increasing rates for private and semi-private patients, and from 1942 on the private rooms were maintained at rates ranging from $7.50 to $12.00 a day. When the special nurses were to be paid $5.00 for their eight-hour day very few patients could afford their services. As a result the hospital undertook to provide a graduate nurse for every four patients in the Pavilion. In 1944, to meet the demands of the Canadian Nurses Association, it was agreed to pay these nurses $110 a month, with an annual increase of $5.00 up to $120. But in spite of this the demands of active service and of industry were such that there was a constant shortage of forty-five to fifty nurses for floor duty. At one time it was reported that eighty-six nurses were doing the work of 135. This forced the closure of floors in the Pavilion, and was responsible for large operating deficits.

With the end of the war Carey Fox felt that he could lay down his burden. His final report presented the same old problem—an operating loss of $210,000, only moderately affected by the endowment income. But the services to patients had improved immeasurably. The battle to retain the status of the teaching hospital had been successful, and in 1945 a new grant was established by the provincial government in support of such institutions. This provided an extra $164,000 for the General Hospital which, however, still fell far short of meeting the increase in wages for the year.

The Chairman's optimism with regard to social postwar measures was tempered with a warning:

> Many social post-war measures will be passed to keep mankind healthy, wealthy and wise and free from care from swaddling clothes to the shroud. I raise and endeavour to discuss the following question. . . . Will the various prospective public health measures, if they become law, change the character of clinical hospitals and if so what will be the essential nature of the change? I have felt that unless great care were taken that a general hospitalization insurance scheme would tend to reduce all hospitals to a general level: that clinical hospitals would be brought down to the level of curative institutions and that consequently the medical profession would be regimented also and confined to a strait-jacket. There are sound reasons to hope that the Provincial Department of Health is fully aware of this danger and the clinical hospitals will continue to function as they have been doing, that is, not only as teaching hospitals but also in setting up and maintaining high standards of practice for the example and benefit of all hospitals and the medical profession throughout the Province.

He welcomed the increased provincial grant but added that there were still great challenges to be met:

> While it is obvious that it does not relieve clinical hospitals from the financial dilemma in which they have been for many years, the encouragement that one takes out of it is the satisfaction that there is being aroused official interest in the cost of operating hospitals. I have repeatedly pointed out to the Board that the indigent public bed rate is basic to the determination of all bed rates. It is grossly unfair for the state to pay less than the per diem cost of a public bed. It is economically unsound and socially unjust. That the vital question of medical education and leadership is also involved can easily be demonstrated. In order to increase the revenues clinical beds may become converted to semi-public use. Each bed thus converted means one less clinical patient for teaching purposes and the natural tendency is to steadily increase the number of semi-public beds.
>
> This city is one of the world's recognized medical centres. It has not reached this stage by accident or fortuitous circumstances. All the gains of a generation can be lost in a ten year period unless we keep abreast of the best in the medical and surgical world!

> Hospitals have had one prolonged depression since 1932. There was first the economic depression and then the bad economic conditions created in the hospitals during the war caused by depleted staffs and advancing costs. The first problem is to get back on to an adequate organizational basis. The second problem is to implement the organization with buildings, equipment and staff to meet the new requirements which the depression and the war have so badly delayed. I am quite confident that the Toronto General Hospital is in excellent shape to adjust itself to the new conditions providing that the basic cost of public hospitalization is met from the proper governmental sources.

He paid tribute to the great industry of Mr. Chester Decker. Through Dr. W. E. Gallie he extended his thanks to the medical staff for their unfailing service and he emphasized the manner in which Miss Mary Macfarland, the Superintendent of Nurses, had risen to every occasion despite a greatly depleted staff of nurses. In retrospect, his own contribution was such that it might be said the accolade of praise never rested on a more worthy shoulder than that of Edward Carey Fox.

In July 1939 the National Executive of the Canadian Association of Medical Students and Internes informed the Medical Advisory Board of the General Hospital that it was prepared to establish a Canadian Interne Board which would be associated with the Department of Hospital Services of the Canadian Medical Association. The intention was to develop a routine procedure for the appointment of interns, so that applications would be submitted by mid-October and appointments could be announced by December 1. The advantage to both the applicants and the hospitals concerned was emphasized. Sir Frederick Banting was the Honorary President and Chairman of a national advisory committee, and two Toronto students, D. H. Copp and W. K. Kerr, were the Vice-President and Secretary-Treasurer of the Association.

As might be expected, from the start the war caused a great shortage of residents and interns. Students in the earlier years, putting country before self, enlisted in large numbers in the Army, Navy and Air Force. Graduates accepted for internships either did not take up their appointments or left after a few months to join the medical services. By March 1940, senior-year students were being appointed as summer interns and, shortly after, the various services were forced to modify the demands for senior appointments, surgery being prepared to accept six instead of nine, medicine three instead of six, pathology one instead of three, and obstetrics and gynaecology, anaesthesia and radiology one instead of two. By 1942 even some of these positions were left vacant. It was particularly difficult to fill senior internships from among the graduates in obstetrics and in gynaecology: some Americans were appointed and at times recent graduates from other provinces. Extern appointments of senior students helped with routine service on the wards, and in spite of possible medical-legal difficulties in some procedures, specially trained nurses for the first time undertook venous section, the introduction of intravenous saline and glucose solutions, routine blood pressure readings, urinalysis and the supervision of oxygen-carbon dioxide inhalation under emergency conditions.

One of the most important decisions made by the Medical Advisory Board during these years was to establish the Hospital Blood Bank. In October 1926, the Hospital Superintendent had reported with some satisfaction that Dr. George Wilson and Dr. Roy Thomas of the Emergency Hospital had organized a blood bank at the Emergency Hospital and that a supply of 1,200 c.c. of blood obtained from universal donors was available. This bank was not maintained very long, however, as with the methods then in use it was not possible to keep blood for more than twenty-four hours, and the alternative of providing fresh blood from professional donors or from patients' friends became the accepted practice at the General Hospital. The control of safety factors for the transfusions became the responsibility of Dr. Philip Greey, the hospital bacteriologist and serologist.

In December 1938 Dr. F. A. Logan, the Medical Superintendent, suggested that the Medical Advisory Board should give some thought to establishing a blood bank, but it was not until December 1941 that a committee was set up to discuss the question with Professor William Boyd and Dr. Greey. Following considerable discussion, the board established a Committee on Blood Transfusion under the chairmanship of Dr. R. I. Harris, with representatives from the Department of Medicine, the surgical specialties, and the Department of Obstetrics and Gynaecology. This committee recommended that Dr. Greey be asked to assume control of a blood bank to be accommodated in the basement of the Private Patients' Pavilion. At the same time, on the advice of the committee, the hospital undertook to approach the Ministers of National Defence and of Pensions and National Health to request that the plasma then stored by the Red Cross in the Connaught Laboratories should be made available to the General Hospital and other city hospitals in case of a great emergency.

The blood bank, under Dr. Greey, began its operations in May 1943 with the services of Mr. Wakefield and Dr. Greey's own technician. It was planned to store 30 flasks of blood and 150 units of plasma, to be issued by the bank for use of patients on a quid pro quo basis. Interns on duty in the Pavilion were responsible for obtaining blood from donors, though the actual bleeding might be done by trained technicians under the doctor's supervision.

One of the outstanding wartime organizations in Canada developed in the Red Cross Society Blood Transfusion Service. Volunteer donors from coast to coast gave 2,500,000 bottles of blood to save the lives of many Canadian servicemen and casualties in the bombed cities of Britain and Europe. Towards the end of the war the Red Cross was approached by a number of hospitals and provincial departments of health to extend this service to civilian hospitals as well as to military and veteran institutions. Although the relations between the Toronto General Hospital and the Red Cross Society were very cordial and many of the nurses serving with the society had received training in the hospital's blood bank, the hospital preferred to retain its own transfusion service. It was felt that this was essential in a teaching hospital, and that the proximity of blood transfusion services to the Hospital for Sick Children was of the greatest importance in connection with the Rh immunization problem as it affected both mothers and new-born infants. By the end of the war, there were approximately 4,000 transfusions taking place each year at the General Hospital.

Of equal importance to the development of transfusion services was the development of methods for the production of penicillin in sufficient quantities to meet the demands of the active services and, later, of the civilian population. The discovery of penicillin by Alexander Fleming in 1929 and its establishment as an effective therapeutic agent by Howard Florey of the Oxford School of Pathology in 1940 still left the problem of developing massive production in the early years of the war. In July 1941 the Rockefeller Foundation brought Professor Florey to America and, through the studies and conferences which resulted in the research laboratories of the United States Department of Agriculture in Peoria, production methods were developed to meet the demands that the war had precipitated.

In the fall of 1941, studies began in the Department of Pathology and Bacteriology of the University of Toronto with the collaboration of biochemists working in the Department of Medical Research under Professor C. H. Best. Dr. Philip Greey and Dr. Ronald Hare visited Peoria and, through the generosity of the American investigators, brought back with them cultures of the mould that gave the greatest yield of penicillin. During the early months their work was facilitated by that of the nurses on duty at the General Hospital, who sterilized culture material in the hospital autoclaves. Eventually a penicillin plant was established at the Banting Institute.

Early in 1943, penicillin was produced which was successful in treating staphylococcic septicemia. The sub-committee on infection advised the director general of Medical Services that large-scale production should be undertaken, and arrangements were made with the Connaught Laboratories of the University of Toronto and with Ayerst, McKenna and Harrison of Montreal to establish penicillin plants under government auspices. In August of that year a joint-services penicillin committee was established at the Christie Street Military Hospital under Wing Commander R. F. Farquharson. Its function was to supervise the use of penicillin and to train medical officers in this special therapy.

The small plant at the Banting finally produced sufficient penicillin for some civilian needs—Dr. Greey recalled later that in those early days it was rushed across the country by the Royal Canadian Air Force and Trans-Canada Air Lines. Then, within the short space of three years, through the combined efforts of scientists and manufacturers, the problems of supply and demand were overcome: penicillin, soon to be followed by an ever-increasing family of similar agents, had come within reach of all on a permanent basis. The Connaught Laboratories rose to the occasion, taking over the old Knox College building on Spadina Crescent, Toronto. Here, by early 1944, in remodelled quarters and with a staff working twenty-four hours a day, facilities were organized sufficient to meet the demands of both the Armed Forces and the civilian population.

The life-saving properties of antibiotic therapy were established by the vast experience of the war years. The General Hospital had considered the treatment of pneumonia in 1938 with the sulphonamide dagenan to be the first important break-through, but this was almost forgotten when penicillin proved its worth in the control of septic lesions in the work of R. A. Cleghorn, John Hamilton and L. A. Chute of No. 1 Research Laboratory, R.C.A.M.C., working in Italy and Northwest Africa.

In September 1938, the Board of Trustees offered its congratulations and felicitations to Miss Jean Gunn on her twenty-five years of service as Superintendent of Nurses, expressing their indebtedness to her for raising the prestige of the hospital and its teaching school to international prominence. It was only a few months later that a similar tribute was paid to Miss Helen Locke, the loyal and efficient Assistant Superintendent of Nurses. Within three years Miss Gunn died, and her tribute recalled that "her gracious leadership, her gentle guidance and her rare understanding, coupled with an unswerving loyalty to individual and to institution had made her an inspiration to all who worked with her." Tributes were also paid to her by the Canadian Nurses Association, the Registered Nurses Association of Ontario and the Canadian Red Cross Society, in recognition of a leadership long acknowledged by international as well as national nursing authorities.

Miss Helen Locke served as Acting Superintendent of Nurses until September 1942, when she retired after twenty-nine years of service. The hospital now lost another strong proponent of high ideals and inspiring ethics: the chairman said that there were graduate nurses throughout Canada and the United States, in the war zones in Europe and Asia, in Palestine and South Africa, who would cherish memories of the kindliness and unfailing sympathy of Helen Locke. It may well have been due to the inspiration of these two women that the hospital received the benefit of invaluable long service from many supervisors and head nurses.

By the time Miss Helen Kelly retired in September 1948, she had completed thirty-four years as Supervisor of the Burnside Obstetrical Department. The high standard of maternal care which had resulted from her appointment was maintained through all those years with the approbation of the professional staff, especially of Alan Brown who was never satisfied with anything but the best.

Miss Elizabeth Purdy was another who had given long and unfailing service. She retired in October 1944, after forty-two years of nursing service. During her time as Superintendent of the Private Patients' Pavilion, she had generated and maintained a warm atmosphere that was thoroughly appreciated by both the professional staff and the patients under her care.

There was also one whose name had become synonymous with the Social Service Department—Miss Mabel Knisely. In November 1945, after twenty-six years of nursing service, during nineteen of which she had been the Director of the Department, she retired, ending an association with the hospital which dated back to her graduation in 1905. As the department extended its services, her work had increased to the point where she was called upon to interview 15,000 individuals annually, and her efficient service to patients, physicians and to the hospital was beyond praise.

Miss Jean Yuill was the Night Superintendent of Nurses from 1915 to 1935. She came from Glasgow, and with her Scottish burr and night light she seemed the veritable "Lady of the Lamp" to patients, nurses and house surgeons. Her control was absolute as she visited the seriously ill, encouraged the younger nurses, and even advised the house staff when a crisis arose. Her death was a great loss to the hospital, and the Nurses Alumni, recalling their undergraduate days, placed a memorial to her in the Nurses' Residence.

With the end of the old regime, Miss Mary Macfarland was appointed Superintendent of Nurses in September 1942—the first graduate of the Toronto General Hospital Training School to hold this position. After serving as a head nurse at the hospital for a number of years, she had also spent a year at the University of Toronto School of Nursing. She was therefore well prepared to meet the challenge of wartime conditions. At this time the training school was filled to capacity, and an average of ninety-two nurses were graduating yearly; while the administrative staff were losing valuable personnel, retired graduates were encouraged to take refresher courses so that they might assist in staffing civilian hospitals.

In addition to these professional services, the whole body of General Hospital nurses were involved in extra-mural activities. In October 1939, the Red Cross Club of the Toronto General Hospital was organized. The Alumni Association, the Social Service Department, the staff and student nurses worked constantly, preparing and packing supplies for overseas. Courses of instruction for V.A.D.s were given, and first aid classes for the ground service personnel in the R.C.A.F. were undertaken in the Emergency Department.

The proportion of staff from the General Hospital who volunteered for overseas service was as impressive as it had been during the First World War.

On September 15, 1939, a week after the declaration of war, C. A. Rae, Associate Surgeon in the Department of Otolaryngology, was the first of the hospital staff to be granted leave of absence for active service. He was appointed Officer Commanding No. 15 Canadian General Hospital, and as the unit was organized he was followed by W. P. Warner, H. H. Hyland, H. E. Rykert, J. A. MacFarlane, Carl Aberhart, F. G. Kergin, H. W. D. McCart, S. M. Campbell, Arthur Singleton, and the original pathologist, Sir Frederick Banting, who was soon replaced by Desmond Magner. Enlistments were continuous, and by early 1942 the list of those on service from the General Hospital had expanded to include P. E. Ireland, J. A. Dauphinee, R. B. Kerr, R. Ian Macdonald, Clifford Richardson, W. R. Little, A. H. Squires, C. W. Young, D. R. Mitchell, J. V. Tilley, G. A. Hendry, B. L. Sparks, W. E. L. Sparks, E. H. Botterell, S. D. Gordon, J. R. F. Mills and M. C. Watson. The Superintendent reported that eighteen of the twenty senior interns were leaving for active service. A little later, R. A. Cleghorn and J. W. Graham, R. I. Harris, W. K. Welsh, J. R. MacArthur and H. M. Macrae left the hospital for wartime posts.

Although members of the staff and interns served with the Medical Corps of the three services in many capacities from the front lines to base hospitals, there was always a feeling of close association between the General Hospital and No. 15 Canadian General Hospital. Miss Agnes Neill was the first Matron, and a large percentage of the nursing sisters of No. 15 were graduates of the Toronto General Hospital School for Nurses. The hospital was mobilized in the Toronto Exhibition grounds where a large number of soldiers of all branches of the services were quartered, and before it left for overseas the Board of Trustees passed a resolution of appreciation to the individual members of the staff who were enlisting for service overseas.

> The Members of the Board of Trustees of the Toronto General Hospital extend their best wishes to the Doctors and Nursing Sisters of the Institution who have enlisted for service for overseas and express to you their deep sense of pride and gratitude in the knowledge of your service for Our King and Country and for the cause of freedom and democracy in all lands.
>
> Such service they know will be rendered in the same faithful and unselfish spirit that has marked your loyalty to the Science of Medicine and to this hospital and its patients through the past years.
>
> It was the gallantry of the officers and men who fought in the War of 1812 that made the existence of this great institution possible. Because of that loyalty and sacrifice, your own contribution to the healing and comfort of the battle stricken, as reflecting the training and experience of years in this hospital becomes a vital reality.
>
> As you have honoured the Toronto General Hospital so the Trustees honour you in their hearts. They wish you Godspeed and an early return to the ranks of your esteemed profession.

During the years in which No. 15 was in England, the wards were constantly filled with patients suffering from a great variety of medical conditions, including a surprising number of cases of pulmonary tuberculosis. Blackout conditions contributed to many accidents, and the surgeons were kept almost as busy as the physicians. Ward rounds and clinical teaching were organized to provide instruction for the recent medical graduates engaged in various non-hospital duties within the Canadian military area in England.

The first battle casualties treated by No. 15 were from the attack on Dieppe by the 2nd Canadian Division on August 19, 1942. After evacuation of the wounded from the beaches had been carried out with great heroism, 230 patients were admitted to No. 15, including many who were in a very poor state and some who had been in the water one or more times. Those who were lightly wounded and could travel were sent to other hospitals, but 125 of the severely wounded were kept at No. 15. The success of treating chest wounds at this time indicated the great advances which had occurred in thoracic surgery, to which the team-work of physicians, surgeons and nurses had greatly contributed. This experience proved that the physician's aspirating needle and penicillin often obviated the use of the surgeon's knife in the treatment of haemothorax.

When the Canadians became involved in the campaign in Sicily, No. 15 was moved to North Africa. In July 1943 it arrived at its new location at El Arrouch, a short distance inland from the port of Philippeville. Security regulations governing this move had been so tight that no tropical dress had been supplied, and the unit landed in temperatures of 105°F dressed in tin hats and battle dress. In spite of these and many other difficulties, tents were erected and the hospital was prepared to receive patients within twelve days of landing. By the end of August 2,200 patients had been admitted. Battle casualties were relatively few, but nearly 1,200 cases of pandemic malaria were treated by the First Canadian Division within a six-week period. During the time spent in North Africa, the staff mastered the art of protecting the hospital area from the mosquito menace, and Captain W. A. Oille combined his service as qualified internist with that of Malaria Control Officer.

A major problem in the Mediterranean theatre was infective hepatitis, which reached epidemic proportions in 1943 and 1944. This caused the most serious wastage of manpower of any disease, and although fatalities were few there was permanent liver damage in some cases. Everybody seemed to have dysentery, but only the severely ill were considered unfit for duty.

It was not until the hospital moved in July 1944 to Casserta, about forty miles from Naples, that it began to receive many fresh battle casualties. The heavy fighting in the attacks on the Hitler Line filled the wards, and during the bitter struggle in which the Germans were driven from one defensive position to another, young surgeons on the hospital staff served in advance surgical units. Prompt evacuation resulted in many seriously wounded patients being admitted directly to the hospital, and at times No. 15 could not handle all the patients who were sent to it. Between August and the end of 1944, No. 15, with over 1,600 beds, had a daily occupancy of 1,390 patients. Finally, with the removal of Canadians from Italy to Northwest Europe in March 1945, No. 15 returned to England and was disbanded.

Another closely related hospital was No. 1 Canadian Neurological Hospital, which was mobilized in December 1939 and went overseas in June 1940. The importance of psychological problems affecting the soldier had been clearly evident in the First War, and the great advances made since then in neurosurgery more than justified a special hospital of this type. During the years of its operation this hospital, which became the Basingstoke Neurological and Plastic Surgery Hospital in May 1943, treated 16,753 patients, of whom 3,774 were neurosurgical cases. The Toronto General Hospital was represented on the surgical and medical staffs by E. H. Botterell, H. H. Hyland, J. C. Richardson and Allan Walters, and R. A. Gordon and George Boddington were the anaesthetists. Stuart Gordon, who was originally with No. 15 General and had been in charge of the first plastic surgical unit in the R.C.A.M.C., joined No. 1 Neurological when his service was combined with it. By means of the services of these men, the closest collaboration was maintained between plastic surgeons, dental services, radiologists and laboratory services. On the medical side, the staff acted both as neurologists and as psychiatrists. As a result, the fully developed, combined services made this hospital outstanding in Britain. Here the first Canadian mobile neurosurgical unit was organized early in 1944 and here Norman Delarue, one of Gallie's recent surgical trainees, and a young physician, Cameron C. Gray, received the experience which prepared them for months of service with the mobile surgical unit in Flanders, Holland and Germany.

E. H. Botterell, who became the senior surgeon at Basingstoke, had already established himself as an outstanding neurosurgeon. His training in general medicine and general surgery, as well as in neurology and scientific investigation, had been a prelude to his appointment by K. G. McKenzie as his associate in Toronto. Now, thanks to the opportunities of this unique hospital, he was able to formulate highly successful routines of procedure. Hyland, Richardson and Walters all had benefited by prolonged training at Queen Square, London, before their appointments to the Department of Medicine at the Toronto General Hospital, and their contributions to the medical side of the Basingstoke Hospital made it an efficient centre not only for treatment and clinical investigation but also for the instruction of medical officers, nurses and other ranks.

Although No. 15 General and No. 1 Neurological seemed to be the units most closely associated with the General Hospital, by 1944 members of the staff of the Toronto General Hospital were holding senior ranks at many hospitals in Northwest Europe. The list included Lt.-Cols. J. A. Dauphinee, J. C. Richardson, R. I. Macdonald, R. B. Kerr, R. C. Dickson, W. A. Oille, E. H. Botterell, S. D. Gordon, F. G. Kergin and Majors J. A. Walters, A. E. Parks, A. H. Squires, K. J. R. Wightman and W. F. Greenwood.

Surgeon Lt.-Commanders W. K. Welsh, D. R. Mitchell, and J. R. MacArthur were with the Navy, and Col. R. I. Harris and Col. P. E. Ireland were consulting surgeon and consulting otolaryngologist respectively to the Canadian Army Overseas. R. P. Farquharson, W. J. Gardiner and A. C. Singleton were consultants to the R.C.A.F., and Surgeon Commander J. W. Graham served as Chief of Medicine at St. John's Naval Hospital in Newfoundland.

History repeated itself and, in addition to those who were involved in hospital service, the staff of the General Hospital was represented in many capacities. Col. Melville Watson was the Assistant Director of Medical Services of the Third Canadian Infantry Division when it was the spearhead of the Canadian Army in the invasion of Normandy on June 6, 1944. He has left a graphic description[1] of the months of planning before the assault, and of his experiences during the time when Montgomery was fighting to close the Falaise Gap. During those critical days conditions were often desperate, calling for services in keeping with the best traditions of the Medical Corps. In spite of battle conditions and adverse weather, there was seldom delay in coordinating first aid with the expert surgical care of the wounded, and this proved the practical value of the staff work from the unit commanders to the over-all director. An exceptional achievement won a Military Cross

[1]"Medical Aspects of the Normandy Invasion," *CMAJ*, LIII (1945), pp. 99–111.

for Capt. G. E. Woodhouse, who came back after the war to a junior appointment in Medicine at the Toronto General Hospital—with his collecting post under heavy fire and the number of casualties mounting, he had carried on in the open, giving transfusions to the more severely wounded and organizing their steady evacuation from the area.

Col. Charles Gossage, who had been an anaesthetist and had served in the Surgical Out-Patient Clinic at the General Hospital, went overseas as Medical Officer of the 48th Highlanders. He finally became A.D.M.S. of the Fourth Canadian Armoured Division in February 1944, and served with the divisional staff during the last year of the war while the Division was engaged in the battles which were to clear the Germans from Northwest Europe.

Others of more junior rank had experiences that almost made history. Allan Graham was seconded to the Royal Army Medical Corps and served in the defence of Tobruk in Cyrenaica in 1942. He was taken prisoner when this so-called fortress fell to Rommel, and was later awarded the Military Cross. His subsequent journey to Italy was in such a dilapidated aircraft that he doubted they would reach their destination.

J. A. G. Reid had the harrowing experience of spending nearly five years as a prisoner of war in Hong Kong, and later in Japan. He was one of Professor Duncan Graham's senior interns at the Toronto General Hospital in 1939–40 before he joined the R.C.A.M.C. to serve with the Canadian Brigade in the forlorn effort to defend Hong Kong in December 1941. For his service during this action and throughout the long years when he cared for his fellow prisoners of war under almost hopeless conditions, he was awarded the M.B.E. On his return home he became resident physician in the Wellesley Division of the Toronto General Hospital.

A. L. Payne, who interrupted his training as resident in obstetrics and gynaecology to serve with the Royal Navy, was on board a British destroyer on that day in 1942 when Admiral Vian's little fleet of light cruisers and destroyers drove off an Italian battleship and heavy cruisers when they dared to attack a convoy en route to Malta.

Douglas P. Bryce had just started his training at the Toronto General Hospital when he went overseas. He served as a medical officer to the Canadian Argyll and Sutherland Highlanders for a year in Northwest Europe, and had the unique experience of being the only Canadian medical officer who took part in the Victory Parade in Berlin.

These are only a few of many, for Dean Gallie reported that over five hundred medical graduates from Toronto were on active service, many serving in the front lines and on those repeated long journeys across the North Atlantic on convoy duty.

Brigadier J. A. MacFarlane was well qualified for the post he held as Senior Consulting Surgeon to the Canadian Army Overseas. He had interrupted his undergraduate training to serve as a sergeant in the Canadian Field Ambulance during the First World War, so he had personal knowledge of the long weary miles the stretcher-bearers had to carry the severely wounded, and of the non-existent facilities at the front. He maintained his interest in the army during the interval between the wars, serving as Medical Officer to the 48th Highlanders. He went overseas as the Senior Surgeon in No. 15 General Hospital, but was chosen to be Consulting Surgeon when the medical services were expanding in England. His reports from Italy and Northwest Europe during 1943–45 show how he grew in wisdom and understanding, largely through his first-hand view of the care of the wounded from the front lines to the base hospitals. He realized with enthusiasm the tremendous value of the skilled teamwork that saved the lives of so many Canadian soldiers as well as the value of forward surgical units, and during the fighting in Sicily he organized the first Canadian Field Dressing Station, in which Major J. R. F. Mills of the Toronto General Hospital was the surgeon-in-charge, assisted by a young anaesthetist, Captain Bruce Tovee. MacFarlane's six years of service prepared him well for the leading role in Canadian medical education which he was to assume on his return home.

On the home front, Duncan Graham and W. E. Gallie set an example of untiring service. Professor Graham had been appointed Consultant in Medicine to the Royal Canadian Army Medical Corps with the understanding that it should not interfere with his duties in the Faculty of Medicine or at the General Hospital. The results more than justified the appointment; older officers were brought back after service to their teaching appointments, younger replacements were specially prepared for their service overseas, and base hospitals, soon to be veterans' hospitals, were organized. Many of the staff of the General Hospital received decorations to commemorate their service, and the contribution of Duncan Graham was rewarded with the C.B.E.

W. E. Gallie filled the dual role of Dean of Medicine and Professor of Surgery, and as such he was the coordinator of special wartime postgraduate training. The departments of both Medicine and Surgery maintained six-month appointments for senior interns. This included intensive training for young surgeons from across Canada or others like F. P. Dewar, E. B. Tovee and W. G. Bigelow, who came home on leave and then returned to active service and major surgical duty in the front lines. R. I. Harris gave special courses in the treatment of fractures and Walter Wright and A. E. MacDonald in ophthalmology. The Department of Anaesthesia ran special courses in an ever-broadening field of techniques, and the Department of Radiology trained twenty-nine radiologists and eighty-five radiological technicians. Before the war ended, the Director General of Medical Services voiced his whole-hearted approval of these important contributions made by many of the staff of the Toronto General Hospital.

In keeping with the record of the physicians and surgeons of the General Hospital, a tablet in the Nurses' Residence bears the names of 227 graduates of the school who served in many capacities and on many fronts. Although they did not suffer any casualties on land or water, those with casualty clearing stations, field dressing stations and field surgical units provided high standards of professional service while they shared many of the hardships of the troops in the front lines. The place of honour on the plaque is given to Col. Agnes Campbell Neill, R.R.C., O.B.E., LL.D., who became Matron-in-Chief to Canadian Military Headquarters in 1942, for under her direction during the final years of the war the nursing services reached a high standard of efficiency.

Along with its triumphs, the war brought its tragedies to the General Hospital. All of Canada was shocked by the almost unbelievable news that Major Sir Frederick Banting had died in a deplorable aeroplane crash in Newfoundland on February 21, 1941, while on his way to England on "a mission of high national and scientific importance." At the outbreak of war he had rejoined the Royal Canadian Army Medical Corps, in which he had served as a battalion medical officer during the 1914–18 war and had been severely wounded and had won the Military Cross. He had become a member of the National Research Council in 1937 and since the beginning of the war had been Chairman of the Associate Committee on Aviation Medical Research and a member of the War Technical and Scientific Development Committee. In November 1939, he had gone to England to take part in conferences with regard to medical and aviation research, and on his return to Canada had been appointed Adviser to the Director General of Medical Services.

For over ten years he and Charles Best had been the "Gog and

Magog of the building on the other side of College Street," where there was always something worth while going on and where young men of imagination were learning the value of hard work in solving a wide range of problems in medical science. Despite the sorrow which met the news of Banting's death, it was felt that it was somehow fit and proper for him to go as he had lived, in the service of his King and Country and of mankind, and be spared the unproductive years of old age. Those who crowded Convocation Hall for his memorial service went back to their tasks stimulated by the spirit of a great Canadian.

Three young men on the threshold of their careers died while on active service. George A. Hendry, the son of Professor W. B. Hendry, had been appointed to the staff of the Department of Obstetrics and Gynaecology in 1939, but had joined the Royal Canadian Naval Medical Service shortly after and was lost at sea when the Canadian destroyer *Ottawa* was torpedoed on September 13, 1942, while on convoy duty. He was an outstanding athlete and captain of the University of Toronto hockey team, and during his short professional career he seemed to personify all the best attributes of the young physician.

Surgeon Lt. William Lyon Mackenzie King, a nephew of the Prime Minister of Canada and of Dr. Harold Wookey of the Toronto General Hospital, went down with his ship H.M.C.S. *St. Croix* in October 1943 when she was torpedoed in the North Atlantic while on convoy duty. He had been a brilliant student, graduating with the Silver Medal in 1937, and after serving as house surgeon at the General Hospital had trained at the Mayo Clinic. He was resident surgeon at St. Michael's Hospital when he joined the Royal Canadian Navy, and had already shown great aptitude and promise for a surgical career.

Dr. Jacques Bourgeois was killed in 1942 while serving with the Royal Navy in the attack on Oran in North Africa. He had come to the General Hospital for surgical training under Dr. Gallie in 1939, largely as a result of the great friendship between Dr. Gallie and his father, Professor B. B. Bourgeois of the University of Montreal. The first of a long line of French Canadians who have been trained at the Toronto General, Dr. Bourgeois had won the respect and friendship of his associates during the short time he had worked there.

The sudden death of Dr. Frederick Logan on February 8, 1942, came as a shock to all who worked at the General Hospital. He had been appointed Assistant Medical Superintendent in January 1938, in which post he had quickly established himself through his keen interest in the house staff and an appreciation of the value of good nursing and efficient service to the welfare of the patients gained from his own experience in the practice of medicine. The four years during which he had held this important position were full of problems, and he had given clear evidence of his ability to meet them. There is no doubt that had he been spared he would have been a leader in hospital management in the years of progress which were to follow.

XVI

The Captains and the Kings Depart

WITH THE END OF THE WAR IN EUROPE IN JUNE 1945, A second great metamorphosis occurred at the General Hospital. In a community which had become accustomed to great challenges and achievements, the hospital would never be the same again—socially, economically or professionally. The problems that faced the institution in the new postwar era had to be confronted in a radically different environment, for the government controls and industrial relations accepted during the past few years were here to stay. In response to the winds of change, older men who had carried on beyond their normal years of service were generally ready to lay down their responsibilities and younger men, returning from their war services in Canada and overseas, were anxious to assume the positions waiting for them. This time, in contrast to 1919, even those serving in the active war zones had enriched their skills as physicians and surgeons. Armed with that broad experience they were ready to make contributions to the service of the hospital that would alter it materially in the coming years.

Duncan Graham and W. E. Gallie terminated their services with the hospital in June 1947. Their combined departure was a fitting climax to an era in which together they had dominated the Faculty of Medicine and the General Hospital. Duncan Graham had never faltered in his absolute control of the Department of Medicine, demanding what he himself gave: complete loyalty and effort to the Medical School and its great teaching hospital. The system he had created bore his imprint, and produced—not only for his own department and the other associated university hospitals in Toronto, but also for Canadian medicine in general—men who never lost the mark of his inspiration. To a great extent, his success had depended on the judgment he showed in choosing his disciples, as these men were to share his mission. Under his direction another door had been added to the triad which Osler had said should lead to the seats of the mighty. The advent of the specific therapy of the sulphonamides and antibiotics gave new importance to the sub-department of Therapeutics, and an opportunity for Ray Farquharson, K. J. R. Wightman, and Robert Kerr to prove their worth before assuming leadership in the department of medicine.

Duncan Graham's influence on medical education extended far beyond Toronto. He was a member of the original Council of the Royal College of Physicians and Surgeons, and President of the College from 1933 to 1935. His influence was strong in the development of regulations governing acceptable postgraduate training for the Fellowship and for specialist certification by the College, an integral feature of which was the recognition of hospitals capable of providing resident appointments for postgraduate students. In recognition of his contribution, the Canadian Medical Association gave him its highest honour, the Frederick Newton Gisborn Starr Award, in 1957.

In the history of the Toronto General Hospital no one has left a greater tradition than William Edward Gallie. His earlier years at the Hospital for Sick Children were featured by the research he carried out with Dr. A. B. LeMesurier, which brought world-wide recognition. When he became Professor of Surgery and Surgeon-in-Chief to the General Hospital his greatest accomplishment was the establishment in 1931 of a systemic course of training in surgery. Under this system his residents first gained adequate experience in the basic sciences as applied to surgery, followed by training in urology, neurology and orthopaedics, as well as in general surgery. It was the first course of its kind in Canada, and by 1940 it had been extended to include appointments at St. Michael's and the Toronto Western Hospital. The efficiency of this postgraduate training proved its value during the war years, and as Dean of the Faculty of Medicine Gallie also organized the accelerated course for undergraduate students. This produced a steady flow of young doctors for intern service in the hospitals, where they received the training which would fit them to meet the demands of active service.

Time has shown that Dr. Gallie's interest and pride in the accomplishments of his students has been rewarded by the life-long gratitude of a widespread group of surgeons who were inspired by the magnetism of his personality. His readily available advice to the trustees, while he was chairman of the Medical Advisory Board was invaluable, yet despite all these demands he served as President of the American College of Surgeons for the unprecedented period of six years. In 1947 he was awarded the Gold Medal of the Royal College of Surgeons of England for "distinguished labours, researches and discoveries eminently conducive to the improvement of natural knowledge and of the healing art," the greatest honour bestowed by this ancient college, and one that had been awarded only twenty times in 150 years. On receiving the award he delivered the Moynihan Lecture to the Royal College of Surgeons on the subject of "Recurring Dislocation of the Shoulder."

The session of 1945–46 marked the end of Gallie's service as Dean of Medicine at the University of Toronto and, in his own words, brought to a close a period in which one of the departmental heads had always acted as chief administrative officer. He would now be replaced by a full-time dean whose major interest would be the study and solution of the problems of general medical education. This progressive move had been made necessary by the growth of the faculty and by the need to keep abreast of changes which were taking place in medical education throughout the world. Dr. Gallie announced the appointment of Dr. J. A. MacFarlane as Dean, and paid tribute to the invaluable service of Dr. Stanley Ryerson on his retirement as Assistant Dean and Secretary.

Dr. Ryerson, for many years a surgeon on the staff of the Toronto General Hospital, had started his long association with the Faculty of Medicine as a demonstrator in anatomy in 1903. He had been Assistant Dean and Secretary ever since the time of Dr. Alexander Primrose's appointment as Dean of the Faculty of Medicine. On the basis of this long experience he had an authoritative knowledge of medical education at both undergraduate and postgraduate levels, which had been of inestimable value in the formative years of the Royal College of Physicians and Surgeons of Canada and to the Toronto Medical School during the trying years of the war.

William Albert Scott retired as Professor of Obstetrics and Gynaecology and as Obstetrician and Gynaecologist-in-Chief to the Toronto General Hospital in 1946, after having held these appointments for eleven years. He had been a Gold Medallist in 1913, and was Professor B. P. Watson's first appointee to the department. He had succeeded Dr. W. B. Hendry in 1935, and made great contributions to both obstetrics and gynaecology at the General Hospital. Besides raising the standard of gynaecologic surgery in his department, he had organized postgraduate training to meet the requirements of the Royal College of Physicians and Surgeons, so that special examinations were set up in the Division of Surgery of the College for obstetricians and gynaecologists. In cooperation with Dr. Gordon Richards he had established joint clinics served by his department representatives working at the Institute of Radiotherapy. As a result, his interns and undergraduate students had learned the important part which radiotherapy played, not only in the treatment of pelvic malignant lesions but, in those days, of some benign tumours and in the control of some major disturbances of female physiology. At the same time, work in these clinics established the increasing role of radical pelvic surgery in the treatment of a large number of patients incurable by any other means. During the war years his department had suffered more than any other from the lack of efficient senior interns and residents, but due to his organizing ability the standard of patient care never failed, though the hours were long and the patients many. He was also very influential in founding the Society of Obstetricians and Gynaecologists of Canada in 1944, and in developing the strong national influence that it has had on major problems of health and welfare.

Dr. H. B. Van Wyck succeeded W. A. Scott as Head of the Department of Obstetrics and Gynaecology at the hospital and the university, and his lifelong service to the hospital was climaxed by four years of outstanding achievement. Having gained an exceptional training in the classics before even entering medicine he had established himself as an outstanding teacher with a philosophical approach to the problems of medicine, which both appealed to his undergraduate students and gained him nation-wide recognition by the medical profession. He served as chairman of the Medical Advisory Board during the postwar period, and his advice to the trustees was of great value, particularly in dealing with the organization and control of the medical services of the Wellesley Hospital and the relationship of the General Hospital to the organization of the Ontario Cancer Institute. With the cooperation of Alan Brown of the Hospital for Sick Children, he combined the teaching of paediatrics with that of obstetrics for the final-year students and the keen interest which he took in his interns and residents, many of whom were preparing for postgraduate degrees, was the basis for a widening of postgraduate training in obstetrics and gynaecology. Two of his senior interns, F. T. Bryans and William McGarrity, returned from postgraduate training in the U.S.A. to careers leading to professorial rank in British Columbia and the University of Texas.

Two surveys of major clinical importance were undertaken at this time. Dr. D. M. Low, working with Dr. Philip Greey, the director of the blood bank at the Toronto General Hospital, surveyed over 20,000 obstetrical patients in the Toronto area to determine the incidence and significance of the Rh sensitization reaction. Dr. D. N. Henderson made a detailed study of material from five hundred patients in his pathology laboratory to determine the nature of in situ carcinoma of the cervix, and was responsible for organizing routine Papanicolaou smears to be taken on all outpatients in the clinics of the department.

Another departmental head who retired in 1946 was Dr. Walter W. Wright, one of the pioneers in modern Canadian ophthalmology. He had graduated in 1904 from the University of Toronto, and after interning at the Hospital for Sick Children had engaged in general practice in Toronto. In 1914 he had gone to London, England, where he studied ophthalmology and received the Diploma from the Royal London Ophthalmic Hospital in 1915. He had gained considerable experience in ophthalmic surgery during the First World War, and on his return from overseas service had been appointed to the staff of the Hospital for Sick Children, becoming Chief of the Department of Ophthalmology in that hospital in 1929.

One of Wright's chief interests had been the early diagnosis and detection of amblyopia in children with strabismus, and he had also developed an original operative procedure using fascia lata for the correction of ptosis. At the time of his appointment as Professor of Ophthalmology at the University of Toronto and Ophthalmologist-in-Chief to the Toronto General Hospital, the staff at the General Hospital had consisted of Dr. Mortimer Lyon, Dr. Frederick Aylesworth and Dr. Clarence Hill, all of whom had gained wide recognition in ophthalmology. More recently appointed were Drs. A. E. MacDonald, W. R. F. Luke, Harry Macrae and J. F. A. Johnston, who had returned from various postgraduate centres in the U.S.A. and Europe to broaden the interests of the department.

Dr. Wright had also organized the first postgraduate training in ophthalmology in Toronto, a feature of which was an interchange of senior interns between the Children's Hospital and the Toronto General Hospital. He had become actively interested in the rehabilitation of blind patients at the Canadian National Institute for the Blind, and during the war had set up special training for medical officers in the R.C.A.F.

Dr. A. J. Elliott was appointed to succeed Walter Wright in 1946 as Professor of Ophthalmology and Chief of the Department at the General Hospital. A graduate of the University of British Columbia, Dr. Elliott had received his postgraduate training in ophthalmology in Toronto and New York. During the war he had been Senior Consultant in Ophthalmology to the R.C.A.F. overseas, and he brought with him a keen appreciation of the problems peculiar to his special field.

Immediately prior to and during the war years, there were many changes in the direction of the Department of Otolaryngology. Dr. Perry Goldsmith, who had succeeded D. J. G. Wishart, continued as Department Head until 1937. During his tenure in that position, the outpatient department grew steadily busier and there were few vacant beds on Ward E, which was shared with the ophthalmologists. With no antibiotics available, acute and chronic infective lesions accounted for the majority of cases. General surgeons, proficient in head and neck surgery, were treating the malignant tumours. However, it was the introduction of bronchoscopy by junior members of Goldsmith's staff which opened the field of thoracic surgery. His reputation as a teacher and surgeon gained him many honours, the chief of which was his election in 1934 as President of the Triological or American Society of Otology, Rhinology and Laryngology. During the First World War he had served with distinction in the Canadian Army Medical Corps, receiving a C.B.E.

Goldsmith was succeeded by a senior member of his staff, Dr. George M. Biggs, who carried on his duties during the war years in spite of the ill health which forced his retirement in 1941. The next Head of the Department was Dr. Angus Campbell, whose association with the Department dated back to 1912. He became well aware that changing conditions were altering the practice of otolaryngology, and that a better organization of postgraduate training was necessary if the specialty were to survive. Wartime experience was showing the importance of investigative studies of the function of the middle and internal ear, and young surgeons were returning home with a broader knowledge of general surgery. He could see the great strides that the major departments were making in the systemic training of graduate students, and in spite of discouragements he initiated improvements which were only to gain recognition during the time of his successor.

Dr. Percy Ireland, who was chosen to be the head of the Department of Otolaryngology at the University and the General Hospital in 1946, had received his major postgraduate training at the Massachusetts Eye and Ear Infirmary. During most of the war he had served overseas and was Consulting Otolaryngologist to the Canadian Army Headquarters from 1944 to 1946. Through this wartime service he had come to appreciate the great changes which were facing his specialty—as well as the necessity of major developments in research and in the training of the new generation of otolaryngologists.

Many of the old guard, whose services bridged the gap from the old hospital on Gerrard Street, had reached their time of retirement. Two of the most distinguished of these were Norman Shenstone and John Oille.

In 1945 Shenstone terminated a service of thirty-six years to the hospital and to the University of Toronto. Since the early years when he had returned from New York to serve with C. L. Starr and W. E. Gallie on the service of Professor I. H. Cameron, his contribution to the hospital, its patients, and his students had been outstanding. In addition to the skills of surgery, his house surgeons had learned from him the techniques of a good physician in the care of the sick and they looked up to him as the ideal personification of the comprehensive general surgeon. Under his control Ward C had become not only the birthplace of thoracic surgery but also the location of a service that left a hallmark on all those who had worked for him.

Another link with the old General Hospital was broken when John Oille retired just before the war, after more than thirty years of service to the Hospital. Through all these years, without fail, the local father of cardiology had carried on his daily inquisition on Ward I. His firm adherence to principles had won the admiration of junior associates, interns and patients, as well as those who owed a better life to him as an unknown benefactor; and he passed those principles on to a generation of students.

Ernest Cleaver, one of Duncan Graham's first appointees, retired in 1946 because of failing health. He had come from a good basic training in New York to establish himself as the senior gastroenterologist at the General Hospital. In his hands clinical observation and continuous therapy had often been found to be a reasonable alternative to surgical treatment of digestive tract disorders and, with his colleagues E. J. Maltby and Robert C. Dickson, he had developed an appreciable co-operation with the surgical department in the over-all treatment of gastrointestinal lesions.

An unexpected tragedy occurred on January 17, 1948, when Dr. Roscoe R. Graham died while skiing at Collingwood, Ontario. At the time of his death he was one of the most distinguished surgeons on the staff of the General Hospital, and was recognized internationally as a master abdominal surgeon. As the Head of the First Surgical Division he had been an inspiring teacher of undergraduate students and a guiding spirit to his interns as they learned the skills of their profession. He had been the youngest surgeon ever to be elected to the American Surgical Association, and had held high offices in leading societies in both Canada and the United States. It was a shock for his associates to realize that this vigorous enthusiast would never be seen again on the wards or in the operating rooms.

Dr. Roy Thomas retired in 1947 after thirty-four years' service to the General Hospital. He had been a close associate of Dr. N. A. Powell since the opening of the Shields Emergency Hospital, and had eventually succeeded him as the senior surgeon in the Emergency Department. He had become a tradition in this department as an ever-available and much-admired mentor to the younger members of the staff, interns and students alike.

Robin Pearse and Robert McComb, two senior urologists, also reached their years of retirement at this time. Under Pearse the Department of Urology had developed diagnostic and surgical standards that put it in the forefront of Canadian medicine, and McComb, who had entered his specialty after valuable years in general practice in a small town in Northern Ontario, had never lost his kindly interest in the patients who came under his care.

Robin Pearse had been in charge of the Department of Urology for thirteen years. During this time surgical techniques had become more comprehensive and the work at the veterans' hospitals, Christie Street and later Sunnybrook, had increased the scope of urological surgeons. Two of these who were particularly outstanding were Carl Aberhart, who had served with No. 15 General Hospital, though at great cost to his health, and David Mitchell, who had earned his F.R.C.S. (England) before joining the staff of the General Hospital. Shortly before he retired, Robin Pearse reported the results of treating 370 patients with cancer of the prostate which showed the favourable trend in survival due to earlier diagnosis and improved methods of treatment. Dr. J. C. McClelland succeeded Robin Pearse and although he retired in 1949 after only three years' service, he succeeded in integrating the service at Sunnybrook and the Weston Sanatorium, to the benefit of his staff and of postgraduate training in Urology.

Dr. Gordon Richards died in January 1949 from leukemia, considered to be the result of his years of exposure to irradiation. Throughout his career there had been very little appreciation of this danger, and practically no thought given to the need for adequate protection of the radiotherapist and his immediate associates. Richards' interests had not been confined to the General Hospital: with the cooperation of Dr. A. H. Sellers, the statistician to the Department of Health, a record system covering all the radiotherapy clinics in the province was developed during his period of service. As the managing director of the Cancer Foundation he had organized support for cancer research in Ontario, and when the National Cancer Institute was established in 1947 he had become its first president.

During Richards' final years the treatment facilities and accommodation in the Dunlap Building had been overtaxed. A total of nearly 2,000 new patients were treated in 1948, with 1,255 patients being admitted and treated for cancer. It was not surprising that Gordon Richards had plans for a greatly enlarged major centre. He felt that the centralization of radiotherapy and newer forms of treatment could not be confined to a department in one of the general hospitals in Toronto. The whole idea, however, was controversial—the Medical Advisory Board of the General Hospital felt it was essential that radiotherapy services be available in the treatment of many surgical patients, and that the development of an ever-widening range of carcino-therapeutic agents not be dissociated from the departments of medicine and therapeutics. Another phase of the impending change was the dissociation of radiotherapy and diagnostic radiology. While Richards was the University Professor of Radiology and Radiologist-in-Chief at the hospital, A. C. Singleton, his senior associate, had taken over the diagnostic services. Two groups were becoming clearly separated: Vera Peters and Clifford Ash with Richards, and Malcolm Hall with Singleton. At the same time there was a growing waiting list of young radiologists all over Canada who wished to train at the Dunlap, under the acknowledged leader of Canadian radiotherapy.

Prompted by the demands of Gordon Richards for improved facilities, the Provincial Minister of Health early in 1949 requested Sidney Smith, President of the University of Toronto, to set up an advisory committee consisting of Professors H. B. Van Wyck, R. F. Farquharson and R. M. Janes. This President's Committee recommended that the new Toronto Institute of Radiotherapy be erected on the site of the Toronto General Hospital or adjacent to it. Two factors governed this choice of location: the ready availability of the facilities to a large number of patients being surgically treated for malignant diseases, and its proximity to the Banting Institute for purposes of research investigation. The criticism of the other university teaching hospitals, that Toronto General was being given preferential treatment, would, it was felt, be overcome by inviting their staffs to cooperate in the consultative clinics and by the return of patients to the referring hospitals if further surgical treatment were required.

After Gordon Richards' time the whole perspective widened. The Ontario Cancer Foundation, through the sponsorship of the Ontario government, became actively involved with the University of Toronto and its teaching hospitals in developing plans for a new Ontario Cancer Institute, to be erected on the grounds of the Wellesley Division of the Toronto General Hospital. A provincial grant of $2,000,000 was made in 1951, but plans for the new institute progressed very slowly since they involved the purchase of adjacent property and the provision and development of major services for both the institute and the Wellesley Hospital.

Dr. Clifford L. Ash, while remaining Radiotherapist-in-Chief to the General Hospital, was appointed Director of the New Cancer Institute. There was a steady increase in the volume of work at the General, over two thousand new patients receiving treatment in 1952. At this time, largely as a result of the work of Professor Harold Johns in Saskatoon, cobalt beam therapy units became available. In November 1953, an Eldorado type of unit, produced by Atomic Energy of Canada, was installed in a specially prepared location in the old building of the Hospital for Sick Children on College Street. Within eleven months 238 patients had received treatment by this unit.

It was as a direct consequence of the prolonged records which Richards had maintained for radiotherapy that a tumour registry was organized to cover all patients treated for malignant disease at the hospital. In 1950 the Ontario Cancer Foundation undertook to cover the expense of maintaining records under the supervision of Mrs. Shirley Gordon, at that time Records Librarian to the Department of Radiotherapy, and a special committee was set up by the Medical Advisory Board in cooperation with the Director of the Radiotherapy Institute. This registry has proved valuable from the time of its inception, producing a continuous flow of publications from the staff of the Toronto General Hospital.

In 1948 Dean J. A. MacFarlane set up a Faculty Radioactive Isotope Committee authorizing Professor J. A. Dauphinee to organize a laboratory at the Banting Institute, where radioactive isotopes could be stored and made available to the University teaching hospitals. Dr. William Paul, physicist to the Faculty of Medicine, was put in charge of making cooperative studies with physicians, surgeons and radiotherapists. On this basis considerable work was carried out in various departments of the General Hospital. Dr. M. W. Johnston and his group of collaborators became involved in one of the most extensive of these, for by 1955 they had used radioactive iodine in the investigation of over five thousand patients, as well as in the treatment of over nine thousand patients suffering from hyperthyroidism. An interesting side-issue was the work of Dr. W. F. Greenwood, using the same isotope in an attempt to control severe angina pectoris. Dr. K. J. R. Wightman and his co-workers in the Department of Therapeutics were soon using radioactive phosphorus in the treatment of leukemia, as well as a means of studying the metabolic disturbances of acromegaly. Neurosurgeon T. P. Morley and Ophthalmologist G. A. Thompson were investigating features of diagnosis in tumours of the brain and of the eye.

Dr. O. B. Miller and Dr. J. C. F. McDonald, a physicist at the Institute of Radiotherapy, published the first report in Canada of a series of patients treated with radioactive gold for malignant pleural and peritoneal effusions. Probably the most outstanding development of the work of Dr. William Paul was the assembling in 1954 of a brain scanner embodying some modifications of the equipment then in use in Boston. This was readily available to the neurosurgeons and for the first time provided the staff at the Toronto General Hospital with a routine pre-operative procedure for determining accurately the location of brain tumours, eliminating the hazards inherent in pneumoencephalography and arteriography.

Dr. Harry J. Shields terminated his active service with the General Hospital in 1952. During his seventeen years as Anaesthetist-in-Chief many changes had taken place in anaesthetic techniques to keep pace with developments in the special fields of surgery. Whereas Dr. Samuel Johnston had been resistant to newer methods of anaesthesia, Harry Shields had contributed to the work of thoracic surgeons, neurosurgeons and cardiovascular surgeons by developing methods more acceptable to them. Although he, himself, was the only full-time anaesthetist on the staff, his department had never failed to meet the unremitting demands of surgeons and obstetricians at both the General Hospital and the Wellesley Division. Harry Shields' long wartime experience with No. 4 Canadian General Hospital during the First

World War had perfected his knowledge of endotracheal anaesthesia and the use of rectal ether anaesthesia for thoracic operations. During these years, too, Dr. W. Easson Brown of his Department, working with Professor Velyien Henderson in the Department of Pharmacology, had done pioneer work with anaesthetic gases—ethylene, propylene and cyclopropane.

The first resident in anaesthesia had been appointed in 1936, and with the outbreak of war two members of the staff, Stanley Campbell and R. A. Gordon, as well as a recent resident, Dr. George Boddington, went overseas. In spite of constant demands at home, Shields and his depleted staff carried on a six-month residency training program to provide anaesthetists for the armed services. Once again the wartime experience of many young anaesthetists prompted them to confine themselves to the special fields of anaesthesia with an increasing interest in basic research as it applied to the problems of respiratory function and the factors contributing to shock and collapse. In 1948 R. A. Gordon became involved in the preliminary studies of Dr. W. G. Bigelow on the use of hypothermia for cardiovascular surgery.

Dr. Stanley Campbell succeeded Harry Shields as Anaesthettst-in-Chief to the General Hospital. He had joined the department in 1926, and therefore had not only a thorough practical knowledge of clinical anaesthesia but also an awareness of the problems which were to face the department in the immediate future. Up to this time Anaesthesia had been recognized both at the University and at the General Hospital as a sub-department of Therapeutics, but the appointment of Stanley Campbell was as an Associate Professor of an independent department. This allowed him the opportunity to extend postgraduate training routines to all the university teaching hospitals, which eventually led to standards acceptable for certification and Fellowship in the Royal College of Physicians and Surgeons of Canada. As plans developed for the hospital extension, Dr. Campbell had a large part to play in placing specific needs before the Medical Advisory Board. These included accommodation for equipment rooms, induction room and a post-operative recovery room with facilities for twenty-four beds, all of which he felt were essential to service the planned centralized operating rooms, and all on a scale unthought of previously. The close association of the group of anaesthetists on a continual rotating duty basis led to the establishment of a partnership association in October 1952. After this all receipts were pooled in a central office located outside the hospital, and the two groups of anaesthetists, full-time and part-time, received their remuneration on a predetermined scale. This represented the first group practice among the staff at the Toronto General Hospital.

Dr. W. L. Robinson retired as assistant professor of pathology and as pathologist to the Toronto General Hospital in September 1953, ending a distinguished service of thirty-eight years. He had begun his career under Professor J. J. Mackenzie and from the primitive methods of that time had developed a surgical pathology service unsurpassed in Canada or the United States. The surgeons of the General Hospital had come to rely on his prompt and authoritative opinion on living pathological material and interns and young assistants, realizing that it provided a clear understanding of disease processes, carried his methods of teaching across Canada and even to centres in the U.S.A. Robinson's reputation as a forensic pathologist made him a national authority, but his greatest attribute was his ability to cooperate with all who worked in the Department of Pathology at the Banting Institute. Eric Linell, the neuropathologist, had already established a special sub-department, but in addition D. N. Henderson from Obstetrics and Gynaecology, A. E. MacDonald from Ophthalmology, and Norman Wrong from Dermatology developed a mutually advantageous liaison with W. L. Robinson—a unique feature of the service available to the clinicians at the Toronto General Hospital. Finally, the teamwork of Professor William Boyd, the great teacher of pathology, and the down-to-earth practicality of W. L. Robinson made a combination unsurpassed among Canadian or American university hospitals.

Although he never accepted an appointment to the staff of the General Hospital, William Boyd made a great contribution through his services on the Medical Advisory Board during the years he was professor of pathology at the University of Toronto (1937–51). The link he forged between the Banting Institute and the hospital influenced many of his colleagues. The wards of the hospital provided the material with which he built the museum that bears his name, and the whole professional community of the hospital was elevated by the magic touch of a great teacher. His students, both undergraduate and graduate, learned much from his approach to the basic problems of disease, and on leaving to take up his appointment at the University of British Columbia he had the satisfaction of knowing that he had won the affectionate regard of his many colleagues in Toronto.

By the time Kenneth G. McKenzie retired in 1953 his neurological service at the Toronto General Hospital had gained international recognition. In later years it was difficult to appreciate the challenge he had originally faced with the primitive facilities available—at a time when diagnosis depended entirely on meticulous clinical observation and there was no suction apparatus or electrocoagulation.

McKenzie's era in neurosurgery was the era of cranial-cerebral injuries, brain tumours and brain abscesses, with surgery of trigeminal neuralgia, glossopharyngeal neuralgia and intractable pain. Towards the end of his active career, with the cooperation of the superintendents of the various Ontario mental hospitals, McKenzie reported the final results of bilateral frontal lobe leukotomy, which he had performed on a considerable number of patients with mental diseases. The surgical complications were minimal, and the end results satisfactory in the vast majority of the patients.

McKenzie's teaching covered a broad range: his guidelines to general practitioners impressed upon them the life-saving value of prompt treatment of cerebral injuries, and through his inspired training his residents took their places across Canada as outstanding neurosurgeons.

Dr. Harry Botterell, his successor, first joined him in 1936. He had had a remarkable postgraduate training after coming from Winnipeg to be W. E. Gallie's resident at the General Hospital in 1933. A year in neuroanatomy at Johns Hopkins and nine months at Queen Square in London were followed by a year of neuropathology at Yale. As a result, in addition to his surgical post, he was appointed lecturer in neurophysiology by Professor Charles Best. His work with Dr. Donald Solandt at the Banting Institute led to his great interest in spinal core injuries and paraplegia. In cooperation with a urologist, Dr. Carl Aberhart, he perfected tidal wave irrigation of the bladder which was to transform the lives of paraplegics.

During the war years while Botterell was at Basingstoke, McKenzie and he were constantly planning the future of neurosurgery in Toronto by long-distance communication, and when Botterell returned in 1945 they made steady progress in evolving a comprehensive service to cover the whole field of neurology. Conditions could not have been more opportune, for their colleagues Herbert Hyland, J. C. Richardson and Allan Walters were uniquely prepared to represent medical neurology in a close liaison. Eric Linell and his associate, Mary Thom, were firmly established in neuropathology by that time and John W. Scott, physician and physiologist, was ideally suited to contribute a knowledge of electroencephalography.

Electroencephalography had been introduced at the General Hospital through the cooperation of the physiologists working at the Banting

Institute. The first equipment had been installed in the Department of Neurosurgery in connection with the original operating room in the basement under Ward D in 1937, but during the war years the equipment was removed as the result of the lack of trained personnel and other demands for its use. After the war Dr. J. C. Richardson returned to the hospital and insisted that the service be re-established. K. G. McKenzie and Herbert Hyland joined with Professor Charles Best and Professor Ray Farquharson in choosing John Scott to undertake the training necessary to become both a physiologist and a clinical electroencephalographer. After spending six months at the Montreal Neurological Institute he went as a Nuffield Fellow to Queen Square in London, where he worked for a year under George Dawson and William Cobb. On his return in August 1949 he was appointed to supervise a re-established electroencephalography department, as a member of the staff of both the Department of Medicine and the Department of Physiology.

Finally, Dr. Douglas Eaglesham, who had served with Harry Botterell at Basingstoke, was prepared to raise the whole standard of neuroradiological diagnosis at the General Hospital and to re-introduce cerebral angiography as a diagnostic procedure.

It was simply a matter of course that Dr. John Oille's successor should be Dr. John Hepburn, for no one in the hospital was held in higher regard: everything he said or did was based on the solid and unshakeable foundation of sincerity. He had grown up in the Orkney Islands and entered Edinburgh University Medical School when he was sixteen years of age, but left after two years to come out to British Columbia "to earn his living by the sweat of his brow." Here he learned much about all sorts and conditions of men, and when the war broke out he joined the Canadian Seaforth Highlanders. As a company sergeant-major he was very severely wounded near Vimy Ridge early in 1918, and returned to a prolonged convalescence in Canada. Dr. Herman Robertson, whose son was later to be Principal of McGill University, was on the board that discharged him from the army, and was responsible for his resuming his medical studies.

Hepburn led his year when he graduated from Toronto in 1921, then worked in Physiology under Professor J. J. R. MacLeod at a time when Banting and Best were involved in their insulin studies. After a year as an intern in medicine at the Toronto General Hospital, his great qualities of mind and character were recognized by Professor Duncan Graham, who appointed him to his staff at the General. From a broad interest in medicine, under the influence of John Oille, he came to confine his practice to cardiology. In this he was closely associated with another of Duncan Graham's chosen physicians, Harold Rykert.

Rykert, like Hepburn, not only showed great promise in his special field but was also a strong personality, and it was obvious that their association was a valuable one—even their pre-war publications showed important contributions to cardiology at the General Hospital. Unfortunately, Harold Rykert returned from his service overseas with No. 15 General Hospital in broken health. In spite of this he never faltered, and when he died in 1954 he was remembered as one who gave his best service to the end of his short life.

As a teacher and lecturer, John Hepburn presented his knowledge with unusual brevity and extreme clarity in the Scottish burr that he never lost. Although he kept abreast of the advances of science, his careful examination of his patients always gave a reassurance that otherwise would have been lacking. He retired from the active staff of the hospital in 1951, when he was the supervisor of Ward I and in charge of the cardiovascular clinic in the Out-patient Department.

John Hepburn rose to high office in the Royal College of Physicians and Surgeons of Canada, being Vice-President of the Division of Medicine from 1949 to 1951 and President of the College from 1953 to 1955. His health, however, was failing, and to the great sorrow of hundreds of his old students, undergraduate and graduate, to his colleagues and to his many patients, he died of a ruptured abdominal aneurism early in 1956.

Dr. Gordon Murray continued to be a major surgical pathfinder. In 1946 he assembled the first artificial kidney ever used in North America, and soon reported the successful treatment of a small number of patients with acute kidney failure. This was the basis of the first Alexander Simpson-Smith Lecture, which he delivered at the Great Ormond Street Children's Hospital the same week that he presented the Moynihan Lecture on "Surgery of Congenital Heart Disease" before the Royal College of Surgeons in London. The work which developed the artificial kidney was clear evidence of the value of the collaboration between surgeons, physicians and biochemists which was then possible at the General Hospital. Gordon Murray had four great assets: he was an exceptionally skilled surgeon in every phase of surgical practice; he was indefatigable, surmounting the lack of good facilities; he was constantly penetrating the hinterland of "how" and "why"; and he kept himself constantly aware of world-wide advances, particularly in cardiovascular surgery, which he adapted as he broadened the scope of his work in Toronto. Shortly after his work with the artificial kidney he performed the first kidney transplant in Toronto.

Murray's wide experience with the use of heparin in thrombosis led to his use of embolectomy and venous arterial grafts, and he was the first surgeon in Canada to undertake the Blalock-Taussig operation for the blue-baby syndrome. Within a short time this latter operation had become a major feature of Ward C operating room, where under his direction more than six hundred patients were operated on for this condition. He carried cardiovascular surgery as far as was possible without the means of open-heart operations. His work included the first closure of an intraventricular septal defect, to be followed by the successful closure of an intraauricular defect which he reported before the American Surgical Association in 1948. He was the first to transplant a homograft aortic valve, but his interests went even wider, for he was also the first to demonstrate the successful treatment of un-united fracture of the scaphoid bone in the wrist by bone graft, which he had performed on 175 patients by 1946, and this was reported before the Orthopaedic Association. He was also one of the first to adopt peritoneal resection of the rectum for cancer, an operation which obviated colostomy and preserved the function of the sphincter ani.

In addition to his association with the Toronto General Hospital, Murray was appointed Director of the Caven Memorial Research Centre when it was opened in November 1949 by Lord Webb-Johnson, President of the Royal College of Surgeons in England. This centre was established by Mrs. W. P. Caven in memory of her husband, a member of one of the most distinguished medical families in Toronto and Associate Professor of Medicine under Professor James E. Graham. Caven's brother, John Caven, had been Professor of Pathology back in the 1890s at the old hospital on Gerrard Street. On his appointment Murray launched himself enthusiastically into the serum treatment of cancer of the breast, seeking a specific control to overcome the experience of accepted surgical and radiological treatment. While the verdict remains negative, the approach was reasonable and the investigation well founded.

Gordon Murray was joined by W. G. Bigelow as his junior associate on the staff of Ward C in 1948 and retired from the General Hospital staff in 1953. By this time it was obvious that although the specialties of cardiovascular and thoracic surgery were still not officially defined in practice at the General Hospital and at the other teaching hospitals of the University of Toronto, they were to be separate entities, and with the development of plans for the hospital extension the cardiovascular service became as distinct an entity as the sub-departments of urology, neurosurgery and orthopaedic surgery.

Two very distinguished surgeons retired almost simultaneously. Harold Wookey, who had introduced radical surgical treatment of laryngeal and oesophageal cancer at the General Hospital, was in charge of Ward B, which in spite of being the centre for head and neck surgery had remained a general surgical service. It was fortunate for all concerned that he had three young surgeons working with him on his service: W. Keith Welsh, Frederick Kergin and Robert Mustard. Two of them became skilled head and neck surgeons and the third, Kergin, who took over the service from Dr. Wookey in 1951, maintained his special interest in thoracic surgery as a result of his earlier association with Norman Shenstone and Robert Janes. Welsh had also served under Shenstone, and all three approached their special fields from the basis of a thorough knowledge of general surgery. The choice of Keith Welsh to succeed Dr. George Wilson as Surgeon-in-Chief of St. Michael's Hospital in 1947 was another proof of the calibre of surgeon developed in this environment, and no one maintained the Shenstone tradition to a greater extent than Welsh did throughout his surgical career.

Every hour was accounted for in the working day of Robert I. Harris. Under the critical eye of W. E. Gallie he rose to international fame in the growing field of orthopaedics. During the war years, in addition to his military service, he continued on duty at the General Hospital, where he supervised the work of Dr. Warren Stoddart in carrying out the routine service of the hospital.

According to W. E. Gallie, the report which Harris prepared for the National Research Council of Canada regarding the foot problems in the army was the most comprehensive study he had ever known. But Harris's numerous publications from 1919 to 1965 all showed the same master's touch. He had a special interest in medical history, and various addresses in this field showed the painstaking thoroughness typical of him. In 1940 the Division of Orthopaedic Surgery was formally recognized at the General Hospital, and Harris became the head of this service. But his work at the hospital did not lessen his interest in the services for the Department of Veterans Affairs, the Crippled Children, and Weston Sanatorium.

Harris was the recipient of many honours. In 1948, as President of the American Orthopaedic Association at a joint meeting of the American, British and Canadian Orthopaedic Associations in Quebec, he was instrumental in organizing the exchange travelling fellowships program in which the three associations became involved. In 1949 he gave the Hunterian Lecture before the Royal College of England, his subject being "Spondylolisthesis," and he was made an Honorary Fellow of the College. In 1955 he was the first Canadian to be appointed Sims Commonwealth Professor by the Royal College of Surgeons of England, and in this capacity he visited New Zealand, Australia, India and England. In 1957 he became an Honorary Fellow of the Royal College of Surgeons of Edinburgh. His tireless energy was evident even after his retirement from the active staff of the Toronto General Hospital in 1952: he continued to go on rounds at both the General and the Hospital for Sick Children.

In 1947, the resignation of so many distinguished members of the profession and the imminent retirement of others resulted in the Joint Relations Committee's extending the retirement age for surgeons and physicians alike to sixty years. In 1950 it was decided that, under exceptional circumstances, members of the clinical departments might continue their appointments on a year-to-year basis until they reached sixty-two years of age, and in 1956 this by-law was amended to allow another year of service to a Chief of Service or a senior staff member.

XVII

Reorganization

NORMAN C. URQUHART BECAME CHAIRMAN OF THE BOARD OF Trustees of the Toronto General Hospital in May 1946. He had considerable experience in commerce and finance, having been Vice-President of Noranda Mines and a member of the boards of several mining companies, and he also had a special interest in the Robert Simpson Company of Toronto. During the Second World War he had taken a prominent place in the activities of the Canadian Red Cross Society and was Chairman of the Central Council. Retiring from his business interest in January 1941, he had become Chairman of the Prisoner of War Package Division of the Red Cross, a responsibility which continued until the end of the war and which had won him many honours and awards, including the C.B.E. and the French Legion of Honour. With his appointment the provincial government amended the Toronto General Hospitals Act so that the Chairman became a direct appointee by Order-in-Council, and at the same time Urquhart became a Governor of the University of Toronto. A year before his appointment to the General Hospital he had been the Honorary Chairman of the Executive Committee of the fund-raising campaign for the erection of the new building of the Hospital for Sick Children. So, once again, a gentleman of high ideals was accepting the responsibility of high office at the Toronto General Hospital.

Mr. C. J. Decker resigned as superintendent of the General Hospital after thirty years' service in January 1947. In his long association with the hospital since taking over from Mr. Horace Brittain, he had rendered faithful service to the trustees during very trying times. With

Mr. E. C. Fox he had faced the severe financial problems of both the Depression and the war period and, anticipating the long-delayed expansion which was about to occur, he now felt that the time was opportune for him to lay down his responsibilities. In accepting his resignation, the board paid tribute to his contribution in maintaining the role of the General Hospital in the life of the community.

A few months later Dr. Charles Parker, the Medical Assistant Superintendent, also retired. Dr. Parker had had a relatively short period of service but prior to his appointment, on the death of Dr. Frederick Logan, he had been a staff surgeon under Dr. C. B. Shuttleworth. This experience had resulted in a special concern for the conditions of the professional staff of the hospital, prompting him to present in his final report to the Medical Advisory Board the problems which he saw arising from indemnity insurance and prepaid medical insurance plans as they applied to many public ward patients. He had foreseen the eventual disappearance of the public ward patient, and had intimated that this would demand a re-appraisal of available teaching material at the hospital. In addition, the provision of fees for attending surgeons and physicians would necessitate consideration by the hospital of an acceptable routine for the collection and disbursement of such money. He left these observations as a legacy to those who followed him.

One of the first problems which faced Mr. Urquhart and the trustees was the replacement of these two executive officers. A special committee was convened, representing both the Hospital and the University, and consisting of Messrs. Norman Urquhart and H. M. Turner, Lt.-Col. W. E. Phillips, President Sidney Smith and Dr. W. E. Gallie. After due consideration by this committee, Dr. John E. Sharpe was appointed Superintendent of the Toronto General Hospital in September 1947.

Dr. Sharpe's whole career had prepared him in an exceptional manner for the duties he now assumed. After graduating from the University of Western Ontario in 1930, he had served for nearly ten years in various posts at psychiatric hospitals in the province, including that of chief of staff of the Toronto Psychiatric Hospital for the two years prior to the outbreak of war. During the war he had served for five years in the Royal Canadian Air Force Medical Service in various parts of Canada, finally being appointed Officer Commanding the Rehabilitation Hospital in St. Thomas, Ontario. For his war service he had received the O.B.E., and from 1945 to 1947 he had been Assistant Deputy Minister of Health for Ontario.

After carrying on in a dual capacity for over a year Dr. Sharpe recommended, with the support of Mr. Urquhart, that the board should appoint Dr. H. S. Doyle as Assistant Superintendent, Medical. Henry Doyle had graduated from Toronto in 1936, spending the major portion of his postgraduate training on the staff of the Riverdale Isolation Hospital and serving during the war with the Medical Branch of the Royal Canadian Air Force. On his return to civilian life, he had earned his D.P.H. and become epidemiologist to the Department of Health of the province of Saskatchewan, where he worked from 1946 to 1949, serving as a member of the Provincial Health Services Planning Commission. As a result he brought with him first-hand knowledge of the most advanced government involvement with the medical profession existing at that time in Canada, which was of considerable interest to his colleagues at the Toronto General Hospital.

The radical changes which had occurred in the senior professional staff appointments at the end of the war brought an entirely new group of medical advisors to work with Norman Urquhart and the trustees as they undertook the long-overdue rehabilitation of the hospital and the reorganization of many of the hospital services. In 1947 Ray Fletcher Farquharson succeeded Duncan Graham as the Sir John and Lady Eaton Professor of Medicine at the University and as Physician-in-Chief to the Toronto General Hospital. The son of a Presbyterian minister, he had been born in the little village of Claude in Peel County, Ontario, in 1897 and had received his secondary education at Harbord Collegiate, Toronto, prior to serving with the Royal Canadian Artillery during the First World War. Following graduation in medicine from Toronto in 1922, he had spent six years of postgraduate study, including a year at the Massachusetts General Hospital, before he was appointed to the Toronto General Hospital staff in 1928. He had soon established himself as an idealistic teacher and open-minded clinician through the readiness with which he discussed problems of diagnosis and treatment with interns, residents and Fellows of the department. From him they learned the primary value of clinical observation and the importance of realizing the psychological impact of all serious organic diseases. In 1934 he had become Assistant Professor of Medicine and Head of the Department of Therapeutics, and served during the Second World War, first as consultant to the Royal Canadian Air Force and later as Physician-in-Chief consecutively to the Christie Street and Sunnybrook veterans' hospitals. For these services he had received the M.B.E. He also sat on the council of the Royal College of

Physicians and Surgeons of Canada, and was just completing his service as President of the Royal College at the time of his major appointment to the Toronto General Hospital.

Robert Meredith Janes succeeded Edward Gallie as Professor and Head of the Department of Surgery and Surgeon-in-Chief to the Toronto General Hospital. He had already won international recognition and had established himself as a leader in Canadian surgery through nearly twenty-five years' service on the staff of the hospital. His colleagues, his students and many grateful patients bore testimony to the qualities which he brought to the Chair of Surgery and the control of the Department at the hospital.

Janes had come from a farm in southwestern Ontario and had stood at the top of his class as an undergraduate. He had benefited from an early association with Professor C. L. Starr and had been his first resident at the Toronto General Hospital. With Norman Shenstone he shared great contributions to the early developments in thoracic surgery, but this was only one phase in his record of achievements, for he remained a general surgeon in the broadest and best sense of the term. His original contributions showed a great breadth of application from parotidectomy to the treatment of pancreatic fistula, diverticula of the oesophagus and repair of diaphragmatic hernia with fascia lata. He was a superb technician in whatever field he applied his skill, and brought to his task a thorough understanding of the problems which were to be faced by his staff as they made advances in an ever-increasing diversity of surgical specialties.

Professor H. B. Van Wyck, who had been appointed Chairman of the Medical Advisory Board in 1946, represented the professional staff on the Board of Trustees of the Hospital. Although the Medical Advisory Board now had entirely new personnel, its members had nearly all worked at the hospital for years and it was well prepared to support the Chairman in the advice he gave regarding the many problems facing the hospital administration.

One problem that remained to be solved was the question of fees for services to public ward patients, which Dr. C. B. Parker had referred to in his final report. Shortly after Dr. Doyle was appointed, he and Dr. Sharpe presented the whole matter to the Medical Advisory Board. The situation facing the hospital was entirely new, for up to this time there had not been any question of payment to the staff for their services to public ward patients. The only situation where a third-person payment had been made was for patients who had been in hospital under the Workmen's Compensation Board. In this program, which had been initiated in 1914, the General Hospital had eventually provided a block of sixty beds on a floor in the Private Patients' Pavilion for which it received payment on a mutually acceptable basis. Payment for professional services was established on a fee-for-service basis, paid directly to physicians and surgeons, and was acceptable to the board but not necessarily to members of the hospital staff. Now for the first time a situation was developing which was in direct contravention of an agreement between the Governors of the University of Toronto and the trustees of the General Hospital, signed in December 1910, that "there should be no remuneration to members of the visiting staff" for the care of public ward patients. After due consideration, the trustees gave notice to the University in December 1949 that they desired an amendment to the by-law, permitting the visiting staff to charge a public ward patient for professional services "where the patient has insurance against such charge or has a claim for indemnity for such charge against a third person." These charges would be collected by the hospital "in the name of the individual member of the visiting staff" and deposited in a special trust managed by the trustees, "free from any claim of the individual member of the visiting staff."

The governors of the University agreed to the amendment, and in October 1950 Mr. Urquhart reported to the trustees that the desired changes had been approved by Order-in-Council of the provincial government. On this basis it was decided that the trustees and the Heads of the Departments of Medicine, Surgery, and Obstetrics and Gynaecology should form a committee to control the distribution of third-party payments. It was fortunate that J. S. D. Tory, Q.C., of the Board of Trustees was available to advise the trustees and the Medical Advisory Board as to the legality of any plans which they might develop. The Medical Advisory Board gradually came to the opinion that the accumulated money should be used to establish a pension fund. This met with the approval of the trustees, and as a result arrangements were made in November 1954 to transfer the funds to the University of Toronto Pension Plan. It was ruled that pensions would only be available to members of the staff who were under fifty years of age, but annual travelling grants to a maximum of $250 over a yearly period would be available to those who, because of their age, were ineligible for the pension benefit. By the end of 1956, $142,000 was held in a trust fund by the University, and in 1957 Dr. Doyle reported that fifty per cent of the patients with public ward accommodation were covered by some form of insurance and that only twenty per cent were indigent.

The yearly increase in the accumulated funds far surpassed the amount necessary to maintain the pensions. On Mr. Tory's advice the decision was made to allow all the in-patient departments to share in the benefits of the plan, and early in 1962 the University agreed to allow the yearly contribution to be doubled in amount as it applied to the pension fund.

In 1963, at a meeting of the professional staff of the hospital, it was decided to organize a partnership—the Toronto General Hospital Staff Association—and Dr. T. P. Morley was appointed President. As Mr. Tory was now seriously ill, M. V. L. Ash became Advisor to the Association from the Board of Trustees. There was strong feeling on the part of the staff of the Out-Patient Department that they should participate by closer relationship to the Medical Staff Association and that this should apply to physicians and surgeons irrespective of having a university appointment.

The fact that financial support from the Ontario Hospital Services Commission did not apply to the Out-Patient Department—where in 1964 the care of nearly 100,000 patients had resulted in a deficit of $275,000—was of major concern to the Board of Trustees. In 1965, the per diem rate approved by the board was $36.25 and the Ontario Hospital Services Commission was presented with the argument that if diagnostic services in the Out-Patient Department could be supported it would greatly decrease demand for hospitalization. Two major factors which demanded top consideration were the universal coverage to be provided by Medicare by July 1966 and the home care program that was developing for Metropolitan Toronto. Although the faculty and the hospital had not accepted the request of the College of General Practice to establish a Department of General Practice, Dr. Spaulding had already accepted some applications for Out-Patient appointments from general practitioners, and plans were developing for a General Practice Clinic with consideration of remuneration of the physicians involved. It was obvious that service in the Out-Patient Department on a voluntary basis was coming to an end. Dr. Doyle suggested that the Medical Advisory Board should be prepared to advise the trustees as to the cooperation of the General Hospital in the Home Care Programming, which might involve payment for drugs, X-rays and laboratory services—this would contribute to the earlier discharge of patients from the wards, and to a decrease in the number of patient days, which reached an all-time high of over 425,000 in 1965.

The changing relationship of the professional staff, many of whom were now full-time, to the hospital prompted Dr. F. P. Dewar to have the Medical Advisory Board consider the provision of a clinic building. The introduction of Medicare, he felt, would make the difference between private patients and so-called ward or teaching patients a thing of the past. New techniques had already increased the number of procedures, both investigative and therapeutic, which could be done on an out-patient basis. Already the trend was for patients to come directly to the Out-Patient and Emergency departments without reference. The hospital service was becoming an alternative to attending a private physician, and it was uneconomical and inefficient for physicians and surgeons of the hospital staff to be disassociated from the prompt final analysis of any problem by maintaining a consulting office apart from the hospital. The Planning Committee under Mr. A. J. Little, however, replied that for the present the hospital would not be involved in erecting a clinic building or renting space to the staff doctors.

The shortage in nurses at the General Hospital did not improve as might have been expected in the years following the war. A survey in 1948 showed that the situation applied not only to Ontario, where 2,800 were needed, but proportionately across the whole of Canada. The Medical Advisory Board of the hospital set up a committee consisting of Doctors J. A. Dauphinee, F. I. Lewis and D. M. Low to study the situation, and their thorough review identified the factors contributing to it. The advances in medical science particularly demanded greater nursing services as well as a major change in the training routine. While the committee recommended that there was every reason to continue hospital training schools, it was felt that the final year of the three-year course should be an intern year, during which a salary should be paid. It was evident that industry and nursing agencies, Public Health, St. John Ambulance and the Red Cross all provided better working conditions, contributing to the fact that only 20 per cent of Toronto General Hospital graduates continued their association with the hospital. The committee warned that the expected Federal Health Programme, expending $65,000,000 within the next five years, would result in an increase of 43 per cent, or from 40,000 to 60,000 hospital beds in the province. They also felt that steps should be taken immediately to overcome the loss of 40 per cent of the nurses within a year of graduation, including the 20 per cent who left for greener pastures in the U.S.A.

While the situation was under consideration in October 1950, the trustees received a letter from the nurses on general duty at the hospital, requesting better working conditions as an alternative to their resignation. The answer of the board was given by Dr. Sharpe a few weeks later when the starting salary was raised to $165 a month for a 44-hour week. A major change was also to be made in the instruction of undergraduate nurses, and in the resulting reorganization the Training School for Nurses became the School of Nursing of the Toronto General Hospital. In recognition of the double function of the hospital the Director of Nursing was to have under her both an Assistant Director of Nursing Education and an Assistant Director of Nursing Services. In keeping with the marked changes taking place in the treatment of patients, courses of instruction were becoming more specialized and concentrated, with small classes conducted by nursing instructors assuming a major role. Coincidentally, it was a good omen that 121 nurses graduated in 1952, this being to date the largest class in the history of the General Hospital.

In 1954 the trustees established a Staff Pension Plan, to the great satisfaction of the nursing staff, and a year later, on the recommendation of Dr. Sharpe, a bursary and loan fund was organized for the benefit of the pupil nurses. The bursaries awarded during the first year did not have to be repaid, and the interest-free loans were repayable a year after graduation. This plan proved so successful that ten years later the Bursary and Loan Committee was able to report that 107 nurses had received $21,000 through it, and that of these "nearly all the loans have been repaid and also an appreciable number of the bursaries."

In 1956 a new course was announced, consisting of two years' instruction followed by an intern year. For two years the nurse instructors were constantly in control of the students on the wards and in the classrooms. As a consequence, the head nurses could not count on their service on the wards, but the result of the training was seen in the efficient nursing interns, who had a knowledge of nursing and paramedical services previously unknown. The salaried interns, who were free to live outside the hospital, also presented a thoroughly professional attitude towards their duties at the hospital.

Province-wide changes in the control of training schools were influenced by the Registered Nurses Association as well as, eventually, by the establishment of the College of Nurses in 1961 and by the government working through the Ontario Hospital Services Commission. Uniform salary levels were established and regular inspection of nursing organizations carried out. While this program provided the basis for a satisfactory level of training, it unfortunately fell short of appreciating developments at the university teaching hospitals, where it was necessary to keep abreast of the progress in clinical investigation and treatment, both medical and surgical.

In 1961 the staff of the General Hospital included 600 registered nurses, 115 registered nursing assistants, 15 operating room technicians, 261 ward aides and 171 orderlies. The opening of the Norman Urquhart Building and the Gerrard Street building, together with the modernizing of the old buildings of the hospital, brought a great increase in routine nursing care. The addition of 450 beds and twenty-one centralized operating rooms with their ancillary services, along with the enlarged emergency department and the major developments of the highly specialized units, presented unrelenting problems to those whose duty it was to provide nursing services, increasing in quality as well as quantity. Inevitably there was criticism regarding nursing shortages, especially on weekends and during the holiday season, but those involved could appreciate the work of the heads of the school of nursing in the face of a serious situation. Everyone realized that nurses from the Registry would no longer provide a satisfactory replacement for those on duty in so many of the highly specialized services.

Miss Mary Macfarland retired as Director of Nursing in 1960 and was succeeded by Miss Jean Dodds. Miss Dodds, a graduate of the Toronto General School of Nursing, had spent a postgraduate year in Nursing Education at the University of Western Ontario. She had served both as supervisor of the decentralized operating rooms in the College Street building and as supervisor of the new central building when it was opened. She had then become Assistant Director of Nursing Services, and was Acting Director of Nursing during the year before her appointment was confirmed. She was, therefore, well aware of the problems confronting her and of the likelihood of their increasing in the future with the constantly changing demands of the hospital.

It is impossible to refer to all the nurses whose long and distinguished service did so much to maintain the reputation of the General Hospital during the time of Miss Macfarland and Miss Dodds, Miss Bertha Woolford, under various titles, was the night superintendent for thirty years. She had graduated from the General Hospital school in 1917 and had joined the staff of the General after some years spent in New York. Her whole career emphasized once again how essential to the hospital is the service of those capable of meeting every eventuality with unshaken judgment. It was said that over two thousand student nurses had had their night terms under Miss Woolford's guidance. One of her contemporaries was Miss Margaret Dulmage, for many years the instructor at the School for Nurses. She set standards of excellence in patient care which produced graduates who established the reputation of the General Hospital wherever they went.

The name of Margaret McGibbon will always be associated with the centralized operating rooms of the Norman Urquhart Wing.[1] Her appointment was well justified by her experience. Night duty in the Emergency and then supervision of the neurosurgical operating rooms had been followed by three years with the Royal Canadian Naval Nursing Service. On her return in 1946 she had become supervisor of the operating rooms of the College Street building before taking on supervision of the cardiovascular operating rooms as well as those in the central block. From this responsible position she had been transferred to that of Supervisor of the Emergency Department at a time when the burden of work was constantly threatening its organization, but wherever she worked her guidance brought efficiency.

Finally, there was Miss Florence Kelsey, a graduate of 1923. She had been in control of the toxaemic patients under study by Professor V. J. Harding and Dr. H. B. Van Wyck in 1929, and therefore was the first nurse at the General Hospital to work in a clinical investigation unit. She continued as Assistant Head Nurse at the Burnside Hospital, and by the time of her retirement in 1962 had seen the name Burnside lose its association with the Obstetric Department—it was shortly to become the designation of a building to accommodate psychiatric patients.

As the General Hospital took the lead in developing special services, nurses came from hospitals in every part of the country to learn new techniques. A Department of Staff Development was created in 1962, under an Assistant Director of Nursing, to orientate the large numbers of graduate nurses coming from Britain, the West Indies, India and the Philippines. There were students from across Canada taking post-graduate university courses and receiving practical training at the hospital. Special training was also organized for male hospital assistants to keep them aware of changes in patient care.

The enrolment of pupils increased, and to comply with the regula-

[1]Following Mr. Urquhart's death the centre block was renamed in his honour.

tions of the College of Nurses students in 1963 began the 35-hour week, so that they had two and three days off a week. In 1964, 130 nurses enrolled at the School and seventy per cent of the graduating class joined the staff of the hospital. By this time plans were developing for a new building for the school and a residence, not only for the large number of nurses in training and on duty at the hospital but also for the resident house staff. Conveniently located property had already been acquired with the support of the Ontario Hospital Commission in the block bounded by Gerrard, Hayter, Elizabeth and LaPlante streets. This building would provide living accommodation for 450 student nurses and would allow the annual enrolment to increase from 125 to 200 students. In addition to the most modern classroom facilities, recreational features would be provided, including a swimming pool, squash courts and a large gymnasium where basketball could be played.

In June 1965, Dr. Matthew Dymond, the Provincial Minister of Health, convened a meeting of executive directors and directors of nursing and placed before them the problem of the health needs of the province. The decision he had reached was that by 1970 the General Hospital, with other training centres, would have to double the number of graduating nurses, and to meet this situation he had decided that in the near future the course of training was to be limited to two years.

Changes were also taking place in the Social Service Department: in January 1954 the trustees had decided that it should come under the direction and control of the hospital. It was somewhat remarkable that up to this time the department, a quasi-independent organization which had been founded forty-three years before by the Social Service Association, had carried on with such efficiency. Its personnel had been recruited on a voluntary basis, largely from graduate nurses of the hospital, whose interest had been stimulated by the instruction which its members gave to the nurses in training. Its financial support had originally come entirely from the Social Service Association, but in recent years the money that had maintained it had come from the Community Chest of the Greater Toronto area. Over the years the influence of the service had spread to more and more departments, especially to the clinics in the Out-Patient Department, and in 1954 it consisted of fifteen social service workers and two secretaries working under Miss Isabel Deeth from an office in the Out-Patient Department. The time was obviously overdue for the hospital to become responsible for the growing demands for social service; in the ten years up to 1955 out-patient visits had increased from 66,000 to nearly 100,000. In 1955 Mrs. Margaret Reid, who had been trained at the School of Social Work at the University of Toronto, took over from Miss Deeth. Within three years the staff increased to twenty-five workers, many having university degrees, and five secretaries. Progress was encouraged by the large number of patients receiving ambulatory care and the broadening concept of government involvement in community health services.

The department provided an outstanding opportunity for field work to students enrolled in the School of Social Work at the University, and up to six students served for three days a week for forty weeks to help qualify them for a Master's degree from the University. The central department maintained a unifying influence, but as the workers became more closely associated with various departmental services there was an increasing tendency for their interest to become localized. When the Princess Margaret Hospital opened, two workers were detailed to that institution. Regular staff meetings were held so that all would be aware of the work that others were doing, and since 1964 the section of social work of the Ontario Hospital Association has been a source of satisfaction to social workers otherwise isolated in smaller centres and hospitals. A natural result has been that many have left this well-organized department to take up senior appointments at hospitals across Canada.

Naturally this re-organization had a profound effect on the personnel of the Social Service Association, and it was fortunate that the President, Mrs. W. A. Oille, provided efficient leadership to those who were interested in planning the future of volunteer services at the hospital. The result was that they organized themselves, with no loss of time or enthusiasm, as the Women's Auxiliary of the Toronto General Hospital. New committees were formed and new services undertaken in keeping with the great expansion which the hospital was undergoing. Under the guidance of Mrs. J. M. Godfrey, who succeeded Mrs. Oille, and with the help of Mrs. R. F. Farquharson, the auxiliary became not only self-supporting but prepared to provide funds for many of the needs of the hospital. One of the first fund-producing activities was a "Shop on Wheels" organized by Mrs. Ian Crookston. Miss Anne Blaire and Mrs. Robert Maxwell undertook the coordination of various activities, and Mrs. F. P. Dewar began the publication of a new bulletin to keep everyone aware of the work that was going on. A major development was inaugurated in 1956 when Mrs. Roscoe Graham opened a new Pavilion workshop which had been organized by Mrs.

Dewar. Mr. Norman Urquhart's interest in the volunteers was constant, and senior members of the medical and surgical staffs acted as advisors. But it was the guidance of Dr. J. E. Sharpe and Mrs. L. R. McCloskie that renewed the close association with the care of patients, which from the first had been a primary objective of the ladies' organization.

A voluntary professional hairdressing service provided by Miss Ida Heaton and six associates to cancer patients in the Dunlap Building proved to be so successful that it was extended to long-term patients in the public wards. By means of mobile carts, the service soon became available to all patients at the hospital. Finally, a fully equipped beauty salon was opened in 1964, and during its first year of operation the auxiliary received $3,760 from patients who patronized it.

With the support of the consular corps a group of thirty-eight interpreters speaking seventeen languages was organized to help overcome the bewilderment of many new Canadians. The oldest of all the women's services, the Burnside Sewing Committee, which over the years had provided hand-knit baby clothes for indigent mothers, had adapted itself to modern conditions and undertook to provide baby feeding formulas to mothers leaving the Burnside. The mobile patients' library, another service maintained from the old days, was also expanded, so that by 1960 14,000 books and 20,000 magazine loans were distributed to the patients by eighteen volunteers two days of every week.

A few months after the lecture hall had been completed in the centre block, Mrs. C. J. Carter, the Auxiliary President, opened a snack bar and lounge where students could obtain refreshment at cost, but even in commodious quarters this was many times a crowded, though highly appreciated service.

Miss Mary Macfarland followed in the footsteps of Miss Jean Gunn, and the Executive Committee profited by her advice. Support was given to the bursaries set up for the student nurses, and an academic school was organized for the instruction of child patients at the hospital. All the hospital departments benefited from the financial strength of the auxiliary, and were invited to present requests for equipment not readily available. Naturally the Social Service Department held a high priority.

A further improvement came with the modernization of the medical wards on College Street, for which the ladies provided coloured drapes to transform the huge windows and the smaller rooms. This was also done in other areas as they were modernized.

The greatest contribution that was made by the auxiliary was the $15,000 given to the Farquharson Clinical Investigation Unit to transform a basement area into a unique model of patient comfort for those who were under intense and uninterrupted biochemical investigation.

A second Women's Auxiliary shop was opened for business in October 1959 in the centre block, and the success of the shops and the carts was evident in the profit of $10,000 they earned in 1960, which was turned over to the hospital. In the same year, the Executive Committee decided to organize a junior auxiliary where teen-agers could learn how valuable their services would be to the patients of the hospital.

The golden anniversary of the auxiliary was featured by a luncheon at which Mrs. Clara McEachern reviewed the progress over the years. The success of the auxiliary was self-evident, not only through the way in which so many anonymous ladies had made their contributions of time and money, but also through its ability to adapt itself to the ever-changing demands of a great downtown teaching hospital. Apart from the great comfort which its services brought to the patients of the hospital, the business acumen of the organization was evident in the report which the Treasurer, Mrs. W. K. Kerr, presented to 660 members of the auxiliary in 1965, in which she stated that the auxiliary had raised over $20,000 during the previous year.

Another service which had proven its value ever since the influenza epidemics in 1918 and 1919 was that of the Red Cross volunteer nurses, who had firmly supported the hospitals in Toronto by providing home and auxiliary nursing help. Regular classes of instruction were organized in 1925 to raise the standard of care provided, and during the war years the volunteers made it possible to maintain good patient care despite a shortage of graduate nurses. In 1945 the Nursing Director and the Red Cross decided to continue the service in the Dunlap Building and on the public wards, and routine evening care under supervision freed professional nurses from many time-consuming duties. Volunteers worked in the central supply room, in many of the out-patient clinics, and even with the physiotherapists in caring for disabled post-poliomyelitis patients. In 1953, a nursing supervisor was appointed to oversee the services of the volunteers, and for ten years Miss Vera Hull was an invaluable aid to the Toronto General Hospital as she worked tirelessly to maintain a quality of service acceptable to the directors of nursing at the hospital.

In 1952, Dr. Sharpe paid a particular tribute to the volunteers from the Cancer Society, who were bringing many comforts and services to the patients receiving radiotherapy in the Dunlap Building. Every year emphasized the increasing value of the ladies of various organizations who contributed so much to the welfare of the patients at the Toronto General Hospital.

The hospital was also faced with the immediate need to consider the remuneration of interns and residents. Before the war, apart from the residents in Medicine, Surgery, and Gynaecology and Obstetrics, members of the house staff had been satisfied to receive their board and lodging while they spent the first two years of their postgraduate training at the hospital. Recompense for their services was not considered at that time, but now many factors were changing this situation.

During the war years, when short eight-month junior internships were undertaken on graduation, those who had volunteered for active service received pay on this basis. When the war ended, interns returning from service received allowances from the Department of Veterans Affairs—accentuating the fact that recent graduates received no monetary return for their services. The situation prompted Dr. R. A. Mustard, then a resident in surgery, to present a submission to the Medical Advisory Board in October 1946, requesting that it consider the situation of young men and women who had just completed six to eight years of university training, depending on the support provided by their parents or guardians. Presenting statistics as they applied to eighty interns on duty at the hospital that year, of whom thirty-nine were sponsored by the D.V.A., he showed that on a yearly basis paying junior interns $25 and senior interns $50 a month would only increase the yearly cost per patient by one dollar. He was confident, he added, that within ten to fifteen years the interns would be receiving an adequate allowance, but as their spokesman he requested that something be done immediately.

The serious nature of the financial problem of senior interns and residents was further emphasized in 1954 by the Anaesthetist-in-Chief, Dr. Stanley Campbell, when he attributed the lack of desirable trainees to the great discrepancy between the remuneration granted by the Toronto teaching hospitals and other general hospitals in the city. He made a comparison between the $50 a month paid by the former group and the $200 to $250 a month then being paid by the veterans' hospitals across Canada.

Although response to these demands was sympathetic, material progress was very slow. Ten years later Dr. Robert Janes, the Chairman of the Medical Advisory Board, reported that the trustees and Medical Advisory Boards of the teaching hospitals in Toronto had approved a schedule of yearly remuneration of $500 for junior interns, while the senior interns were to receive $1,000, increasing to $1,400 and later $1,800 on the basis of yearly increases up to the fourth year of service. The University increased the maximum to $3,000 in recognition of the teaching responsibilities of these senior men at the resident level undertaking another year of service. A committee set up to consider the shortage of interns coming to the hospital emphasized the problem of the large number of married students in the graduating year, which had increased from ten per cent to fifty per cent in the ten years under consideration, and they also noted that there were more students anxious to receive a rotational service in general practice than a junior year, which was merely a stepping-stone towards prolonged hospital training in a special field. This viewpoint was influenced by a regulation which was proposed to come into force in 1958, demanding such a year of hospital service before a licence to practise could be obtained.

The establishment of the Division of Postgraduate Medical Education by the University of Toronto in December 1955 brought about a fundamental change in the status of the resident staffs of the teaching hospitals. It coordinated training in the basic sciences and centralized the facilities for research during postgraduate training. The Head of the Division became an assistant to the Dean of Medicine, as well as chairman of a board with representatives from all the clinical and basic science departments and from all the teaching hospitals. It confirmed the program of postgraduate training as it affected the Royal College of Canada, which had been organized with the help and advice of so many members of the staff of the General Hospital.

To the satisfaction of all concerned, Professor R. Ian Macdonald was appointed director of the new division. He had come to the Department of Medicine of the Toronto General Hospital in 1936, having previously been involved in the practice of internal medicine in Halifax after graduating from Dalhousie University in 1930 and receiving his M.R.C.P. (Lond.) in 1933. He had served with the R.C.A.M.C. in England and Northwest Europe from 1940 to 1945, retiring with the rank of Lieutenant-Colonel, and was appointed Chief of the Medical Service at Sunnybrook Hospital when he returned to his duties at the Toronto General Hospital after the war. He was well aware of the importance of combining laboratory investigation with the care of patients at a teaching hospital, and of the inevitable increase in the demand for full-time appointments.

One development which involved the General Hospital as well as the other teaching hospitals was the first planned internship for general practice offered in Canada. This started in 1948 and became the responsibility of the Postgraduate Division, embodying a second year's internship which included emergency surgery, medicine, paediatrics, obstetrics and gynaecology. The division also developed a variety of postgraduate refresher courses, which brought to the hospitals special lecturers from the United Kingdom and the U.S.A., as well as from other centres in Canada.

Even before the appointment of Ian Macdonald, the Hospital and the University had come to agree on a new designation of the staff:

University Rank	*Hospital Appointment*
Professor (Head of Department)	Physician (etc.)-in-Chief
Associate Professor	Senior Physician
Assistant Professor	Physician
Clinical Teacher	Assistant Physician
Fellow	Resident
	Clinical Assistant
Graduate Student	Voluntary Assistant

The junior members of the staff represented appointments made possible by fund-granting foundations and societies; and the responsibilities and duties of the residents, both as physicians or surgeons and as teachers, were recognized by the Joint Hospital Relations Committee. From this time on, three interrelated factors contributed to the increasing demand for residents and assistant residents by the heads of the various divisions of medicine and surgery and by the clinical departments: more highly specialized therapy necessitated more responsible service; progressive clinical research required constant correlation between wards and laboratories; and the recognition of specialists' degrees by the Royal College influenced those who sought the training which only a great general hospital could provide.

By 1963, in addition to the Chief Resident Physician, there were three Residents and twenty Assistant Residents in Medicine. In Surgery, the Chief Resident was supported by eight Residents and fourteen Assistant Residents. The growing responsibility of the Department of Anaesthesia was acknowledged in the positions of a Chief Resident, two Residents and nine Assistant Residents. Obstetrics and Gynaecology had both Residents and Assistant Residents, while Ophthalmology had three Assistant Residents and Otolaryngology two. But it was in the Departments of Laboratories and Diagnostic Radiology that the greatest changes had taken place, with ten Assistant Residents in the subdivisions of Pathology, Clinical Pathology, Haematology, Neuropathology, Chemistry and Biochemistry, and Microbiology, and twelve Assistant Residents in Radiology. There were also a Resident and Assistant Resident in Dentistry. Everyone realized that this was only the beginning of an expanding system to accommodate the growing numbers coming to the General Hospital for postgraduate training, and also to meet the demands of the Health Services which were to be inaugurated in July 1966.

Dr. John Hamilton succeeded J. A. MacFarlane as Dean of the Faculty of Medicine in July 1961. MacFarlane's fifteen years in this position had already proven the function of a full-time dean to be essential to the application of progressive instruction in the changing world of the medical practitioner. One of the first principles that governed John Hamilton was that the young graduate-in-training should not suffer from lack of financial security and his influence was strong in that area. Gradual increases were made, and in 1965 an Intern Committee under Dr. T. A. Doran and consisting of younger members of the staff was convened to consider especially the criticism of the junior interns with regard to their service at the General Hospital. Salaries had been approved for the university teaching hospitals, beginning with $3,050 for the first year with increases of $600 a year for Assistant Residents during the next three years and $5,750 for the fourth year, which might apply to either an Assistant Resident or a Resident. The interns themselves, however, felt that this was inadequate: the hours of service seemed frequently too long and the features of the rotating program varied considerably in terms of value of experience gained. They most appreciated Out-Patient and Emergency Surgery, Out-Patient Orthopaedics, Neuro-surgery and Otolaryngology. General Medicine and especially Haematology, Psychiatry, Obstetrics, and Anaesthesia were all of value to them in reviewing future possibilities in private and group practice.

With the rapid growth in the size of the intern staff, living conditions were quickly becoming inadequate. Beginning in 1947, quarters which had been available on the ground floor of the Private Patients' Pavilion had been gradually taken over to provide offices for departmental heads and a growing resident full-time staff. The house staff lived on the top floor of the College Street building, in two old houses on

University Avenue which came to be known by them as "Blunder Inn," and in the old servants' quarters of the so-called Burnside Annex, which were so crowded that many residents became non-residents and others lacked the amenities that had made the old "Non-Pay Era" a happy comradeship.

Closely related to consideration by the Medical Advisory Board of the practical training of the junior interns were the rules established at this time with regard to the work of undergraduate students on the wards of the hospital. Although there was as yet no recognition of clinical clerks, senior students under close supervision were to be permitted to do some routine procedures such as needling of veins, male catheterization, lumbar punctures, paracentesis and thoracocentesis, and minor suturing. The Out-Patient Department, as it developed an even more important function with the preparation for Medicare, continued to present the direct approach to the problems of sick persons so essential to the knowledge of the medical student.

Professor Ray Farquharson appointed Dr. Trevor Owen to succeed Fletcher McPhedran as Chief of the Medical Out-Patient Department in 1947. Owen had spent the early years of his professional career in general practice at St. Catharines before becoming a resident physician at Johns Hopkins Hospital in Baltimore in 1926. On the advice of Duncan Graham, he had trained further in London, England, where he became a member of the Royal College of Physicians. On his return he was associated as a general physician with Dr. C. B. Farrar when he was in charge of the Toronto Psychiatric Hospital. This experience had a marked influence in later years on his relationship with his patients. He came to be known as a sympathetic listener and his interest went even deeper than the diagnosis and treatment of disease, to studying the psychological problems which were often associated with them. His students and interns were influenced by this characteristic of a good physician, and the fact that many of them later became his patients was evidence of their appreciation of his character as well as his ability. On his retirement in 1956, Professor Ray Farquharson acknowledged Owen's great value to the Department of Medicine as both physician and teacher, and his younger associates recalled the great benefit of the monthly out-patient rounds which he had organized.

During this time the staff of the medical clinic included, as it always had in the past, a group of practising physicians outstanding in Toronto. G. W. Lougheed, Valentine Stock, R. Ian Macdonald, Robertson Caven, Barnet Berris, John E. C. Cole, Arthur Parks and Wright Young all served at this key clinic. The chest clinic, dating back to the time of Dr. Harold Parsons, numbered among its members Albert Crowther, Edgar Sexsmith, Cameron C. Gray, Herbert Pugsley and William Oille. The Diabetic Clinic, which had had its origin with the first use of insulin, was under the direction of Dr. Edward S. Jeffrey until his retirement in 1948, and served over one thousand patients through observation and treatment by Albert Crowther, Eleanor Robinson and Barbara Hazlett. The Haematology Clinic, which had always held a particular interest for Ray Farquharson, benefited from the services of Arthur Squires, K. J. R. Wightman, Irving Rother and James Watt, and its patients received the highest quality of clinical investigation.

The clinics of the Departments of Surgery, Obstetrics and Gynaecology, Otolaryngology and Ophthalmology were largely serviced by members of the in-patient staffs, but in addition H. F. Robertson, D. R. Bohnen, G. E. P. Wilson, A. G. Shaw, Magnus Spence, Herbert Tait, and L. J. Harris were among those who gave their time to teaching and the care of patients, enriched by a long experience of the art, as well as of the science, of medicine.

The Department of Dermatology, with its out-patient clinic where 3,500 patients received treatment each year, had an old association with the treatment of syphilis and this was revived by Emerson Trow and Hammett A. Dixon, who worked with Gordon Bates in the Special Treatment Clinic at the end of the war. Dixon, who succeeded Emerson Trow as Head of the Department in 1949, held appointments both at the General and at the Hospital for Sick Children. In 1954 he in turn was succeeded by Norman Wrong, who had always taken a keen interest in the pathology of certain lesions, and with Dr. R. C. Smith carried on an extensive clinical investigation of the value of oral cortisone in the treatment of certain dermatoses. With the assistance of colleagues at the Hospital for Sick Children and at St. Joseph's Hospital, Wrong gave the first report in Canada of the use of griseofulvin in the treatment of superficial fungus infections. During his time teaching in the department aimed at providing a practical knowledge for general practitioners, and when he retired in 1962 he continued to aid his successor, Dr. James Trow, in establishing postgraduate teaching in Toronto to meet the requirements of the Royal College of Physicians of Canada, with the hope that in the near future the department would be given a specific area in the hospital where their in-patients could be kept under continuous observation while undergoing treatment.

Dr. W. B. Spaulding succeeded Trevor Owen as Physician-in-Charge of the Medical Out-Patient Department in June 1958. He had been Resident Physician under Ray Farquharson in 1950–51 and served on the staff of the Out-Patient Department from that time on, except for a year at King's College Hospital, London, England. He was a Markle Scholar, and as such he spent a year in the Department of Psychiatry under Professor A. B. Stokes, which resulted in his appointment as an Associate of that department in addition to his appointment as an Associate Professor of Medicine.

While still in control of the Medical Clinic, Dr. Spaulding was appointed Assistant Dean of the Faculty of Medicine in 1964. His contact with medical students had been both prolonged and intimate, and when he left Toronto the next year to undertake administrative duties at the new school of McMaster University, he carried with him not only the high regard of his old colleagues but also a practical efficiency born of his years of service.

XVIII

A Metropolitan Hospital

EARLY IN 1944, THE MEDICAL ADVISORY BOARD REQUESTED THE various heads of services to discuss plans for the expansion of the hospital with the members of their staffs. At this time, however, wartime conditions prevented any positive effort, and it was not until the fall of 1949 that a Planning Committee was appointed and the trustees were made aware of the opinions of the staff with regard to the need for modernizing and extending the facilities for patient care as well as the teaching and research facilities.

Among the more urgent priorities were the need to establish a complete neurosurgical and neurological unit, more lecture theatres, centralized operating rooms, separation of radiotherapy and diagnostic radiology, major extension of the physiotherapy and occupational therapy accommodation, a new women's department, separation of the departments of ophthalmology and otolaryngology, with the department of ophthalmology being located in a separate building, reorganization and expansion of the admitting and emergency departments, and greatly increased administrative accommodation. The chairman, Mr. Norman Urquhart, and Dr. John Sharpe were authorized to consult with the architects Mathers and Haldenby so that they might develop preliminary plans to meet these demands.

The Hospital for Sick Children had just completed its move to the new buildings on University Avenue and Gerrard Street, south of the General Hospital, and some thought was given to the possibility of renovating the old buildings at College and Elizabeth streets, but it was obvious that they were too old for any possible use. However, the

Medical Advisory Board felt that the site should be used for the erection of the separate buildings that were under consideration at that time.

A survey was made in regard to a fund-raising campaign by John Price Jones (Canada) Limited and at the request of the Board of Trustees Mr. E. P. Taylor accepted the appointment as Chairman of the Toronto General Hospital Building Fund Campaign in July 1951. The objective for the campaign was set at $11,000,000, with the understanding that grants of $2,500,000 would be available from the province and from the city of Toronto. A management committee was appointed consisting of:

Chairman—E. P. Taylor		Honorary Treasurer—S. M. Wood
Edgar G. Burton	Dr. D. E. Cannell	S. A. Duke
Dr. R. F. Farquharson	J. G. Godsoe	J. G. Hungerford
Dr. R. M. Janes	D'Arcy Leonard	George McCullagh
Mr. Frank Prendergast	Benjamin Sadowsky	Dr. J. E. Sharpe
H. M. Turner	J. S. D. Tory	N. C. Urquhart

The appeal stressed the importance of the hospital not only to the 1,100,000 citizens of Greater Toronto but to the province at large, and the Lieutenant-Governor and the Prime Minister of Ontario, as well as the Mayor of Toronto, became Honorary Chairmen of the fund.

After further consideration, the objective was raised to $14,000,000, and during the fall of 1951 committees were organized to approach every group of citizens. Edgar G. Burton of the Robert Simpson Company became Chairman of the Commerce and Industry Division, and J. G. Hungerford, Executive Vice-President of the National Trust Company Limited, Chairman of the Division of Personal Gifts. The Women's Division had Mrs. Clara Flavelle McEachern as Honorary Chairman, Mrs. A. G. Baldwin as Chairman, and Mrs. Fraser Coate as Vice-Chairman. Dr. F. I. Lewis was Chairman of the Doctors' Committee and the trustees, undergraduates, staff nurses and alumni all gave generously both of their time and of their money to the campaign.

The press, theatres and radio gave wide publicity to the project, and the medical staff, under the chairmanship of the Physician-in-Chief, Dr. R. F. Farquharson, presented lectures and demonstrations to show the advances in science which had taken place in the various departments. W. E. Gallie, still pre-eminent, reviewed the progress he had seen within the past fifty years, which had led to applicants coming from all over the world to be trained at the General Hospital. He emphasized the great value of the centralization of the operating rooms, and the new lecture theatres which were planned. During eighteen years there had been phenomenal progress in thoracic surgery, since Norman Shenstone and Robert Janes undertook the first lung resections in 1933. Now over 150 resections, one-third of them total pneumonectomies, were being done annually. K. G. McKenzie's Department of Neurosurgery was gaining international renown. Dr. F. P. Dewar had achieved the first successful use of the Kuschner nail in the treatment of fractured femurs, resulting in a decrease in hospitalization of 120 to 25 days. Orthopaedic surgery was bringing about the practical rehabilitation of many cripples. Dr. H. M. Macrae reported that during the past twenty years electro-coagulation in the treatment of retinal separation had resulted in an increase of from 15 to 75 per cent in the saving of the sight of afflicted patients. Dr. Bruce Tovee reported on the increasing efficiency of the emergency department, where 21,000 accident cases had been treated during the previous year. Dr. J. Wallace Graham demonstrated the rehabilitation of arthritic patients. Dr. Joslyn Rogers pointed out the great increase in live births resulting from the treatment of diabetic mothers. Another important report showed the rehabilitation of patients crippled with poliomyelitis: the Department of Physiotherapy, reporting on the treatment of 4,000 patients the previous year, showed the justification for great expansion of the department facilities to include a swimming pool and remedial gymnasia.

In March 1952 Mr. Taylor presented the final report, announcing that as a result of the work of 2,500 volunteers, from heads of business and finance to school children, $16,128,000 had been raised through gifts from 113,000 donors. The public information committee, under the chairmanship of W. F. Prendergast of the Imperial Oil Company, was to be commended, and he thanked the Confederation Life Insurance Company, the Manufacturers Life Insurance Company, the Massey-Harris Company, the Royal Trust, the Canadian Bank of Commerce, and the Robert Simpson Company for lending their employees on a full-time basis to augment the work of the professional fund-raising organization. In addition to $8,686,000 coming from voluntary gifts, capital grants of $3,000,000 had been received from both the province of Ontario and the city of Toronto, $1,000,000 from the Dominion government and $500,000 from the county of York.

The great success of the campaign ensured the future of a large-scale program for expanding and modernizing the hospital, which it was originally thought would include 75 beds for the chronically ill, a 250-bed women's building and a 75-bed all-inclusive eye service building, as well as a new residence to accommodate 200 nurses. A building committee was appointed consisting of H. M. Turner, Chairman, Dr. R. M. Janes, Lt.-Col. W. E. Phillips, E. P. Taylor and N. C. Urquhart; and J. H. Collins, formerly with the firm of Mathers and Haldenby, was appointed to the hospital staff so that he might be readily available to advise on the details of the program as it developed. It was decided to seek the advice of Dr. Arthur Bachmeyer, at that time Consultant to the University of Chicago, in reviewing the plans for the new buildings and the renovation of the old. After a three-day visit, Bachmeyer reported to Dr. Sharpe that in his opinion the plans to that date would have to be completely revised. The main structures of the General Hospital, with their large wards and high ceilings, were now obsolete and would not lend themselves to contiguous connection with a modern construction. The new separate buildings for obstetrics and gynaecology and ophthalmology would further decentralize the institution, and make the service facilities—already inconveniently located—even more inefficient. He advised, therefore, that a central structure should be constructed of sufficient size to accommodate the administration and services and to meet the demands of the expanding departments. There would be an entrance to the Admitting and Emergency departments from Gerrard Street and to the centre block from University Avenue. A new tunnel system for freight and pedestrian traffic should be constructed and a new nurses' residence should be built of sufficient size to accommodate all in training or at work at the hospital. With these developments it would then be possible to undertake the re-allocation of space in the old buildings on an efficient basis.

One of the qualifications restricting the design team was that the new construction not interfere with existing accommodation, at least until the new facilities were ready for occupancy. The basic configuration of the new concept consisted of a T-shaped element with a multi-storey wing extending eastward from University Avenue and a north-south wing extending as far north as existing buildings would permit and southward to connect to the new building block fronting on Gerrard Street. This new building was to connect by tunnel with the College Street building on the north and directly to the Private Patients' Pavilion and the Gerrard Street block on the south.

The first sod was turned by Mr. Walter C. Laidlaw, the senior member of the Board of Trustees, on Wednesday, June 2, 1954, on the property then lying behind the Dunlap Building. Construction began shortly after this, and in 1955 the structural steel for the main central block and the Gerrard Street building was completed. The wing to provide teaching facilities was ready for occupation by the end of 1957: it consisted of a lecture theatre with a seating capacity of 280 and two classrooms, each accommodating 75, capable of opening into one large room. A students' lounge, a snack bar, washrooms and locker accommodation were also provided.

The formal opening took place on May 15, 1959. The Prime Minister of Ontario, the Hon. Leslie Frost, officiated in the presence of the Lieutenant-Governor, the Hon. J. Keiller Mackay. The program to this date had cost approximately $15,000,000. The thirteen-storey main block provided accommodation for diagnostic radiology, neurology and neurosurgery, obstetrics and gynaecology, the centralized operating rooms and the recovery room, the central supply service, central receiving room and warehouse, the medical records department, and the hospital administration. The four-storey Gerrard Street building contained the emergency and admitting departments, accommodation for rehabilitation and physical medicine, ophthalmology, urology and therapeutic radiology. Fortunately the opening in 1955 of the Ontario Cancer Institute, the Princess Margaret Hospital, had made it possible to demolish the Dunlap Building in order to allow the construction of the entrance from University Avenue to the central block.

As they viewed the great buildings, all who had taken part in the years of planning were well rewarded, and early reports from several authorities showed what was being accomplished. Five hundred new beds and two hundred bassinets met, for the time being at least, the growing demand for accommodation which reached the level of 30,000 admissions in 1960. The day for large public wards was past, and accommodation was now provided in four-bed, two-bed and single rooms, with a toilet and basin in every room. In every department it was obvious that the double-corridor construction with a central area for service contributed immensely to comfort and efficiency. The admitting department on Gerrard Street had X-ray facilities convenient to the examining rooms and the emergency department had a twelve-bed recovery ward, three minor operating rooms, and a small laboratory. With the tunnel system there was ready transportation to any part of the hospital.

The centralized operating rooms for the whole hospital were located on the second floor of the centre building. Twenty-one operating rooms and a 26-bed recovery room under the control of Miss Margaret McGibbon were prepared to meet the continual demands of progressive surgical technology. Two rooms with ceiling X-ray, special neurosurgical equipment, and an arteriogram room were set aside for the neurosurgeons. A well equipped pathology laboratory provided on-the-spot service, and glass-enclosed observation galleries with microphones provided for teaching and demonstrations.

The central supply room, conveniently located on the floor above, was highly mechanized to meet the demands of the new techniques in medication; trays and equipment were prepared for the whole of the hospital, with dumbwaiters serving the operating room and obstetrical delivery room floors. Three types of sterilizers were installed—autoclave, dry heat, and ethylene gas. Instruments and glass were washed automatically. One evidence of the volume of work carried on under the supervision of Miss Marjorie Brown was the provision of 1,000 to 1,400 pairs of sterilized gloves every day.

Originally it had been planned that the seven floors above this would be occupied by the obstetrical and gynaecological services, thus replacing the private accommodation that had been available in the Private Patients' Pavilion, and the public and semi-public services at the Burnside Hospital. The fourth floor was specially prepared for obstetrical patients. Here were located the first stage and delivery rooms, a special feature being the provision of two rooms reserved and available at any time for caesarean section, capable of being prepared for operations within a matter of twenty minutes. A two-bed recovery room was also of considerable value, as it permitted supervision of complicated post-partum conditions, and a radiological unit was available to aid in the diagnosis of patients with ante-partum haemorrhage or questionable dystocia. There was sleeping accommodation for the attending and anaesthetic staff, as well as resident quarters for the house staff. A small laboratory was available for routine and investigative procedures. On two of the patient floors, teaching space was provided for clinics, with examining rooms and a small lecture room. An outstanding feature was the nurseries, with equipment for the routine and emergency care of the newborn and especially of premature infants.

Miss Margaret Ketchen was in charge of the dietary services which were now centralized for the whole hospital. The main kitchen, located in the basement of the centre block, was soon serving 7,000 meals a day. A tray service was organized with regular and special diets being delivered to patients anywhere in the hospital. Besides this, a large cafeteria and 24-hour-a-day snack bar were available to the staff, with 1,500 meals being served at noon and 2,000 people visiting the snack bar daily.

A major development was the new Medical Records Service under Miss Margaret Wilson, and every effort was made to provide facilities for the maintaining of good liaison between doctors, medical secretaries and the staff of the Medical Records Department. Many new features made it possible to process 2,000 records daily and to keep 10,000 records in circulation. A pneumatic tube station was connected with 26 other stations throughout the hospital, and records were transmitted by dumbwaiter, conveyor belt, and by messenger to wherever they might be required. A telephone system allowed the doctor to record directly to the central bureau twenty-four hours a day, and an electrically operated file made it possible to locate a patient's record among 1,000,000 numerically filed records. A quiet study room was provided for the convenience of the staff and resident physicians and surgeons.

The move to the new buildings made it possible to completely dissociate diagnostic radiology from therapeutic radiology. Dr. Arthur Singleton, the Diagnostic Radiologist-in-Chief to the hospital, had joined the Department of Radiology in 1924 and since the opening of the Dunlap Building in 1933 he had become more and more responsible for diagnostic service. In twenty-four years the annual volume of work had grown tremendously—1,632 cases increasing to 40,257. Not only were more routine examinations done, but each year the work involved more complicated fields. This was particularly true in the postwar period, when advances in chest surgery, neurosurgery and cardiovascular surgery required more complex procedures and the installation of more specialized X-ray equipment. As the department moved into the centre block, Singleton felt that he must plan for twenty years into the future, although he realized that this would fall far short of the demands of time. There were four general diagnostic rooms, four for gastrointestinal radiology, and one for laminography. In addition, there were three cystoscopic rooms available to the Department of Urology. In all, there were twenty-one installations. Automatic film processing had become a reality, and a large automatic processor was installed. A new and enlarged film library and secretarial pool were built, and an area was set aside for long-term film filing. Singleton was also responsible for the installations in the surgical operating rooms and in the obstetrical department. Within three years the case load had risen to over 58,000, and a notable addition to the equipment, again due to Singleton, was the image amplifier provided for the cardiovascular department.

Arthur Singleton retired as Radiologist-in-Chief in 1962. His distinguished career had included wartime service with No. 15 Canadian General Hospital from 1939 to 1943, and on his return to Canada he had become Consultant to the Royal Canadian Air Force, a post in which he had continued up to the time of his retirement. He had gained international repute, and a large percentage of young Canadian radiologists had been trained in his department. He had also organized a system of training for radiotherapy technicians which was outstanding in Canada.

One of Arthur Singleton's unique presentations, which he delivered at the Sixth International Congress of Radiology in London, England, in July 1950, dealt with the identification of victims of the *Noronic* disaster in September 1949. During the early hours of the morning, this pleasure steamer was totally destroyed by fire while docked in Toronto. Of 527 passengers, 119 lost their lives and 136 were treated in hospitals. It was a busy night in the Emergency Department at the General Hospital, filled with a crowd of patients and refugees. Two young resident surgeons, Doctors Donald Robertson and Cameron Harrison, with the help of Miss Bertha Woolford, organized two operating rooms for the burned and injured and a diet kitchen which supplied hot coffee for the cold and the wet. Within a few hours of hard work everything was under control, with 35 patients having been admitted to the General Hospital.

It took some time to realize the full extent of the tragedy, and a morgue was opened in a building at the Toronto Exhibition grounds. One hundred and ten persons actually died on the ship, with many bodies so destroyed that seventy-eight were unrecognizable. At the request of the Attorney General, Arthur Singleton organized three mobile X-ray units in the morgue. These were served by radiologists and radiation technicians from various city hospitals, and within forty-eight hours over one thousand roentgenograms were taken. As missing individuals were reported, these were compared with previous X-ray films which were found in medical records, mostly in Detroit and Cleveland. The end result of weeks of work was that positive identification was established for twenty-four individuals out of thirty-five for whom comparisons were available. This was by far the largest group reported anywhere to this date. As Arthur Singleton said, "The conformation of the bony structures of an individual is a permanent characteristic of the individual and is not subject to change by plastic operations, the growth of beard or putting on a wig or dyeing the hair." In the case of the *Noronic* disaster, roentgenological identification was of much greater value than fingerprint identification.

As a result of the *Noronic* incident, the hospital undertook to develop a disaster plan so as to mobilize quickly and handle efficiently the reception and treatment of any large group of casualties resulting from a local catastrophe such as an explosion or fire. The administrative control was to be the responsibility of the Assistant Medical Superintendent, Dr. H. S. Doyle, and Doctors R. A. Gordon and R. A. Mustard were to direct the services which would be initiated by the resident surgeon. A booklet was prepared defining the duties of all the hospital services which would be involved. A little later, further consideration was given to the possibility of a larger catastrophe which might develop from "enemy attack," and this extended to the actual evacuation of the hospital. It was even suggested that this might result in a move to as far away as Barrie.

A more practical development occurring at the same time was the establishment of rules by the Anaesthetist-in-Chief regarding operating room precautions. Proper footwear was specified, and the constant danger of explosion from anaesthetic equipment was clearly defined for all who worked in and about the operating room areas.

During the planning of the new buildings, Dr. Clifford L. Ash submitted his recommendations to the Medical Advisory Board in regard to accommodation for the Department of Radiotherapy. He had hoped to have fifty beds available for patients under his care, but when it was decided to locate the Department in the Gerrard Street building, the only space provided was for treatment facilities. The cobalt unit was moved from the old Sick Children's Hospital building on College Street to the Ontario Cancer Institute, and all the patients requiring major curative therapy were transferred from the General Hospital. It took some time to organize the new clinic, but in 1960 a major treatment unit was installed. This was a caesium unit designed specially by Dr. Harold Johns. The radioactive source was a by-product of an atomic energy pile, and although it lacked the intense power of cobalt it delivered energy of approximately 600 KV and did not require the great shielding necessary for the more powerful source. This particular unit was designed with two heads, permitting short and long focal distances suitable for the treatment of superficial and deep-seated lesions. As the clinic came to function it proved adequate for all forms of palliative therapy, bone metastases, lung, prostate and breast cancer. With two other X-ray units of conventional intensity, skin cancers, some lymphomas, and some of the patients from the Children's Hospital not requiring the facilities available at the Cancer Institute were treated at the General Hospital. The peak was reached in 1962, with over 6,300 treatments being given to 600 patients. There was also a sufficient amount of radium available to meet the increasing needs of the gynaecologists in pre-operative treatment of cancer of the uterus.

The staff under Ash in 1956 consisted of Doctors Vera Peters, W. E. C. Allt and W. D. Rider. The latter two were British-trained radiotherapists, the first of an increasing number who came to constitute the therapy staff at the Ontario Cancer Institute.

There was, at this time, a physician on the staff of the hospital who had a great deal to do with the development of the medical treatment of cancer. Dr. O. H. Warwick joined the staff of the General Hospital in 1947, and brought with him a particular interest in the haematology and chemotherapy of malignant disease. He had been a Gold Medallist at McGill, with postgraduate training at Oxford, and was the first physician appointed to the staff of a radiotherapy treatment centre in Canada. He was also instrumental in combining the chemotherapy and hormone treatment of both patients in the radiotherapy department and those who were on the medical and surgical wards of the hospital.

In his first report to the Medical Advisory Board from the special committee on chemotherapy for cancer, Warwick detailed his experience in the treatment of about two hundred patients in 1951. Hormone therapy for prostatic and breast cancer had produced striking results, and it was also true that lymphomas and leukaemia were showing sufficient response to antimetabolites such as Aminopterin to warrant the presentation of papers before various societies. Joseph Bardwell, a Research Fellow of the Department of Medicine, was involved in interesting studies of the fundamental effects of the treatment of these particular conditions. As well as important results in the treatment of leukaemia, the committee also reported a gradual replacement of isotope therapy in the treatment of widespread cancer by more easily controlled chemotherapeutic agents.

Prior to the opening of the Princess Margaret Hospital in 1958, when Dr. Warwick left the General Hospital to become Physician-in-Chief to that institution, the chemotherapy committee was merged with the drug committee under Dr. K. J. R. Wightman, who was at that time in charge of therapeutics. Chemotherapy was then well established, and clinical surveys of large numbers of patients with a great variety of malignant lesions were being supported by various research grants. Under Dr. Wightman's over-all control, this relatively new field of therapeutics was constantly expanding, and two young research fellows, E. A. McCullough and D. A. Cowan, were laying the foundations for the work which was to develop so successfully at the Princess Margaret Hospital in the years to come.

Even before it was possible to organize plans for the major developments at the General Hospital, the board of trustees was approached with a request to consider taking over the Wellesley Hospital. This hospital had been developed by Dr. Herbert A. Bruce to meet the demands of his large surgical practice at a time when there was a great shortage of accommodation for private patients. The hospital was ideally situated in a large house, formerly the home of Frederick Nichols, on a four-acre lot at the head of Homewood Crescent, adjacent to the corner of Wellesley and Sherbourne streets.

The work of Dr. Bruce had won the full appreciation of the higher echelons of society, and the hospital had been opened in June 1911 by Sir Wilfrid Laurier, the Prime Minister of Canada. A year later the Governor General, the Duke of Devonshire, had presided at the opening of an additional wing. The hospital was well equipped for that time, with two operating rooms and a labour room, and its 100-bed accommodation was constantly filled with private patients who were mostly either surgical or obstetrical cases. In 1942 it had been decided to build an addition with 100 more beds and accommodation for X-ray and laboratory services, and with one wing on the second floor set aside for offices for the senior members of the surgical and medical staffs and the hospital radiologist. Up to this time the hospital had been intended only for private patients, but now it was planned to provide accommodation for public ward patients with the hope that provincial and municipal grants could be arranged to help cover the cost of this service. Dr. Bruce had retired from active practice by this time, but he continued to serve as an active member of the board of the hospital. The new building was completed in 1946, but expected major donations were lacking and the institution faced a state of bankruptcy.

Dr. Bruce credited the good offices of Col. W. E. Phillips, Mr. J. G. Godsoe and Mr. George McCullagh in finding the solution to the problem, and at a special meeting of the board of trustees of the General Hospital held in April 1948 Mr. Urquhart presented a letter from Mr. Godsoe proposing the possible amalgamation of the operations and facilities of the hospital with those of the General Hospital. This involved the assumption of the liabilities of the Wellesley Hospital, amounting to $2,000,000 with the request that the identity of the Wellesley Hospital should be continued with the designation "The Wellesley Division of the Toronto General Hospital." He requested also that the board consider providing an already planned Nurses' Residence, Out-Patient Department, and the other services necessary to enable the Wellesley Division to function as a teaching hospital of the University of Toronto. Mr. Urquhart made it clear to the Board that the responsibility consequent to the amalgamation would not jeopardize the plans for the expansion of the General Hospital, and that all staff appointments would have to come under the jurisdiction of the present Joint Hospital Relations Committee.

Mr. George McCullagh informed the meeting that both the Prime Minister of Ontario and the Mayor of Toronto were aware of the financial state of the Wellesley Hospital and had agreed with the statement made by the Chairman of the Board. Dr. Sidney Smith, President of the University of Toronto, welcomed the amalgamation as it would provide additional teaching facilities. Dr. H. B. Van Wyck, Chairman of the Medical Advisory Board, brought the Board's endorsement, providing that it did not prejudice plans for expansion and modernization of the Toronto General Hospital and that the Wellesley Division should be administered as an integral part of the hospital. The amalgamation became effective on August 25, 1948, and the chairman of the board of trustees reported that payments had been received from the provincial government covering the indebtedness of the Wellesley Hospital.

One of the conditions which was proceeded with as soon as property became available and planning could be completed was the erection of a new School of Nursing and residence for nurses. The School of Nursing at the Wellesley had a long and enviable record of accomplishment, largely due to the character and control of Miss Elizabeth Flaws, the first Superintendent of Nursing, and her successor Miss Elsie Jones. Wellesley graduates were unsurpassed in their appreciation of good patient care at a time when home nursing was greatly in demand. The school, however, was functioning under a great disadvantage, the student nurses being housed in four former private residences with no proper classrooms and limited library accommodation. The new school and residence was constructed on Wellesley Place and opened in 1952.

The six-storey building provided accommodation for 228 nurses, a suite for the Director of Nurses, and a small infirmary, and it was planned to allow the nurses from the Ontario Cancer Institute to have occupancy of one floor. Teaching facilities were very good and a large lounge and two snack bars made for home-like living conditions.

Immediately after the takeover, Doctors Neill McGillivray, J. L. McDonald and W. A. Dafoe, the Chiefs of the Departments of Medicine, Surgery, and Obstetrics and Gynaecology at the former Wellesley Hospital, met with Dr. Sharpe and the departmental heads of the General Hospital to discuss the allocation of beds for the care of patients and teaching needs. There were no public gynaecological beds at the Wellesley Hospital. The Surgeon-in-Chief was of the opinion that there were sufficient public surgical beds at the General, and he did not require any additional beds at the Wellesley Division. It was decided that the Department of Medicine would add the beds on the second floor of the old wing to its service and that these beds should be used for the treatment of patients with emotional disorders as a psychosomatic service. This was the first service of its kind in any public general hospital, and proved highly successful. Eventually, gynaecological beds were made available as the result of taking over the previous office space on the second floor of the new building, and a post-operative recovery room was also provided in this area. The laboratories were enlarged by taking over the former Board Room and adjacent office space, and a small emergency department and out-patient clinic were organized using part of the east corridor of the basement of the new building, with an entrance on Sherbourne Street. All departments of the Wellesley Hospital were placed under the control of the heads of various departments at the General, with the exception of the Nursing School which continued to have its own Director of Nursing and to function separately from the school at the General Hospital. The special services of urology, orthopaedics, physical medicine, otolaryngology, and ophthalmology were provided on a consultative basis by the General Hospital.

It had been decided that the new Cancer Institute would be built to the north of the Wellesley property. Plans developed so that many services could be carried out on a shared basis by the two institutions. A new power plant was erected which included space for maintenance shops, the laundry was demolished and the staff integrated with that of the General Hospital, and a truck service was organized to meet the needs of the Wellesley Division. Finally, new operating rooms and laboratory, X-ray, kitchen and food services, including a modern cafeteria, were planned to serve both the Wellesley Hospital and the Ontario Cancer Institute.

The sudden death of Dr. Neill McGillivray in June 1949 shortly after the departments were organized at the Wellesley Hospital was a severe loss to all concerned. He was succeeded by Dr. R. C. Dickson. Robert Dickson had graduated from Toronto in 1934 after which he had been thoroughly indoctrinated by Professor Duncan Graham. He had joined the 15th Canadian General Hospital in 1939, and after five years' service returned to Canada as a Lieutenant-Colonel with the O.B.E. Although his particular interest was gastroenterology, he also had broad interests in internal medicine, and in the three years that he was in charge of the Medical Service at the Wellesley he helped to develop an atmosphere of close cooperation between all departments. He had also been chairman of a committee set up to arrange refresher courses for physicians returning from active service, and this committee organized the first intern rotation appointments for the benefit of those who were to go on into general practice. His later career as professor of medicine at Dalhousie University and the prominent part he played in the Royal College of Physicians and Surgeons of Canada were a fitting close to the work of one who always gave his best in everything he did.

Dr. Arthur Squires was appointed as Senior Physician at the Wellesley Division when Robert C. Dickson left to take over his duties in Halifax. Under his guidance the medical service became more definitely organized, and several members of the medical staff of the General were seconded for duty with him for various periods of time. This resulted in the establishment of a treatment and teaching routine, approved by Farquharson, which was to have a strong influence on changing the very nature of the Wellesley Division.

Dr. J. L. McDonald, who was essentially an orthopaedic surgeon, invited Dr. Frank Mills to join his staff in 1947 with the view to improving the standard of general surgery on the wards of the hospital, but Mills' service was terminated after a short period upon the death of Dr. Roscoe Graham. Professor Robert Janes then brought him back to the Graham Service, which was now under Dr. F. I. Lewis.

Mills was succeeded in June 1948 at the Wellesley by Dr. I. B. Macdonald, who had just completed his postgraduate training at the General and at the Wellesley. He not only proved to be a very able surgeon, but also showed considerable ability in organizing the surgical routine, and as a natural result he succeeded Dr. J. L. McDonald when his time came to retire. The volume of work had increased by this time, and together with Dr. Janes he invited Dr. Neil Watters to accept an appointment on the staff of the Wellesley in May 1955. Dr. Watters, trained by Dr. Janes, had been in practice in Galt but his academic ambitions were a paramount influence in bringing him back to Toronto. Working together, Watters and Macdonald set the foundation for a steadily improving surgical service at the Wellesley.

In spite of very inadequate bed accommodation, Dr. William Dafoe, who had been an appointee of Professor William Hendry of the General Hospital, developed a steadily growing obstetric department. Dr. Dafoe retired in 1956 and was succeeded by Dr. J. R. Norris, a British-trained obstetrician and gynaecologist who had been on Professor Cannell's staff at the General. Progress was slow, but out-patient clinics were organized despite inadequate facilities and a public ward service gradually developed in gynaecology, a field of surgery hitherto completely dominated at the Wellesley by private practice.

The Wellesley was very fortunate to have two good radiologists, K. P. Bonner and James Worth. The latter came to the Wellesley Division after the takeover, and although he left Toronto a few years later, he established an outstanding reputation as a perfectionist who sought the ultimate solution in the pathological laboratory and even in the post-mortem room.

The laboratory services were developed by Dr. T. C. Brown. He was a product of the training of Professor William Boyd and W. L. Robinson, and with the moral support which they provided he organized an efficient clinical pathological department which included bacteriology and pathological chemistry. The result was that when the Ontario Cancer Institute was opened it joined with the Wellesley Hospital in profiting from the excellence of the service which he was able to provide. With the large number of patients under treatment for cancer at the Institute, the volume of work increased greatly, and through his close association with so many clinicians and research scientists Dr. Brown's experience was outstanding in Canada.

The years of close association between the Wellesley and the General hospitals resulted in several very important developments. In the first place, under the guidance of Ray Farquharson, Robert Janes, and Douglas Cannell, and the staff at the Wellesley, an institution that bore a close resemblance to the best type of British private hospital was transformed into a general hospital which was soon to be accepted as a teaching hospital of the University of Toronto. Secondly, the post-operative care unit at the Wellesley, the first at a Toronto hospital, proved so valuable that a similar service was organized in the Private Patients' Pavilion at the General Hospital. But the most important development was the forty-bed psychiatric unit under Herbert Hyland, J. C. Richardson and Allan Walters, which re-established psychiatry as a therapeutic department of a general hospital and was the basis for a major change at the Toronto General Hospital a few years after the Wellesley had been re-organized as an independent institution.

At the opening of the new General Hospital buildings in May 1959, the Prime Minister of Ontario chose this auspicious occasion to announce that as of the first of the year the Wellesley Hospital would again become a separate institution with its own Board of Governors. Mr. Harold Turner, who had served as Chairman of the General Hospital Building Committee, became Chairman of the new Board, a duty which he undertook with his well-proven enthusiasm and industry. The administrative responsibilities which had been borne by Mr. Urquhart and the board and by Doctors John Sharpe and Henry Doyle were appreciable; the annual report for the last year (which included the Wellesley Division) showed that with a total capacity of 1,772 beds there had been over 32,000 admissions and that nearly 100,000 patients had been treated in the Out-Patient Department. An over-all deficit of $1,282,000 in 1958 was the largest in the history of the hospital, but the following year the inauguration of the Ontario Hospital Services Commission brought an end to a period when hospital finance had depended on repeated annual requests for support from the municipal and provincial governments.

The hospital lost a very valuable administrator when Mr. R. W. Longmore died in September 1957. His service as administrative superintendent over a period of thirty-six years had earned him the high regard of all who knew him. He was succeeded by Mr. J. H. Collins, who had already provided expert advice on major developments at the hospital, and within a few years the trustees and the medical staff became more and more dependent on him. The new Chairman of the Building Committee, Mr. Norman C. Pearce, faced with the modernizing of so much of the hospital structure, found in him an unfailing guide whose service to the hospital was second to none.

One of the most important questions which the Medical Advisory Board had to consider in the new building expansion was the establishment of centralized laboratory services. In September 1952, a report was submitted by a committee under Dr. John Hamilton, Pathologist-in-Chief to the hospital, consisting of Doctors R. F. Farquharson, P. H. Greey, J. A. Dauphinee and W. G. Bigelow, recommending that such a laboratory provide services in biochemistry, haematology and surgical pathology. It should also have control of the blood bank, and employ a full-time biochemist. It was obvious that scientific progress could only come about through closely related laboratory departments, and that the day was past when basic investigative studies necessary to clinical progress could develop in scattered locations at the hospital and the Banting Institute.

In the years before the war, laboratory services had been very limited indeed. Throughout this period, there were two physicians on the staff of the hospital who had constantly emphasized the importance of biochemical investigation in the treatment of patients under their care. No one rivalled Walter R. Campbell in the reputation he developed. He had graduated with honours in Physiology and Biochemistry in 1911, and serving under Professor J. M. MacCallum had received his M.A. for research on kidney function two years before graduating in Medicine in 1915. During the early years of the First World War he had organized a pathological chemical laboratory, and his studies had earned him his M.D. (Tor.) in 1917. He had served as chemical pathologist and serologist to the Military District No. 2 before joining No. 4 Canadian General Hospital in England, where his special interest was the diagnosis and treatment of kidney disease. As one of Professor Duncan Graham's original research fellows, and together with Almon Fletcher, he had played a very important part in the care of patients during the clinical trials of insulin. From that time on, he had carried out investigations into the biochemical problems presented by many pathological conditions from a laboratory that he maintained at the Banting Institute, and his quiet enthusiasm kept him abreast of scientific advances which augmented the purely clinical knowledge of his colleagues in the Department of Medicine. Naturally, one of his chief interests was the study of new types of insulin being developed as well as the analyses of various types of diet. The wide range of his investigation included many analytical determinations that could not be carried out in the hospital laboratories, and it was with the facilities that Campbell provided that J. A. Dauphinee undertook the study of blood changes of cyanosed patients, and plasma sulphonamide levels of patients under treatment with various sulpha preparations. Even after he retired from the staff of the General Hospital in 1952, Campbell continued to work in his laboratory during the years when he was serving as a consulting physician to the hospital, and he perfected an original and highly accurate method of calcium determination which was used for some years by his younger colleagues.

Dr. James Dauphinee had the most varied career of any member of the medical staff of the General Hospital. He had graduated in Arts from the University of British Columbia prior to coming to Toronto, where he obtained a Ph.D. in biochemistry before graduating in Medicine in 1929. After a year spent in clinical research at St. Bartholomew's Hospital, and two years' internship at the General Hospital, he became a research fellow in medicine and was appointed a junior assistant and attending physician to the hospital in 1933. At this time the laboratory service available to the Department of Medicine consisted of an electrocardiographic laboratory on Ward I, a small biochemical laboratory on Ward H for urine and gastric analyses and some primitive blood chemistry, and a haematology laboratory on Ward G, where all the demands could be met by two technicians. By way of contrast it is worthy of note that at this time Professor A. G. Gornall was organizing an efficient steroid laboratory located in the basement of the Burnside. This unit, under his supervision, provided a very necessary scientific control for the increasing use of cortosteroids on the wards and in the clinics of the hospital.

When the new Private Patients' Pavilion was first opened in 1931, one technician working in a small laboratory on the medical floor was able to provide service for all the patients in the building. But in 1935, at the request of Professor Duncan Graham, Dauphinee organized a new laboratory to meet rapidly increasing demands. Here the first biochemist employed by the hospital, with the help of three or four trained technicians, undertook urine and haematology examinations, some biochemical studies, and even electrocardiograms.

Dauphinee served on the staffs of several hospitals in England and northwest Europe during the war, finally being in charge of the Medical Service in No. 8 and then No. 11 Canadian General Hospitals. He received the O.B.E. in recognition of his service. In 1946 he became Professor of Pathological Chemistry but continued his association with the Department of Medicine at the General Hospital, thus strengthening the bonds between the clinical department and the laboratories and research facilities of the Banting Institute. Under his direction the Isotope Laboratory at the Banting came to provide an outstanding service to the hospital, and during the years preceding the opening of the Farquharson Clinical Investigation Unit the biochemistry for many of the metabolic studies was carried on under his direction.

In 1956 it was decided that the centralized laboratories, including divisions of biochemistry, radioactive isotopes, bacteriology, haematology and a blood bank, and surgical pathology should be located on the thirteenth floor of the central block building. At the same time, special laboratories were to be conveniently located for electroencephalography and electrocardiography and to service cardiovascular, respiratory and metabolic units. Laboratories were also to be available to the Out-Patient Department and for diagnostic team purposes on the various wards of the hospital.

Dr. Murray Young was appointed Director of Laboratories, assuming his duties in August 1957. He was particularly well qualified to undertake this demanding position, as even before embarking on the study of medicine he had received his Bachelor's degree in Agriculture with special training in chemistry, his Master's degree in Biochemistry, and a Ph.D. in Physiological Hygiene. He had graduated in Medicine in 1950, and after serving as an intern at the Toronto General Hospital he was appointed to the Medical Clinic in the Out-Patient Department of the hospital in 1951. His conviction of the importance of comprehensive laboratory services to the hospital was therefore based on a broad knowledge.

Young was faced with two main problems: the development of facilities and the organizing of a staff at both the academic and technical levels. As his plans developed he received constant advice from Dr. John Sharpe, to whom he was personally responsible, and from Professor John Hamilton. It was soon evident that, as the senior appointees were to have academic recognition, their appointments must satisfy the heads of departments of the Faculty of Medicine. For his own part he was convinced that properly developed laboratory medicine would eliminate errors in diagnosis and treatment and in a time of increasing financial support would have a profound effect on the whole practice of medicine. He welcomed an appointment to the Medical Clinic in the Out-Patient Department, as it was a proving ground for his beliefs, and he felt very strongly that the qualified medical staff on duty in the laboratories should have a similar experience.

Dr. John Crookston was appointed to be Head of the Division of Haematology in September, 1957. He had graduated from Toronto in 1947 with the Gold Medal and after a year with Professor Charles Best had received a B.Sc. (Med.). He had spent three years' internship at the

General and Sunnybrook hospitals and had then gone on to Cambridge University on a McLaughlin Fellowship, working under Sir Lionel Whitby in haematology and receiving his Ph.D. in 1956. This was followed by three years at the London Postgraduate Medical School, and he had almost decided to remain in England when Professor R. F. Farquharson influenced him to return to Toronto to organize the Haematology and Blood Transfusion Laboratories at the Toronto General Hospital. Together with Dr. Murray Young, Crookston recruited the technical staff of the new department and arranged to take over the Blood Bank from Dr. Philip Greey. He insisted that a contract be signed with the Red Cross Society, thus relieving the hospital of the necessity of procuring blood donors. From the first the available space on the thirteenth floor was inadequate, and he invaded inactive areas wherever it was possible. His interest in clinical haematology involved bringing together various component activities, and his special laboratory, located close to the Clinical Investigation Unit, was a centre for the investigation of blood dyscrasias, especially as they affected haemolytic anaemia, blood transfusion problems, and blood coagulation. The work of the blood bank, which in the previous ten years had increased from supplying 5,800 to nearly 18,000 units, soon developed to an unprecedented degree. Major achievements in surgery, especially in the cardiovascular division, increased the work load so that by 1965 over 48,000 units were being provided and 20,000 transfusions given.

Another key appointment was made in September 1957, when Dr. Murray Young recommended that Dr. C. J. Porter head the Division of Chemistry and Biochemistry. Porter had already had considerable experience in biochemical research during seven years' work in the research departments of two major drug houses.

In 1957 there was no coordinated biochemistry service. Gradually, however, various laboratories in the hospital and at the Banting Institute were moved to new quarters in the centre block, where obsolete equipment was replaced and a skilled staff recruited. The increasing demands of clinicians and the need to develop methods of proven reliability in the hands of a limited number of technical personnel were met by the transformation of manual to automatic systems. The change on this basis was such that the work-load increased five-fold between 1957 and 1965. The number of tests available tripled, and seventy per cent were carried out by automatic equipment. At the same time, a great deal of effort went into the development of control systems to ensure the quality of laboratory results.

The division presented an excellent base for the education of medical laboratory technicians, as well as that of clinical pathologists and residents in medicine. The first course for technicians was soon followed by an advanced course recognized by the School of Graduate Studies at the University, and Dr. Porter became an Assistant Professor in the Department of Pathological Chemistry.

Invaluable as these laboratory services became to the experienced investigative physician, they threatened to alter, to some degree at least, the perspective of the newer generation. Presented with the means of receiving a biochemical profile on each patient, there was a danger that the doctor might ignore the age-proven virtues of clinical study of patients under his care. It was a temptation which most resisted, however.

A major change took place with the appointment of Dr. Peter Tuffnell to take charge of the Department of Microbiology. Up to this time Dr. Philip Greey, who had played a major role in establishing the Department of Bacteriology at the Banting Institute, had served as Bacteriologist-in-Chief to the hospital. Dr. Tuffnell was a graduate of Sheffield University and had had extensive training at Manchester in pathology and bacteriology. With the increasing demands of all the university teaching hospitals, it was essential that this division of laboratory services develop full cooperation with the clinical departments in the General Hospital. Dr. Greey continued his service as consulting microbiologist while Dr. Tuffnell became an Assistant Professor in Bacteriology at the University of Toronto.

The Department of Surgical Pathology moved from the Banting Institute to the centre block in January 1959. Dr. John Hamilton, Professor of Pathology, was Pathologist-in-Chief to the General Hospital, but Dr. William Anderson was in charge of the laboratories. An Edinburgh graduate who had come from Hamilton to be a protégé of Professor William Boyd, Anderson had served in his department for ten years prior to taking up his special duties at the General Hospital. In addition to the routine work in the main laboratories on the thirteenth floor, a laboratory was located on the second floor, convenient to the centralized operating rooms where an efficient frozen section service became a determining factor in definitive surgical treatment. As a result, the volume rose until as many as forty quick section reports were being given in a working day.

An outstanding development in the Department of Pathology, which was transferred to the centralized laboratories at the General Hospital, was the work of Dr. D. W. Thompson, who became Director of the Cytopathology services in 1957. His postgraduate training, after graduating from Toronto in 1949, had led him to a career in pathology, but the year he spent with Hertig in Boston channelled his interests into cytology. His routine duties brought Thompson to national prominence and he was the first in Canada to apply cytology to a wide field of investigation. Up to 1953 only gynaecological cytology had been done in Toronto, but ten years later this comprised only fifty per cent and by 1965 a third of the total preparations in the field. Thompson's work with Dr. Norman Delarue on the early diagnosis of lung cancer was an outstanding example of his pioneering approach. With the support of the Ontario Cancer Foundation he established a school for cytotechnicians which met the demands of the hospitals in Metropolitan Toronto and across the province, so that cytology services became available to a wider extent than anywhere else in Canada.

The opening of the R. F. Farquharson Clinical Investigation Unit in 1961 was a major step forward in the history of the General Hospital. It marked the culmination of the efforts of a number of men working on the wards and in the laboratories of the hospital and the Banting Institute over a period of ten years. Their common interest had been the metabolic changes effected by disease and the response to specific forms of treatment. Ray Farquharson himself had spent a year in such a unit at the Massachusetts General Hospital, and had watched with great interest the developing work of the younger men in his own and other departments. His small metabolic unit on Ward G, consisting of four specially supervised beds and a small laboratory, had been only a modest promise of things to come. Now the new Clinical Investigation Unit completed in the basement of the College Street building, in the area vacated by the Department of Physiotherapy, provided facilities hitherto unavailable. With a twelve-bed capacity, a special kitchen, a large room for recreation and for conferences, and two offices with examining rooms, it was possible to achieve full coordination of all the members of the staff—doctors, nurses, dieticians, social service and laboratory assistants. The patients, living in a completely controlled environment, could now be studied for three major purposes: first, to establish a diagnosis if this was obscure; second, to improve the method of treatment; and third, to determine the fundamental effect of treatment if this was not clearly evident. The need for such a centre in a major teaching hospital was the result of the achievement of recent years, which had brought the physician powers of definitive therapy almost as absolute as those of the surgeon. It was only by the development of such research studies that the hospital could give its best service to the whole community.

Dr. J. C. Laidlaw returned from Boston to become director of the Unit, and E. R. Yendt became associate director. It was now decided that the Unit facilities would be available to other departments besides the Department of Medicine. Up to this time the graduate training of the chosen members of the staff of all departments had not gone far beyond pure clinical training, and the Unit was soon to emphasize that prolonged experience in laboratory investigations would produce a new generation capable of making outstanding contributions to the science of medicine.

J. C. Laidlaw was involved in endocrine studies. Yendt returned from Johns Hopkins with a special interest in calcium metabolism from which he developed his studies of renal function and the development of renal calculi. Calvin Ezrin's special interest was the pituitary gland, and John M. Finlay studied malabsorption phenomena. J. D. Wilson was involved in renal function studies and the problems underlying successful kidney transplant, and Richard Wilson's interest was gynaecological endocrinology and the problems of reproduction and fertility. N. T. McPhedran, of the Department of Surgery, was working on fundamental features of acute pancreatitis.

Work in the Clinical Investigation Unit resulted in the recognition of several new disease processes and the development of satisfactory therapy for most of them. The most successful fields of investigation were in the aetiology of renal calculi, the diagnosis of hyperparathyroidism, the use of thiasides in the treatment of renal calculi, the diagnosis of renovascular hypertension, the relation of the adrenal cortex to hypertension, the cause of acute pancreatitis and of idiopathic oedema, and many of the causes of female infertility.

The Ontario Hospital Services Commission supported the building of the Clinical Investigation Unit, and various fund-granting bodies provided the money to maintain the laboratory services and the research fellows who were engaged in investigations. When Ray Farquharson, after his retirement, became associated with the National Research Council, support for institutions such as the Investigation Unit took a new lease on life. Farquharson fully appreciated the great advances now possible which before had depended entirely on the dedicated, unselfish labour of those who had sought a corner in the Banting Institute in which to solve the obscure problems of many patients. It was at this time that rooms along the corridor in the basement leading to the Emergency Department were renovated and turned into research laboratories for various departments, where work was done resulting in the establishment of service units for the treatment of acute functional failures.

In 1960 the Committee on Isotopes of the Medical Advisory Board, under Dr. K. J. R. Wightman, recommended that the time had come to centralize a properly organized isotope service. Up to this time hospital laboratories in five locations had surgeons, neurologists, haematologists, endocrinologists and ophthalmologists who were making use of radioactive material supplied by the biophysicist, Dr. William Paul, from the hot laboratory located in the Banting Institute.

The volume of work was increasing rapidly. Dr. John Crookston had given as much over-all supervision as his time would permit, but his commitment to the blood bank and the haematology laboratory precluded any more than a decreasing responsibility, and as Dr. Paul lacked medical qualifications it was essential that a fully qualified director be appointed to take charge of the Division of Nuclear Medicine. The choice made was Dr. Donald Wood who had been trained in Internal Medicine by Dr. Wightman and had served under him as a Fellow in the Department of Therapeutics. On Wightman's recommendation and with his support, Wood had spent two years training in Nuclear Medicine at the Middlesex Hospital, London, England, and had returned in 1964 to receive appointments in the Department of Medicine at the University and in the Department of Laboratories under Dr. Murray Young at the Toronto General Hospital.

Accommodation for the isotope service developed in a somewhat haphazard manner. After considerable delay due to the major nature of the structural changes, accommodation was provided for a total body scanner in the corridor of the basement of the College Street building, leading to the area in use by the photographic department, and a little later in the basement of the Burnside building. Although the location was far from satisfactory, facilities were provided for linear scanning of brain, thyroid, liver, kidneys and pancreas. The unit became an important part of the laboratory service of the hospital with the development of new techniques, and with the availability of new material for research studies there was promise of an even more important future.

Some years of discussion and planning came to an end when the Fudger Medical Library was opened in March 1964 in the south wing of the ninth floor of the Private Patients' Pavilion. Harris H. Fudger, who had served on the board from 1913 to 1922, had maintained a residence on Sherbourne Street for self-supporting business women with the proviso in his will that when the trustees of his estate decided that this could no longer carry out his original intent the property was to be sold and the proceeds paid to the Endowment Fund of the Toronto General Hospital. The legacy was somewhat in excess of $500,000, and the trustees decided to provide an endowment of $100,000 to support a hospital library which was to be known as the Fudger Medical Library. With the approval and support of the Ontario Hospital Commission, the south wing was renovated and furnished and the first librarian, Mrs. M. Robinow, began her duties in May 1964. Dr. Thomas Morley was Chairman of the Library Committee at the time of its opening, and was succeeded by Dr. Norman Delarue the following year. The annual interest from the Fudger beneficence was to be used to provide monographs, but major donations came from the neurosurgical and neurological library, and a considerable number of the hospital staff provided many valuable books and periodicals. By the end of 1965 there were nearly 1,200 books and over 200 periodicals available. Affiliation with the University of Toronto Library, the library of the Academy of Medicine, and the library of the Canadian Hospital Association on an interchangeable basis broadened the scope greatly. With its hard-working staff the library provided a reference service and reading material for staff doctors and senior students alike and frequently—especially towards the end of the academic year—there were no empty seats to be had. Besides the permanent staff, part-time service was given by university students and students from the University of Toronto School of Library Sciences undergoing their practical training.

In December 1957 the Medical Advisory Board endorsed the report of the Photographic Committee that recommended transforming the Ward D operating area in the basement of the College Street building to provide for a properly equipped photographic department. Since the time of Professor W. E. Gallie, sporadic efforts had been made to organize such a service, but more pressing needs always took priority. The University Division of Art as Applied to Medicine had its origin in the work of Miss Maria Wishart, who had studied under Max Broedel of Baltimore, and for many years provided an excellent service to those who desired drawings and other artistic illustrations. Miss Wishart maintained a very satisfactory liaison with the surgeons and others on the staff of the hospital. But until very recently it was mostly individual photographers, working in various departments, who provided a photographic service. Mr. Robert Slater, who was the first medical photographer employed by the General Hospital, designed the new facility made possible by the transfer of the neurosurgery division to new quarters in the centre block. Slater also envisaged the possibility of a much more comprehensive department, but unfortunately he retired before any action took place.

Slater's assistant, Mr. Platon Michaels, was appointed as Director of the new department. The service was centralized with an office for the Director and his secretary, a studio, and processing laboratories, and a staff was employed consisting of several technicians and assistant photographers. It was anticipated that the department would serve the dual purpose of providing visual evidence of certain lesions for the patients' records, and illustrations, including 35 mm film, for teaching purposes and staff publications and lectures. The lack of financial support which had seriously delayed the development of the department was overcome to some degree when the Ontario Hospital Commission accepted responsibility for this feature of the maintenance of patients' records. The long anticipated service was soon overwhelmed by demands, and the future was complicated almost from the beginning by the progressive thinking of the committee established to consider audiovisual services at the hospital.

Renovation of the old Shields Emergency Hospital to provide accommodation for out-patient services in ophthalmology and otolaryngology and in dentistry, as well as administrative offices for the Social Service Department, was completed in 1960, and a name long associated with the hospital now became only a memory. The new Building Committee under Mr. Norman Pearce began to consider the plans which had been presented by the surgical planning committee with regard to modernizing the surgical wing of the College Street building. The purpose of these alterations was to replace the large multi-bed wards with two- and four-bed units, with adequate washroom and toilet facilities and centrally located nursing service. Estimates showed that the cost would be well in excess of a million dollars, and Dr. Kergin as Professor of Surgery and Chairman of the Medical Advisory Board accompanied Mr. Urquhart and Dr. Sharpe in presenting the undertaking to the Ontario Hospital Services Commission. It was agreed that the remodelled wing would be used for at least twenty-five years, and the commission undertook to provide a grant of $750,000 towards the cost of renovation. After some discussion the surgical staff agreed that all three floors should be vacated at one time. Accommodation for patients was provided in the Burnside building (which, itself in preparation, required the installation of added toilet facilities), as well as in Ward F and Ward D.

Work progressed favourably, and when the interior was cleared the basic structure of the old wing showed that a properly constructed building justified renovation. Finally, on December 5, 1962, Dr. Sharpe reported to the trustees that modernization had been completed, and within a period of three weeks the wing was completely occupied. The patient capacity had decreased from 214 to 164, the original operating rooms had been converted to classrooms, and office space became available for the heads of the various divisions and for the routine duties of their resident staffs. Dr. Sharpe also reported that during all the reconstruction and building it was necessary to have 1,100 beds available at all times and credited the cooperation and understanding of all the staff of the hospital in coping with the problem. Extensive alterations were also made in the basement to provide locker and washroom facilities for the non-professional staff, and a new security office and accommodation were also provided for a clinic to be organized under a physician director present in the clinic each morning with full-time nursing and clerical staff to be responsible for the employees' health service. It was opportune that Dr. E. J. Maltby, who had just retired from the active staff of the hospital, was available to assume the duties of this responsible position.

The renovation and modernization of the central portion of the Out-Patient Department was completed in 1965. A new entrance rotunda was built on the site of the driveway which led to the old Emergency and Admitting Department. One floor was added by extending the building westward to University Avenue. It was a major project, the cost approaching $1,000,000, and not only were there many new examination rooms added, but registration facilities and a main waiting-room and offices changed the whole appearance and atmosphere of the institution.

The pharmacy was moved from its old location and became a two-floor department on the north side of the foyer. The volume of work had quite outgrown the old quarters, for by 1964 there had been 134,000 prescriptions filled for in-patients and 58,750 for out-patients. Another phase of its growing importance was evident in the cost of the drugs it supplied, which had risen from $210,000 in 1951 to over $631,000 in 1964. In keeping with the reorganization was the appointment of Mr. Douglas Stuart, an Assistant Professor of Pharmacy at the University, as Director of Pharmaceutical Services. This cast no reflection on the excellent service which the hospital had received for many years from James McDonald and Harold Hicks, but was merely indicative of the opportunity which the pharmacy presented, through its volume of work, to familiarize pharmacy students with the responsibilities they would assume after graduation.

XIX

Combined Operations

DR. H. B. VAN WYCK RETIRED IN JULY 1950 AS PROFESSOR OF Obstetrics and Gynaecology and as Obstetrician and Gynaecologist-in-Chief to the Toronto General Hospital. His successor, Dr. Douglas E. Cannell, had had an exceptionally good preparation for his new appointment. Graduating from Toronto in 1927, he had spent his first postgraduate year under Professor Oskar Klotz in the Department of Pathology and received his B.Sc. (Med.). He then went to Cleveland, Ohio, where he served under A. H. Bill and W. H. Weir, two of the leaders in American obstetrics and gynaecology. Returning to Toronto he completed his training in surgery under Roscoe Graham and in 1936 received his F.R.C.S.(C.) by examination in General Surgery. His first association with the Department of Obstetrics and Gynaecology came when he was appointed to the staff of the Toronto Western Hospital in 1938.

On the outbreak of war Cannell joined No. 15 Canadian General Hospital and, with Frederick Kergin, went to England in advance of the unit in the fall of 1939. He spent four years in England, retiring with the rank of Lieutenant-Colonel, R.C.A.M.C., and rejoined the staff of the Western Hospital in 1943. His appointment as Head of the Service at the General Hospital was evidence of the increasing liaison between the teaching hospitals of the University of Toronto.

In 1954, an endowment set up by Mr. Gordon C. Leech, at one time Chairman of the Board of the Toronto Western Hospital, established the Chair of Obstetrics and Gynaecology on a full-time resident basis, and the new Gordon Leech professor came to have the same stature as the heads of the medical and surgical departments at the hospital and the university. Together they faced a rapidly rising tide of change. The diversity of interests which had already provided the basis for research was to become the *raison d'être* of sub-divisions, particularly in the Departments of Surgery and Medicine. Sharp boundaries between the departments would be broken down as common interests over-rode them. The Medical Advisory Board would represent the viewpoint of the majority of the members of the hospital staff, and special committees would advise on developments within the hospital, whereas the trustees had previously listened to the voice of one representative of the professional staff. Fund-granting bodies and private foundations, as well as the governments, would provide not only for the support of junior members of the staffs working as research fellows, but also for the facilities which would make their work possible within the hospital. A new era was dawning in which the chosen candidates were to receive ample support when they trained at world-wide centres from which they would bring back the knowledge necessary to keep the hospital advised of all the advances in modern technology. The growing volume and complexity of the duties of the heads of all the departments, even those who were not as yet assuming full-time duties, transformed these positions. Clinical excellence was still an essential attribute, but the demands of the departmental offices called for the wisdom of a diplomat to gather the interests of all the teaching hospitals into the orbit of the Faculty of Medicine. Increasingly, departmental heads and their advisors would have to anticipate problems of the future as carefully as they had coped with those of the present.

Two major changes took place on the staff of the General Hospital when both Robert Janes and Ray Farquharson retired from their positions with the university and the hospital. Robert Janes retired in 1957; in the previous ten years he had trained well over a hundred surgeons in the postgraduate course in Toronto, and had expanded the program in both depth and breadth. While he had encouraged those who were concentrating their efforts in highly specialized fields, he never lost the opportunity to train his residents in the essential foundation of good general surgery. Dr. Janes had succeeded Dr. Van Wyck as Chairman of the Medical Advisory Board, and as a member of the Board of Trustees he took an active part in the development of the new buildings and the renovation of the old, especially the modernization of the Out-Patients Department and the Surgical wing of the College Street building.

Janes had never spared himself in whatever service he undertook, and the many honours which came to him only emphasized his characteristic integrity and strength of purpose. After long service on the Council of the Royal College of Physicians and Surgeons of Canada, he was made President of the College and held that position at the time of his retirement. He was also an Honorary Fellow of the Royal College of Surgeons of England, a Regent of the American College of Surgeons and President of the American Association of Thoracic Surgeons. On his retirement he became a Sims Commonwealth Travelling Professor of Surgery appointed by the Royal College of Surgeons of England.

Ray Farquharson retired in 1960. As Professor of Medicine, Farquharson felt that the undergraduate student and the postgraduate trainee should view the practice of medicine as a whole and he had therefore maintained all-inclusive services on the wards of the hospital. As Head of the Department of Medicine he had clearly demonstrated in his practice the value of sound clinical investigation, as well as showing a full recognition of the fact that the future of medicine was inseparably associated with progressive laboratory research. As Chairman of the Medical Committee of the National Research Council of Canada, he had presented a report which was instrumental in establishing the Medical Research Council of Canada, of which, when he retired, he became the first President on a full-time basis. He was an Honorary Fellow of the Society of Medicine of the United Kingdom, six Canadian universities conferred their honorary degrees upon him, and he was a Fellow of the Royal College of Physicians of London and of the Royal Society of Canada. As a special tribute and memorial, the Clinical Investigation Unit at the Toronto General Hospital was named after him.

Frederick G. Kergin succeeded Professor Janes as Head of the Department of Surgery at the University and as Surgeon-in-Chief to the General Hospital in July 1957. The son of a pioneer doctor in British Columbia, Kergin had spent seven years in Biological and Medical Sciences in Toronto, receiving a B.A. in 1927 and graduating in medicine with the Silver Medal in 1930. He was a Rhodes Scholar and had spent three years in Oxford studying physiology and anatomy before proceeding to house appointments in urology and gynaecology, as well as general surgery, in London and Toronto hospitals. He became the resident surgeon at the General Hospital in 1936. His degrees included an M.A. (Oxon.), M.S. (Tor.) and Fellowship in the Royal Colleges of both England and Canada. He was intimately associated with Norman Shenstone and Robert Janes in the field of thoracic surgery, and had succeeded Dr. Harold Wookey in taking charge of the second division of general surgery at the General Hospital before becoming Surgeon-in-Chief. Kergin's war service extended from the beginning to the end in Canada, England, North Africa and northwest Europe, and he retired with the rank of Lieutenant-Colonel, R.C.A.M.C., having served as the Senior Surgeon in No. 15 and later with No. 2 Canadian General Hospital.

Kergin was widely recognized as a very skilled surgeon, and as he assumed his administrative office his extensive knowledge gave full promise of wide and capable leadership. His wartime experience had influenced his reaction to the semi-autonomous nature of the special divisions in the departments of Surgery, and he appreciated the great advantage of developing a closer relationship with similar services in the other teaching hospitals. There was a strong movement at work towards this latter ideal, as a considerable number of the staff at the General Hospital also held appointments at Sunnybrook Hospital, where the camaraderie of wartime service was breaking down outworn prejudices against close interdepartmental relations in finding new answers to old problems.

Dr. K. J. R. Wightman succeeded Professor Ray Farquharson in the Department of Medicine and as Physician-in-Chief to the General Hospital in July 1960. Born and educated in Peterborough, he had graduated in Medicine from Toronto with the Gold Medal in 1937. He had been awarded the Ellen Mickle Fellowship and had spent a year in Cambridge under Sir Alan Drury, the distinguished medical biologist who was Director of the Lister Institute. Returning to the Toronto General Hospital, he had become Resident in Medicine in 1941 and had then served overseas with the R.C.A.M.C. from 1942 until the end of the war. He had been appointed to the staff of the General Hospital in 1945, and in 1950 became Associate Professor and Head of the Department of Therapeutics at the University of Toronto. Besides establishing an outstanding record as a teacher, he was involved in considerable clinical research, especially in the field of cancer therapy. He rose steadily in the regard of his colleagues, and his appointment as the Sir John and Lady Eaton Professor of Medicine was a fitting reward for one who had served so industriously on the wards and in the classrooms of the General Hospital.

Wightman's experience as Professor of Therapeutics had kept him aware of the nature of the hospital wards and their value as a testing ground—especially with regard to the chemotherapy of malignant disease and the rapidly broadening use of radioactive isotopes, not only in treatment but also as an accurate means of measuring many metabolic processes. Although special divisions were not generally located in designated areas in the wards of the department, those of his staff who were responsible for the care of the patients were recognized in the hospital and in the community as leaders in their fields of practice. As the department progressed under his direction, more and more of his appointees followed the example which had been set by W. R. Campbell and A. J. Dauphinee and applied their contributions in laboratory investigation to the treatment of the patients in the wards and clinics of the hospital.

The professional staff of the hospital who were appointed in 1961 (the first year of Dr. Wightman's appointment as Physician-in-Chief) presented many interesting features. An increase in numbers was associated with the assignment to various out-patient clinics in the Department of Medicine. At the same time, some physicians who had served in the Out-Patient Department were included not only in the list of Consulting Physicians but also in that of Senior Physicians, Physicians and Assistant Physicians on the same basis as those serving on the In-Patient Service. The Department of Anaesthesia under the Anaesthetist-in-Chief, Dr. S. M. Campbell, was no longer under the Department of Therapeutics but was recognized as a separate department at the university and the hospital. Included in the list of Senior Anaesthetists was Dr. Shirley Fleming, who was to leave a short time later, the first member of the staff of the General Hospital to join the staff of the University of Lagos, Nigeria, and to establish an association between the teaching hospitals in Toronto and that country.

In the Department of Obstetrics and Gynaecology, the list of voluntary assistants indicated the increased activity in the Out-Patient Clinics and one voluntary assistant in the Department of Paediatrics represented the association with the Hospital for Sick Children which had been inaugurated by Dr. Alan Brown many years before. In the Department of Radiology, the close association with the Ontario Cancer Institute was seen in the designated staff under Dr. Clifford L. Ash, and the changing function of the dental service was indicated by the presence of a Dental Oral Surgeon serving under Douglas Tanner.

The new Neurosurgical Unit at the General Hospital was opened on November 8, 1958. The distinguished audience included the members of the American Academy of Neurological Surgery, which was holding its annual meeting at the hospital in appreciation of the work of K. G. McKenzie and E. H. Botterell. When McKenzie and Botterell spoke, they traced the progress of the neurosurgical service from its birth under C. L. Starr through its growth under W. E. Gallie and its planning under Robert Janes. This was truly the valediction of Kenneth McKenzie, but Frederick Kergin also paid tribute to the major part that Robert Janes had played in establishing the department within the General Hospital and the disciplines which had contributed to its progress: Eric Linell and Mary Thom had established neuropathology; D. Eaglesham and D. G. Wollin, neurological radio-diagnosis; and John Scott, electroencephalography. But it was the close liaison with the neurologists Herbert Hyland, J. C. Richardson, and Allan Walters, that had contributed since the pre-war era to the clinical and research study of the patients and which had established the value of having this surgical division embodied in the General Hospital. The large concentration of patients had provided for good undergraduate teaching as well as the training of many residents coming on rotation to serve in the unit. Further proof of its contribution was seen in the men who had gone from the Toronto General to hold senior university appointments at three Toronto hospitals, and in Vancouver, London, Halifax and even the United States.

Specially equipped operating rooms were set aside on the operating floor, and on the twelfth floor there was accommodation for sixty patients. On the eleventh floor there were facilities for investigation and research available to surgeons and physicians alike, as well as accommodation for mentally disturbed patients and those requiring prolonged and extensive investigation.

Dr. Harry Botterell took charge of the Division of Neurosurgery in 1953, and proceeded gradually to increase the staff by the appointments of T. P. Morley, William Lougheed, and Ronald Tasker. Once again it was the special interests that each developed that strengthened the efforts of the whole. Botterell's own work with the problems of paraplegics has already been referred to and with every passing year the great importance of John Scott became more and more evident. Scott provided the link with the Department of Physiology, and as the younger members of the staff came back from postgraduate training the necessity of a basic knowledge of the physiology of the central nervous system became an established fact.

The work of Hyland and Richardson in 1941 had shown that

spontaneous intracranial haemorrhage was most frequently due to ruptured aneurysms, a far from hopeless condition if diagnosed in time. The challenge was taken up by William Lougheed, a graduate of 1947, who was appointed to the Division in 1956. He had worked under Gordon Murray and had almost chosen cardiovascular surgery for his career. This background continued to influence him, for when he went to Harvard to work under William Sweet he took with him Bigelow's great discovery of hypothermia to be accepted as the means of protecting the brain during operations on aneurysms or vascular malformations. Following this first step, his interest in the field of neurovascular problems continued to grow. In 1965, Lougheed reported his experiences over a ten-year period with carotid endorectomy, and also the experimental work he had carried out which was soon to establish microsuturing techniques in the treatment of small arterial defects.

Ronald Tasker came a little later, in 1961. A Silver Medallist in 1952, he had had a prolonged training in physiology under Professor Charles Best, and Professor Woolsey of the University of Wisconsin had directed his interests particularly into neurophysiology. He had been further prepared for an academic appointment by a McLaughlin Travelling Fellowship which supported two years of intense training. Tasker's interest came to apply to Parkinson's disease and to the electrophysiology observed through steriotactic surgery in the treatment of epilepsy and pain. While engaged in this work he was supported by a Markle Scholarship.

Botterell, in his wisdom, saw very clearly the future which lay ahead for the neurologists, both surgeons and physicians. T. P. Morley, who succeeded Botterell as Chief of the Division in 1961, had worked under Sir Geoffrey Jefferson in Manchester before coming to Toronto. It was he who worked so satisfactorily with William Paul in the scanning of brain tumours, and in addition was a very capable surgeon. Experience impressed him with the value of full collaboration with the neurologists which had been a characteristic of the work in the centre block from the beginning.

The situation in medical neurology was not as clearly defined. As the psychiatric unit was phased out at the Wellesley Hospital, Hyland, Richardson and Walters continued with their eight-bed units on the three floors of the medical wing on College Street. Neurology still included psychiatry at this time, but in his increasing involvement with the neurosurgeons Richardson's interest became more specialized. With his appointment as head of the service in 1961, and with the support of John Humphrey, who had recently returned from prolonged training in London, England, the eleventh floor in the centre block became the location for an investigative unit out of which new developments were to emerge.

John Humphrey established an electromyographic laboratory on the eleventh floor. Along with the electroencephalogram, the isotope scanning, and a little later Dr. J. R. Wherrett's new neurochemistry laboratory, this provided facilities at such a level that full postgraduate training in neurology could be established for the first time at the General Hospital. Humphrey's interest was in the histochemical muscle changes and, like the work of Tasker, involved a previously little-understood biochemistry of the tissues involved.

Another neurologist whose contributions were considerable was H. M. Barnett. His interests were particularly clinical, but in cooperation with A. T. Jousse and William Lougheed he made an interesting study of progressive myelopathy following traumatic paraplegia. Morley, like Botterell, encouraged the intimate involvement of his staff in those cooperative investigations which were now receiving international recognition.

With the loss of the psychiatric unit at the Wellesley Hospital, Farquharson and later Wightman realized the need to provide a similar service at the General Hospital. But it was not easy to find an area of sufficient size for its accommodation. Consideration was given to the Burnside building, now that the Department of Obstetrics and Gynaecology had moved to the centre block, but the renovation of the surgical wing caused considerable delay. In the meantime, Dr. Allan Walters had become the unofficial head of psychiatry at the General Hospital, and he was joined on the staff by three junior appointees. By 1962 an appreciable number of in-patients were under treatment for various psychoses and an active out-patient clinic had been organized. In 1963 a centralized unit was finally established on the seventh floor of the centre block, and Professor A. B. Stokes of the University Department of Psychiatry undertook to coordinate the services of all the Toronto teaching hospitals. In this he received strong support from Allan Walters and Robert Pos, both of whom were ambitious to establish a department whose autonomy would be recognized by the General Hospital.

Apart from his service on the ward and in the clinic, Allan Walters' major research contribution was his study of psychogenic pain. This had its origin in work which he had carried out with Harry Botterell many years before, but the final result was a tribute to the unfailing industry and enthusiasm of an untiring worker.

January 19, 1962, was another gala day for the General Hospital, for it marked the coming of age of the division of Cardiovascular Surgery. It was fitting that the Royal College of Physicians and Surgeons was holding its annual meeting in Toronto, as this allowed many surgeons with both long and short associations with the hospital to be among the audience for the opening of the new quarters for cardiovascular surgery on the eighth and ninth floors of the Private Patients' Pavilion. This achievement, like the conquest of any great peak, was due to a combined effort: physicians, anaesthetists and physiologists, as well as surgeons, had all played their part in the accomplishments of the decade from 1948 to 1958.

Following in the footsteps of his father, William Oille, with the help of Dr. D. P. Murnaghan, had performed the first cardiac catheterization to be done at the General Hospital in 1947. Oille and Murnaghan continued their work under very discouraging conditions, for their efforts were not acceptable to their seniors, and when Dr. Murnaghan was transferred to the Wellesley Hospital by Dr. Farquharson the next year the service was not developed any further. It soon became obvious, however, that if the General Hospital were to keep pace with the progress in cardiology a cardiovascular investigative unit was a necessity, and the return of Doctors W. F. Greenwood and W. G. Bigelow from their postgraduate studies in Baltimore and Boston provided an opportunity which could not be ignored indefinitely.

W. F. Greenwood, who became the key man in the Department of Medicine, had graduated in 1937 and had spent a year in physiology and as a research fellow in medicine before his four years' service overseas during the war. He was appointed resident physician to the Toronto General Hospital by Professor D. A. L. Graham in 1945, and then spent another year in physiology under Eugene Landis of Harvard, which focused his interest on heart disease. It was under his direction during later years that Ramsay Gunton, Douglas Wigle, Harold Aldridge and Kenneth W. G. Brown were first inspired to contribute to establishing the reputation of the General Hospital at the forefront of investigative medicine.

W. G. Bigelow was one of the young surgeons whom Professor Gallie brought back during the war to complete their training. During the time he had already spent overseas Bigelow had become interested in the problem of avoiding the amputation of limbs which had suffered vascular injury, and he had designed a cooling cabinet to maintain viability of tissue while awaiting vascular repair. Although nothing had come of this, it became the basis for his prolonged studies of hypothermia as a means of performing open-heart surgery. William Greenwood and Roderick A. Gordon, the anaesthetist, worked with him in the research laboratories of the Royal Canadian Air Force on Avenue Road in Toronto during the period 1948–50, where they persevered in a cold room, wearing flight suits and boots. A little later, having obtained a cooling machine, they were able to move their work to the Banting Institute. Undoubtedly the prolonged study of hibernating animals was the most unique feature of Bigelow's research. Many answers were not forthcoming, but the principle of the relative safety of preserving tissue vitality during a reduction of body temperature to 30°C. was established, and with this principle open-heart surgery became a routine procedure. One of the side-issues which resulted in an entirely new development was the production of the first electrical artificial pacemaker by John Callaghan, one of Bigelow's collaborators in the years of the groundhog studies, and J. A. Hobbs, a Fellow of the National Research Council.

W. G. Bigelow worked with Gordon Murray on Ward C on his return from Johns Hopkins Hospital in 1948. Murray's reputation and accomplishments attracted many patients, and the volume and variety of work increased so that within two years they were joined by Dr. Donald R. Wilson. Wilson had just returned from a travelling fellowship in Europe, studying problems of peripheral disease, and his work with Murray and Bigelow set the foundation for his future career at the Toronto Western Hospital.

When Murray retired from the staff in 1953, Bigelow took over the service and was joined by Dr. James Key, a Scottish graduate who had previously worked with him on his studies of micro-circulation. Key welcomed the opportunity to work with a leader whose ambitions were never satisfied by mere surgical excellence and who believed that the research laboratory at the Banting Institute was an essential base from which to improve the service evolving at the General Hospital. In 1955 they were joined by Raymond Heimbecker who became the first full-time member of the Department of Surgery at the University of Toronto. Heimbecker had graduated in 1947, and had received an exceptionally good postgraduate training. His primary stimulus had been service with Gordon Murray as a junior intern and then as a research fellow under Bigelow. This had been followed by work under Blalock at Johns Hopkins, William Mustard at the Hospital for Sick Children in Toronto, Sir Russell Brock at Guy's Hospital, and Paul Wood at the National Heart Hospital in London, England.

By the time of Heimbecker's appointment, John Gibbon of Philadelphia had developed the first heart-lung machine to be used in open-heart surgery. Heimbecker and Barry Fairley of the Department of Anaesthesia had developed a similar piece of equipment, and in the fall of 1957, using a heart-lung pump, the first adult open-heart operation in Canada took place at the Toronto General Hospital.

W. G. Bigelow and William Greenwood reached their first objective when the Cardiovascular Investigative Unit, built on the site of the old hospital greenhouse, was opened in September 1956. Bigelow had repeatedly emphasized in his discussions with the Medical Advisory Board, the departmental heads, and the hospital executive that without proper pre-operative investigation high standards of treatment could not be reached. Through his efforts money became available, $35,000 of which had come from John T. Frame and John A. McFadyen in gratitude for his services, and the Heart Foundation and the federal government both made liberal grants to cover furnishings and equipment. Now for the first time an interdepartmental unit was organized, coming under the alternating chairmanship of Bigelow and Greenwood. Doctors Ramsay Gunton and Raymond Heimbecker were appointed as full-time resident members of the staff with offices in the unit. With proper facilities available, left heart catheterization and angiographic studies became routine procedures.

Professor Kergin took over where Professor Janes had left off and strongly supported the centralization of the patients' and ancillary services in one area. With the re-allocation of space which resulted from the opening of the large new buildings, two floors in the Private Patients' Pavilion were available to accommodate the cardiovascular division, with fifty beds on the eighth floor, some offices, and good teaching facilities. On the ninth floor there were twin operating rooms with overhead galleries and a central monitoring room. In addition, there were cooling and pump assembly rooms, laboratories, and additional store-rooms. Of major importance was the acute therapy unit, where nine beds were available to accommodate patients post-operatively for periods of up to five and six days.

The surgical staff at this time consisted of Bigelow, Key, Heimbecker and R. J. Baird, the latter two being on a resident full-time basis. There was also a senior resident, two assistant residents, two juniors, a clinical assistant and three research fellows working in the cardiovascular laboratory at the Banting Institute. At this time there were fifteen to twenty cardiovascular operations being performed each week, including three to four open-heart procedures.

The original cardiovascular investigation unit was enlarged to more than twice its original size, and in 1961 an image amplifier, the first of its type in North America, was installed. To meet the greatly increased volume of work the staff now consisted of seven cardiologists, three on a full-time basis, two peripheral vascular specialists, four surgeons, three radiologists, two anaesthetists, one cardiovascular specialist, and seven research fellows. In such a stimulating atmosphere productive research was a natural result. Dr. Douglas Wigle joined the unit in 1960 and Dr. Harold Aldridge in 1962, and their contributions soon received world-wide recognition. Aldridge's skill with left heart catheterization became proverbial, and Wigle steered a straight course from his Gold Medal on graduation in 1953 through his postgraduate years in Toronto, London and San Francisco to eventually become director of the unit in July 1964 when Ramsay Gunton became Professor of Therapeutics. Gunton later left to head the Department of Medicine at the University of Western Ontario. Although investigative procedures gradually became the function of the physicians, young surgeons still had their offices in the unit and a comprehensive view of the nature and control of cardiovascular disease was thereby common to all.

Another young physician, specially trained in cardiology, was appointed in 1961 as an Associate in the Department of Medicine and a physician to the Toronto General Hospital. Dr. John R. Evans had graduated with the Silver Medal in 1952 and after a year's internship, had spent two years at Oxford on a Rhodes Scholarship, obtaining his D.Phil. (Oxon.), followed by a year at the National Heart Hospital, London, three years at Sunnybrook, at Toronto General, and as an Ontario Heart Foundation Fellow at the Hospital for Sick Children, and a year in research at the Baker Clinic Research Laboratory at Harvard. He became Chief Medical Resident at the Toronto General Hospital in 1959, and held the Markle Scholarship in Academic Medicine at the University of Toronto from 1960 to 1965. His particular interest was in the adolescent cardiac clinic and in studies of the metabolism of the heart muscle as affected by high fat diets. To the regret of his clinical associates, he became involved in the planning committee of the Board of Governors for the new Medical Sciences

Building at the University of Toronto and, soon after, this most promising cardiologist became a medical administrator. After serving as Dean of Medicine at McMaster University from 1965 to 1972, Dr. Evans returned to Toronto to become President of the University of Toronto.

Heimbecker and Gunton made invaluable contributions during the years they worked together. Ramsay Gunton made a long stop-over at the General Hospital during the period between his graduation from Western Ontario and his return there as Head of the Department of Medicine. He was Ray Farquharson's resident physician in 1952, and made an important contribution to the clinical standards of the hospital: the observations he made both pre-operatively and over the long period of follow-up established facts on cardiovascular patients which were to gain universal acceptance.

Heimbecker's skilled research resulted in a standard of patient care in the Cardiovascular Surgical Division that was to gain him many honours. Outstanding examples of his work were the studies in and clinical use of the homograft cardiac valve, its application in mitral valve replacement, and the development of emergency infarctectomy.

James Key earned his place by his utter dependability: as evidence of the standard of surgery in his division, he presented a report of 133 consecutive cases of excision of asymptomatic abdominal aneurysms, with no deaths.

Contributing through their investigative studies and improved techniques to the progress and success of these two great interdepartmental efforts were the departments of Anaesthesia and Radiology. Stanley Campbell, R. A. Gordon, Stuart Vandewater, and H. B. Fairley were involved from the first in seeking solutions to problems which had to be answered, and through their masterful control in the operating room they demonstrated the great strides that had been made and continued to be made in anaesthesia at the General Hospital. It was not surprising that, in addition to the increase in resident staff, the number of post-graduate students who came for instruction rose rapidly. As the inter-hospital services were brought closer together, each institution vied with the others in the contributions they were making.

Dr. Malcolm Hall succeeded Arthur Singleton as Radiologist-in-Chief in July 1962. They had had a long association, both at the hospital and in their private practice in the Medical Arts Building, where so many of the hospital staff carried on their private practices. As a result there was no disruption in the department but merely continued progress, which was featured by the development of specialists within the field. Singleton and Hall were joined by R. B. Holmes and D. E. Sanders, who were both to rise to senior appointments as they participated in the efficient service and good relationships which had characterized the department from its beginning. As more radiologists joined the staff, they became not so much assistants as masters of a special field, and when the department moved to much larger quarters in the central block in order to give service to more patients, it gained from newer and more efficient equipment and techniques. Angio-catheterization revolutionized the techniques necessary to visualize the vascular state of the kidney, liver, pancreas, lungs, thymus and brain. The image intensifier with video-tape equipment transformed the studies of the heart and its blood supply. X-ray pictures at the rate of eight per second showed the flow through the heart and lungs and the great vessels of the chest. Automatic processing units reduced the time needed to provide a finished radiograph from forty minutes to ninety seconds.

With all these features, it was not surprising that the work of the radiologist became increasingly dependent on special procedures, and the long list of patients from the Out-Patient Department came to equal the number from the wards as radiology took its place with the laboratory services as an essential aid to thorough clinical investigation. Dr. R. B. Holmes succeeded Malcolm Hall as Radiologist-in-Chief to the General Hospital in July 1965.

Although there was an obvious common interest, two of the most active services in the hospital did not enjoy the close relationship of the neurologists and cardiologists. While rheumatic arthritis presented conditions which eventually called for treatment by the orthopaedic surgeons, this was only one of their interests, and as Wallace Graham established his specialty of rheumatology it pursued a tortuous path towards cooperation with the orthopaedic surgeons.

Dr. James Wallace Graham was chosen for the staff of the General Hospital by Professor Duncan Graham, but his greatest activity took place under Ray Farquharson (1949–60). He had graduated with honours in Dentistry before beginning the study of Medicine, in which once again he was an honours student. After two years' internship at the General Hospital he spent three years at various London hospitals and received his M.R.C.P. (Lond.) in 1936. During these years he was involved in research which demolished the current belief of a major association between dental caries and focal infection and rheumatoid arthritis. In 1937 he was appointed to the staff of the General Hospital and began a close association with Almon Fletcher on Ward H, in the study of diabetic therapy and arthritis. He served with the Royal Canadian Naval Service during the war, being chief of medicine at the naval hospitals in Halifax and then St. John's, Newfoundland. In 1944 he organized a tri-service rheumatic unit in St. Thomas, Ontario. It followed as a natural result that after the war, when he returned to his service on Ward H, he was appointed Chief Consultant in Rheumatology to the veterans' hospital, Sunnybrook.

Graham's clinical research was a testing ground for therapeutic agents—gold, steroids, antibiotics and various new analgesics—and working at the Queen Elizabeth Hospital he maintained the first long-term study of rheumatic patients. His knowledge and influence were broad in their effects. In 1948 he was a founder of the Canadian Arthritis and Rheumatism Society and became its first president. Through his efforts public interest was organized to provide increased financial support for research. On this basis special centres developed at medical schools and at teaching hospitals across Canada. No longer was rheumatic disease a neglected specialty in internal medicine, but increasing numbers of young men now chose it as a field of special interest. Wallace Graham's tragically early death from coronary thrombosis in December 1962 was a great loss, not only to the General Hospital but to national and international organizations to which he had contributed so much. He was at the height of his career, serving at the time of his death as President-elect of the Pan-American League against Rheumatism, as Chairman of the Gairdner Foundation in Toronto, and as President of the Academy of Medicine, Toronto. He was an idealist, a great teacher and a good physician. Following in his footsteps, Metro Ogryzlo, and later Hugh Smythe, by their combined efforts carried on the investigation and treatment of patients which was to set the stage for the development of the special department at the Wellesley Hospital.

Dr. F. P. Dewar became Chief of the Division of Orthopaedic Surgery at the General Hospital in 1951. He had been serving as Senior House Surgeon to Dr. Roscoe Graham when he left for overseas service with the R.C.A.M.C. in 1940, and was one of the young surgeons brought back by Professor Gallie for a special training period which, in his case, concentrated on the treatment of fractures. Prior to his return after the war he had gained his Fellowship in the Royal College of Surgeons of England, and he completed his postgraduate training at the Hospital for the Ruptured and Crippled in New York. His appointment as a Junior Associate of R. I. Harris began in 1947, and he became involved with him in the training program for orthopaedic surgeons at the General Hospital, which developed during the postwar period. As various new members came to the staff of the division, they became particularly involved in different phases of orthopaedics. Dr. Dewar's special interest was scoliosis, David MacIntosh gained a reputation in the treatment of ligamentous injuries of the knee joint, Ian MacNab's interest was back surgery, and W. R. Harris took a keen interest in amputations and especially in the production of new and better types of artificial limbs.

The advent of antibiotics completely altered the whole practice of orthopaedic surgery. Open reduction of fractures and the use of plastic and metal prostheses were now free from the haunting fear of sepsis. Operations for arthritic joints and various deformities improved in efficiency, and among the developments at the General Hospital was the MacIntosh prosthesis to replace worn-out knee joints suffering from rheumatic destruction. Although close association between the medical and surgical specialties developed slowly at the General Hospital, combined rounds were organized and Wallace Graham and Dewar consulted regularly at the Queen Elizabeth Hospital. As a result, the scope of surgical treatment broadened, to the great satisfaction of the rheumatologists.

The division was fortunate in receiving generous financial support from several grateful patients. Dr. Wallace Duncan, a Toronto graduate who had become a distinguished orthopaedic surgeon in Cleveland, supported a special fellowship during his lifetime. With good financial support, the postgraduate training of residents and fellows produced many who were to fill professorial appointments at other Canadian schools. A number of hospitals in Toronto were drawn into the postgraduate scheme, and eminent orthopaedic surgeons were invited to visit Toronto to take part in postgraduate training programs in a division of surgery that was attracting candidates for training on a worldwide basis.

The renovation of the surgical wing was particularly beneficial to the division which took over Wards C and B, and provided accommodation for 100 patients. In addition, there were many patients on the Workmen's Compensation floor in the Pavilion, and in appreciation of the work of the division the Workmen's Compensation Board undertook to support a research fellow. Dr. John Hall, who was the first of the Wallace Duncan Fellows, eventually became the orthopaedic surgeon to the Boston Children's Hospital, which is the largest children's hospital in the United States.

In January 1959 the Department of Rehabilitation and Physical Medicine moved into its new quarters in the Gerrard Street building, with facilities to provide a maximum of continuity in treatment of physically handicapped patients. The department had developed by degrees from its beginning as a centre of physical medicine under Dr. W. J. Gardiner. In 1948 occupational therapy, which had become an efficient service under Miss Elsie Jackes, was merged with the Department of Physical Medicine; then in 1951, after a conference arranged by Dean J. A. MacFarlane, a committee was set up under Dr. Gardiner consisting of Doctors F. P. Dewar, E. H. Botterell, H. H. Hyland, A. T. Jousse, A. Zinovieff, and Wallace Graham to make plans for a new department to be known as the Department of Rehabilitation and Physical Medicine. This was endorsed by the Welfare Council of Toronto and its committee chairman, Dr. C. D. Gossage, who recommended that the General Hospital receive every assistance in setting up a training centre for various professional personnel who would be involved in rehabilitation services. In 1957 a speech therapist was appointed to the department and, under the over-all director, there were now heads of three sections—physiotherapy, occupational therapy and speech therapy.

The Department of Rehabilitation and Physical Medicine occupied most of the first floor of the Gerrard Street building, with the hydrotherapy units on the ground floor including a pool in which wheel-chair patients could be lifted by an electrically-powered apparatus. Occupation therapy covered a wide range from sewing and weaving to carpentry, even sawing logs and various activities of heavy industry. A gymnasium and the General Hospital Academic School provided help for body and mind in the effort to aid patients to become useful to themselves and to others. Within two years the volume of work tripled, and in 1963 100,000 treatments were given in the various divisions.

In addition to a greatly implemented staff, Dr. Gardiner was joined by A. T. Jousse and A. Zinovieff and a little later by William Geisler and C. M. Godfrey. The arrival of A. T. Jousse brought a new atmosphere of patient care to the department. His earliest interest had been the care of paraplegic patients, which he developed in association with Dr. Harry Botterell. He had been excellently trained in both neurological medicine and in physical medicine. His interest never flagged, and in addition to the patients under the care of neurosurgeons he and Geisler served the patients in the paraplegic ward, which was located separately in the Gerrard Street building. The inspiration of Jousse raised the standard of service to a level unsurpassed anywhere: he was the link between the General Hospital and Lyndhurst Lodge, which was never-failing in its service though it felt it had been deprived of its full status in not having a designated area for the in-patients under treatment by its staff.

XX

The Old Order Changes

THREE DEPARTMENTS WERE MARKEDLY AFFECTED BY THE WAR-time developments of transfusion services and the production of antibiotics: Obstetrics and Gynaecology, Otolaryngology and Ophthalmology all made rapid strides as a result. The latter two departments were particularly influenced by the development of equipment in response to the growing problems of aeronautics.

Douglas Cannell held the post of Professor of Obstetrics and Gynaecology and Chief of the Department at the General Hospital longer than any of his predecessors. His fifteen-year tenure from 1950 to 1965 was characterized by a steadily increasing integration of the work of the university teaching hospitals. Beginning at the General Hospital but soon extending to the other hospitals, a system of full-time staff appointments not only improved the standard patient care but also the teaching of undergraduate and postgraduate students. As junior members of the staff came to realize that an active interest in basic or clinical research was essential to their future careers, contributions of some value became yearly features of the work of the department.

William Allemang spent eighteen months in England on a McLaughlin Travelling Fellowship to become Supervisor of Clinical Investigation. On his return in July 1953 he became the first person appointed in the Department with University support to assist the Chiefs of Obstetrics and Gynaecology in academic and research endeavours. A few years later, in July 1963, Richard Wilson established a division of Steroid Chemistry to support the investigation of endocrine function.

Wilson had previously spent eighteen months training in this field in Canada and the U.S., as well as a year in Sweden as a Markle Fellow.

The department was particularly favoured by the distribution of space and facilities in the Urquhart building, though as a consequence the designation of the Burnside Lying-In Hospital was lost, along with its very old associations. Junior members of the staff profited from the opportunities now available to them to study the factors bearing on fertility and the viability of the child in utero and at the time of birth. J. A. Low in particular was involved in metabolic assessments at birth, establishing a reputation which led to his professorial appointment to Queen's University.

It was a period of great change in both obstetrics and gynaecology. The mortality rate associated with infection, haemorrhage and toxaemia had been reduced to such an extent that on a province-wide basis it was reaching an almost irreducible minimum.

Home deliveries in Toronto had become a thing of the past, for with the development of good peripheral hospitals in the metropolitan area and the standard of care provided by specially trained general practitioners an increasing number of women preferred to have their confinements in conveniently located hospitals. Family planning, birth control and a more liberal justification for abortion were affecting the birth rate and resulted in a decrease in the number of normal deliveries at the General Hospital, but this was counteracted by a relative increase in patients presenting problems of pregnancy and delivery.

Dr. Leslie Watt supervised the obstetrical care of the first large series of patients with mitral stenosis to be treated by commissurotomy during pregnancy. In cooperation with Dr. William Greenwood and Dr. Wilfred Bigelow (the latter of whom performed the operations), they reported the safety of the procedure, which lessened the threat of this serious complication of pregnancy. Abortion and sterilization were no longer primary considerations, and the value of interdepartmental cooperation was proven once again.

Biological investigation was altering the practice of gynaecology, and laboratory-controlled medical care was obviating considerable surgical treatment. At the same time, major surgery was re-established in the treatment of many malignant lesions, and combinations of endocrine and radiotherapy and surgery were the means of controlling hitherto rapidly fatal conditions. In these routines, consultants to the Princess Margaret Hospital carried out special services in the wards and operating rooms of the General Hospital.

Other milestones were reached with changes in staff. The deaths of John McArthur and John Mann brought to an end the career of a very skilful gynaecologist, and that of an inspired teacher and productive investigator. Douglas Cannell retired in 1965. He had proved the value of full-time service by the head of the department, for all who came under his influence received a basic training in the constantly changing problems of research as well as of practice.

Cannell's successor, William Paul, was an outstanding example of the Toronto school. His studies at the Carnegie Institute in Baltimore while on a McLaughlin Fellowship contributed greatly to the knowledge of reproductive physiology, and although his career prior to his appointment in 1961 to the chair of Obstetrics and Gynaecology at the University of Alberta was on the staff of the Toronto Western Hospital, he had received much of his early training at the General Hospital.

When Percy Ireland took over the Department of Otolaryngology in 1946, he was faced with the possibility that it might lose its identity as a separate department. Antibiotics practically precluded the necessity for surgical treatment of the lesions which up to that time had called for the skills of the otolaryngologist, and only Howard McCart was attempting to compete with general surgeons in the treatment of malignant lesions of the larynx and upper air passages. Ireland realized that postgraduate training must be broadened and that a knowledge of basic science as it applied to audiology was essential to meet the problems which wartime experience had shown to be associated with that function.

Within a year Ireland had organized a rotational service of junior and senior interns throughout all the teaching hospitals, and the postgraduate course was extended to include a year of basic science and a year of intern service in medicine and surgery. On this basis D. P. Bryce, who was to have a distinguished career in the department, was one of the first to obtain his F.R.C.S.(C.) when the examination was modified for otolaryngology. Ireland was eventually able to arrange a full year of general surgery for his postgraduate students, and his department became the first in Canada to develop this satisfactory standard of training.

Ireland was also successful in obtaining financial help from a number of generous donors for specially chosen trainees, to support travelling fellowships and appointments in the United States and in Great Britain.

Dr. Joseph Sullivan, the head of the department at St. Michael's Hospital, was a constant stimulus with his original surgical treatment of the internal ear and the research he carried out under the auspices of the Royal Canadian Air Force. Ireland appreciated that the problems of deafness and vertigo demanded facilities not available at the General Hospital. The Workmen's Compensation Board offered its cooperation, as the problem of noise in industry was causing growing concern.

H. O. Barber undertook the study of vertigo, and through combined studies with neuropathologist Eric Linell sought fresh knowledge of conditions of the temporal bone and the internal ear. Barber's clinical contributions led eventually to the development of the Audiology Centre on the second floor of the old emergency building. Air-conditioned and soundproof, it provided for a full range of tests in audiology.

Finally, the appointment of Dr. Walter Johnson in 1966 as Director of Research, with staff affiliation in both Otolaryngology and Physiology, was a strong influence in obtaining support from the Hartford Foundation of New York in the investigation of dizziness and disorientation—additional evidence of the prestige of Professor Ireland's department.

D. P. Bryce, the consultant to the Princess Margaret Hospital, developed a good liaison with the radiotherapists in the treatment of malignant lesions. Careful consideration was given to controlling disease as well as maintaining to the greatest possible degree effective speech without the use of mechanical devices. Further cooperation with the Department of Rehabilitation Medicine resulted in the founding of an efficient speech therapy centre at the General Hospital, and with financial help from Mr. E. C. Fox plans were made for an investigative area in the hospital where, taking advantage of the service of Dr. John Scott and the Electroencephalogram Department, hearing defects of infants and small children could be studied.

Professor A. J. Elliott was Professor of Ophthalmology at the University of Toronto as well as Chief of the Department at the General. As the result of his experience in the Air Force, he was well aware of the need to reorganize the Departments of Ophthalmology at both the university and the General Hospital. He lost no time in adding a year of basic science to the two years of rotational clinical training at St. Michael's and the Toronto Western, as well as at the Sick Children's and the General.

Dr. T. H. Hodgson took over the Ophthalmic Pathology service from A. E. MacDonald and A. L. Ormsby became Ophthalmic Bacteriologist. Hodgson also organized a special glaucoma clinic at the General Hospital.

Dr. Alexander MacDonald retired in 1953 after twenty-nine years of service at the General Hospital. Besides his many contributions to the investigation and treatment of ophthalmic diseases, he had been an enthusiastic advocate of a fully integrated Eye Institute in a separate building within the hospital grounds. Liberal contributions were obtained, but unfortunately the concept did not fit into the new building program, which favoured centralization. With considerable disappointment, the department accepted its new quarters in the Gerrard Street building.

Elliott arranged that each member of the staff should have a special interest. Harry Macrae continued to attract increasing numbers of patients with retinal detachment, and to meet his demands the hospital installed an electro-coagulator in 1960. W. R. Luke, with an efficient tonometry service, developed a routine for the prevention of blindness from glaucoma. G. A. Thompson, working with the isotope service, developed a method of locating malignant tumours of the eye by means of radioactive phosphorus.

A key appointment was that of Dr. P. R. Basu as Stapells Director of Research and controller of the eye bank located at the Banting Institute. The value of this service was such that, at the General Hospital alone, ninety-one corneal grafts had been performed up to 1956.

Professor Elliott retired in 1961 to return to Vancouver as Professor of Ophthalmology at the University of British Columbia. His fifteen years' service had transformed not only the department at the General Hospital but those at all the teaching hospitals. His well-trained residents had been inspired to remain at the forefront of their specialty, and returned regularly to reunions, showing their continuing interest in the department which had trained them.

Dr. Clement McCulloch was chosen to succeed Elliott. He had literally been born into the specialty, in which his father was a skilled practitioner. Following postgraduate training at the Presbyterian Hospital, New York, and war service with the Royal Canadian Air Force, he had been Senior Ophthalmologist at the Toronto Western Hospital for a period of fifteen years. He had always taken a personal interest in research, and one of his early studies on hereditary ocular disease earned him the Reeve Prize for the best research accomplished in any department in the Medical Faculty during the year. He continued his interest in the problems of aviation as consultant to the Royal Canadian Air Force.

Under McCulloch, the staff carried on with their special interests.

G. A. Thompson, besides directing the provincial eye bank, developed a very active corneal clinic, J. S. Speakman took over W. R. Luke's Glaucoma Clinic, and C. B. Mortimer served with Macrae in the retinal clinic. J. S. Crawford directed an Orthoptic Clinic, and Lois Lloyd became responsible for special work in neuroophthalmology.

The work in these three departments was representative of the transformation taking place at the Toronto General. As W. E. Gallie had said years before, the residents were no longer "wayfarers" but chosen apprentices receiving the best training possible. After ten years of reorganizing the training program in Ophthalmology, Professor Elliott reported the production of forty-six trained specialists in Ophthalmology. The ground was now prepared for a firm partnership between the teaching hospitals and the developing Medical Science Centre of the University of Toronto. No longer were the years spent on the wards of the hospital or in research laboratories a sacrifice for the ambitious: young scientists and clinicians from many places now sought the opportunity to work in the productive atmosphere of the university and its teaching hospitals.

In December 1957, on the request of Dr. Stanley Campbell, the Anaesthetist-in-Chief, the Medical Advisory Board appointed a committee under Dr. William Oille to organize a unit for the treatment of patients in a state of respiratory failure. There were, at this time, thirty to forty patients in various departments who required such treatment, and as a start, Dr. Stuart Vandewater was asked to supervise a small three-bed unit where resuscitary equipment was available. This was set up in the old Ward F operating room in the College Street building, and he undertook to train the nurses and residents from the Department of Anaesthesia and the Department of Medicine in the services that would be required.

Shortly after this, on a more permanent basis, a staff was organized consisting of C. R. Woolf, R. A. Chambers, H. B. Fairley, Norman Delarue and H. O. Barber, representing the Departments of Medicine, Urology, Anaesthesia, Surgery and Otolaryngology. In 1958 they reported on their experiences in the treatment of twenty patients, and gave their opinions with regard to the immediate requirements for an efficient service. Their recommendations included the need for a permanent graduate nursing staff, experienced in post-operative recovery room service, and the requirement that the Resident of Anaesthesia should be constantly on call. A Fellow in Urology would be responsible for the day-to-day care of patients. The first patient was admitted to the centralized unit in October 1958, and within six months the unit was functioning in such a satisfactory manner that a request was made for its enlargement to accommodate from ten to twelve beds to meet any emergency situation. Money was now available to permit the appointment of a research fellow from the Department of Anaesthesia and the nursing service had improved markedly under the efficient control of Mrs. Flett. In 1961, the unit moved to the seventh floor of the centre block, and here accommodation was increased to ten beds. Growing clinical experience and efficient clinical research were building a reputation which was attracting physicians, surgeons and physiotherapists for special training. The recovery rate of seriously ill patients was seventy per cent, most of whom would have died without the special facilities and intense care now available to them. One of the most important developments which resulted from the work of this unit, through cooperation between the Departments of Anaesthesia and Medicine, was the emergency box. This was made available to the wards of the hospital and the Out-Patient and Emergency departments, and contained equipment for the management of acute respiratory failure and cardiac arrest. The senior nurses were trained to meet emergencies, and the resident staff received instruction so that the service could be readily available throughout the hospital.

The experience of Dr. Woolf and his associates resulted not only in the establishment of an efficient system of therapy but also in a greatly increased knowledge of pulmonary physiology. When the research laboratory of the Department of Anaesthesia was organized adjacent to the Clinical Investigation Unit, Dr. R. A. Gordon was given the opportunity to centralize the work which would continue to benefit surgeons and physicians alike at the General Hospital.

When he succeeded Stanley Campbell as Anaesthetist-in-Chief in 1961, Dr. H. B. Fairley took over the direction of the work in this laboratory. Dr. Cameron C. Gray assumed Dr. Oille's duties as Chairman of the Respiratory Paralysis Committee in 1962, continuing the record of accomplishments. By midsummer 1964, the Respiratory Paralysis Committee reported on the results of its five and one-half years' service. The admission in 1963 of 183 patients was compared with that of 115 in the previous year. The mortality rate was twenty-five per cent, and it was felt that consideration should be given to embodying the unit in a centralized intensive care area: services common to many critical conditions, such as hypothermia to aid in intracranial anoxia and constant cardiac monitoring, were becoming increasingly available.

A major development, in some degree associated with the respiratory unit, was the installation of a hyperbaric oxygen chamber. This was a joint project of the General Hospital, the Ontario Department of Labour, and the Workmen's Compensation Board. A committee consisting of H. B. Fairley, K. W. G. Brown, and R. J. Baird was set up to consider the organization of the service it would require. The chamber was installed early in 1964, and arrangements were made with the Defence Research Medical Laboratories whereby Lt.-Com. Kidd, R.C.N., organized a team to operate the chamber for a two-weeks trial while the hospital staff became familiar with the duties essential to its safe usage. Dr. Norman Delarue became the representative of the Department of Surgery on the service.

A report was presented to the Medical Advisory Board in September after the first two patients, divers brought up from a depth eighty feet below water while working at Long Branch, had been treated successfully for caisson disease. A year later the use of the chamber was extended to the hyperbaric oxygen treatment of gangrene and gas gangrene infections. The team now consisted of a full-time operator and both a resident and a technician from the Department of Anaesthesia, and staff members from Anaesthesia and Surgery were becoming aware of the hazards and limitations of this powerful therapeutic agent.

One of the most important studies carried out at the Toronto General Hospital was reported in February 1961 by Doctors R. L. MacMillan and K. W. G. Brown. This showed that the generally accepted routine of anticoagulant therapy had failed to show any beneficial effects in the treatment of acute myocardial failure. At this time the mortality rate at the General Hospital was approximately forty per cent in such cases, and very little was known as to the immediate cause of death.

The result was the first coronary unit for intensive care to be organized anywhere in the world. This was accommodated in a four-bed room in the College Street building, recently vacated on the moving of the Clinical Investigation Unit to its new location. The shortage of trained nurses delayed the opening of the unit, but on March 13, 1962, using an old electroencephalogram unit provided by Dr. John Scott, it became possible to maintain a record of each patient's cardiac behaviour. During the first year, lack of nurses forced closure of the unit on many weekends and during vacation periods. Nevertheless, nearly 150 patients were treated during the first year and although there was only a slight decrease in mortality it was found that one-half of the patients died with heart block or arrhythmia and that many of them could be controlled by defibrillation, pacemakers or anti-arrhythmic drugs. As a result of this routine, the mortality rate was lowered to less than half of its previous level and some experience with the surgical treatment of patients with massive infarction gave promise of further improvements in the future. By the end of the first five-year period, 789 patients had been treated and plans were laid for a larger and more centralized unit, made possible by a bequest from the estate of the late Percy R. Gardiner.

The development of the artificial kidney by Gordon Murray came unfortunately at a time when laboratory services at the General Hospital had not developed to the degree necessary to support a full-time service. Also, comparatively few of the staff were convinced of its potentials. The opening of the centralized laboratories altered all this, and also brought to recognition the life-saving properties of dialysis in patients with acute renal failure following shock, as well as some complications of pregnancy and mismatched transfusions. Following a strong plea to the Medical Advisory Board by Doctors Charles Robson, W. T. W. Clarke and D. M. Young, a dialysis service was organized by members of the Departments of Urology, Medicine and the Division of Laboratories in 1958, and the first patient was treated in January 1959. In 1962, a three-bed room was provided in the paraplegic unit, and for the first time nurses received instruction regarding their special duties. The unit then moved to the operating room and College Street wards of old Ward F, where it was possible to have a laboratory adjacent to a four-bed unit.

Peritoneal dialysis became available in 1962, allowing for the treatment of poor-risk patients by a much simpler technique. The following year a Kiil kidney was procured and preparations were made to organize a chronic dialysis program. As might have been expected, one of the biggest problems during the early stages was the provision of a properly trained nursing and technical staff. Dr. Clarke, who undertook the often frustrating spadework on which the unit was established, paid tribute to the help he had received from Dr. George F. Smith of the Wellesley Hospital during this period, and often referred to the team effort which had developed during the seven years in which the service had concentrated on the treatment of acute renal failure. Many problems had to be faced, and the experience gained by the team in dealing with many of these proved more important than the actual technique.

There was no doubt of the importance of the urologist in the surgical aspects of the problems which developed. Clarke observed that it was interesting to see surgeons becoming metabolically orientated and physicians mechanically interfering in the course of disease. He announced the treatment of the first patient to undergo chronic haemodialysis in 1965, with the hope that this would soon become the basis on which to establish a home dialysis program which in other centres had already shown an excellent prolongation of life in patients suffering from chronic kidney failure. Plans were also under consideration for inter-hospital cooperation in a fully coordinated program, and as yet no kidney transplant operation had been undertaken at the General Hospital.

The impact of this important service had a deep if not broad effect: from it there developed nephrologists, few in number but with the investigative zeal necessary to solve many problems. Dr. E. R. Yendt had already added considerably to the knowledge of renal vascular sclerosis as a cause of hypertension and had opened a new field for the vascular and urological surgeon. The young postwar appointments in the urological division of surgery included several whose contributions were to maintain the good reputation of the hospital.

During the time when Dr. David Mitchell was in charge of the Division of Urology (July 1949–June 1966), a marked change took place in the surgical treatment of many lesions. Radical procedures affecting the kidney, the bladder and the prostate came to be accepted as a means of prolonging life and curing many patients. At the time of his appointment, two surgeons of outstanding ability were on the service. J. L. T. Russell was just beginning to develop his skill in important urinary diversive procedures, as well as in the provision of substitute bladders, when he left the General to become Urologist-in-Chief to St. Michael's Hospital.

Dr. Carl Aberhart fortunately had a longer association with the hospital. He had graduated with the Gold Medal in 1932, and his post-graduate training under W. E. Gallie included a close association with Roscoe Graham. After further training in the United Kingdom and Europe, he had received a junior appointment at the General Hospital shortly before leaving with No. 15 General Hospital for overseas service. He was invalided home from North Africa in 1943 with relapsing fever, and on recovery was re-appointed to the General Hospital and also to the staff of Sunnybrook Hospital where, in association with Dr. Harry Botterell, he became involved in the group interested in the control of paraplegic bladders. Although he served on the staff of the General, the postgraduate training which he developed at Sunnybrook became his chief interest, and when that hospital came under the jurisdiction of the University Department of Postgraduate Studies the position as resident to Aberhart became a highly prized appointment. As a clinical teacher he was without peer, and his surgical ability was such that he eventually became Director of Surgery at Sunnybrook Hospital, a post which he held up to the time of his death.

Two younger surgeons who completed their training after the war made important contributions to the Division of Urology. C. J. Robson returned from prolonged service at sea with the Royal Canadian Navy to complete his training with a travelling fellowship in the U.S.A., and W. K. Kerr, who had served with the Royal Canadian Air Force Medical Service, was appointed as a research fellow in the Department of Surgery and joined the division a year later, in 1950. Robson was one of the first Canadian urologists to adopt the thoraco-abdominal approach for radical nephrectomy, and he also took a particular interest in operations required to provide a substitute bladder. Kerr never lost his primary interest in investigative procedures, and made many original observations regarding the aetiology of cancer of the bladder. As a very skilled surgeon, he was capable of undertaking extensive operations for the control of pelvic malignancies and cooperated on a team basis with the gynaecologists in performing exenteration operations within the pelvis in cases of uterine cervical cancer when radiotherapy had failed to produce a cure. During this time the division was preparing many young surgeons for senior hospital appointments, both in Toronto and in many other centres, and they invariably carried with them the desire to seek the why and wherefore of their calling.

Charles Robson held a second appointment as urologist to Sunnybrook Hospital. Here the stimulating atmosphere groomed him to succeed David Mitchell when he retired in 1965. William Kerr, on the other hand, served as the chief urologist at the Weston Sanitorium, and here with the benefit of medical therapeutics he developed a surgical service which made him an authority in the treatment of tuberculous conditions of the urinary tract, which were still surprisingly prevalent.

Urology had been the first of the surgical specialties to establish its separate identity after the hospital moved to College Street, by occupying quarters on the third floor of the Dunlap Building. With the demolition of the Dunlap Building, the division moved to the third floor of the Gerrard Street building, which provided all the features required for the best treatment and comfort of the patients. The cystoscopic rooms were located on the ground floor adjacent to the Department of Radiology, and in addition to one-, two-, and four-bed rooms, small conveniently-located and comfortably furnished lounges, and a central nursing station, there was a lecture theatre. Facilities were available for forty-five patients, but from the first the busy department constantly had to find additional accommodation in other parts of the hospital.

Dr. Stuart D. Gordon completed five years of postgraduate training as a surgical resident to W. E. Gallie in 1930–31, and on Dr. Gallie's recommendation spent the next year in London, England, being trained in plastic surgery by Sir Harold Gillies. He returned to receive an appointment on Dr. Roscoe Graham's service in general surgery, but with the intention that he be responsible for the care of patients requiring plastic surgery—marking the beginning of this subdivision of surgery.

By this time on Ward A, K. G. McKenzie was established in neurosurgery and R. I. Harris, although designated as a general surgeon, was developing his control of orthopaedics. The other two surgeons on the service were F. I. Lewis, who was to succeed Roscoe Graham, and J. H. Couch. Couch was at times a brilliant surgeon, taking a particular interest in the surgery of the hand, and had published a small text on this subject. As a result, Gordon was directed to confine his interests to skin grafting, fractures of the facial bones and burns. Gordon had seven years in which to mature on the Graham service, and although he went overseas in January 1940 as a junior officer with the No. 15 General Hospital, he was soon promoted to lieutenant-colonel in command of the first plastic surgical unit to be set up in the R.C.A.M.C., and he came to share the hospital accommodation at Rocksdown House, Basingstoke, with his old mentor, Sir Harold Gillies. From there he moved on to become Senior Plastic Surgeon at the newly organized Neurological and Plastic Hospital, and after a year was brought back to take charge of the tri-service Plastic Surgical Division at Christie Street Hospital in 1944.

When the Division of Plastic Surgery of the Toronto General Hospital was established at the end of the war, Gordon became responsible for the training of general surgical residents on a six-month rotational basis. Gradually the status of the division became more definitely recognized: a resident was appointed and a training scheme evolved consisting of two years spent at each of the Hospital for Sick Children, the Western and the General, preceded by three years in general surgery. Trainees were soon leaving Toronto to establish themselves across Canada in the specialized field of plastic surgery. Dr. Donald Robertson, first trained as a general surgeon, joined Stuart Gordon in 1951. Their service was constantly busy, largely as a result of motor car accidents, and an increasing number of young surgeons sought training in this active field.

Dr. Stuart Gordon lived up to his obligations regarding applied research, and was involved, among many other projects, in a study with Professor Arthur Ham, in the fate of transplanted cancellous bone. He also undertook to study the effect of quick freezing of dermis grants as well as the problems of surgery involving the tempero-mandibular joint. Shortly after Donald Robertson joined the service an agreement was reached between Dr. Woolhouse of McGill and Stuart Gordon that their residents be traded after a year. This cooperative plan emphasized the great advantage of diversified teaching.

An interesting controversy developed with the Department of Dentistry in 1958. This department had developed greatly under the direction of Dr. D. M. Tanner, who had succeeded Dr. Gordon McLean in 1933. During the war Tanner had gone overseas with No. 15 General Hospital and risen to high rank in the Dental Corps, finally becoming the Senior Dental Officer at Canadian Army Headquarters. He continued as Dental Surgeon-in-Chief at the hospital, and as such he served on the Medical Advisory Board until his retirement in 1961.

Before Tanner's time the department had functioned as little more than a pain-relieving extraction service. The importance of oral hygiene and reparative dentistry as a means of maintaining a healthy mouth evolved as a major contribution of the Dental Clinic, and consequently dental students, interns and finally residents learned much more from their experience at the General Hospital. In 1948 Dr. Robert Janes, recognizing the rights of the dental students at the General Hospital, arranged a curriculum in surgery for them, with Dr. Jessie Gray, Harold Wookey, Stuart Gordon, Clifford L. Ash and Douglas Tanner as the clinical instructors, and Dr. Albert Antoni was later appointed to the staff as a dental oral surgeon.

Antoni had been trained in the United States in procedures involving the surgical treatment of extensive injuries of the jaw and the oral cavity and extending to the reconstruction of the prognathous jaw. According to the Dental Act of Ontario, this was within the law, but the plastic surgeons at the General considered it an unjustifiable invasion of their field and they questioned the right of a non-medically qualified practitioner to undertake major surgical procedures at the General Hospital. At the same time, the wiring of a broken jaw, the splinting of the teeth and the making of models of the teeth, and operations for the prognathous jaw were procedures considered to fall within the skills of a dental surgeon, but the responsibility for the admission and discharge of patients referred to the hospital by dental surgeons was ruled to be the responsibility of the Department of Otolaryngology.

Thus the arguments went back and forth until Antoni's retirement in 1962. The new Chief of the Dental Service, Dr. J. A. Pedler, British-trained and a graduate of both medicine and dentistry, proved more interested in the medical aspects of dental problems. The prejudices disappeared, and dental interns and residents came to assist and to be trained in the operating rooms. A little later, the appointment of a plastic surgeon, Dr. Robert Newton, a Gold Medallist in dentistry as well as a medical graduate of McGill, provided a compromise to differences of viewpoint which had caused some acrimonious discussions. Stuart Gordon retired from the active staff of the hospital in 1965, and was succeeded as Head of the Plastic Surgical Division by Dr. Donald Robertson.

The development of an increasing number of surgical specialties naturally had a profound effect on the practice of general surgery at the General Hospital. In the beginning, those whose interests were concerned with a special field still considered themselves to be general surgeons. When the Royal College of Canada came to recognize fellowship in various specialties in 1944, it demanded a good training in general surgery as an introduction to a more confined practice. Gynaecology, urology, and otolaryngology all represented specialties which demanded resourcefulness in the performance of radical procedures, only possible when the surgeon had had residency training to meet critical situations during the course of operations. The concentration of neurological, plastic, cardiovascular and orthopaedic surgical patients at the General Hospital limited the number of beds available for general surgery, and the steady number of well-trained young surgeons going out to hospitals in the suburbs and smaller cities and towns across the country provided an alternative which challenged the prerogative of the staff at the General Hospital in the treatment of those conditions which required general surgery. It was fortunate, therefore, that the surgeons not involved in special divisions showed an outstanding ability to attract patients to the hospital and to train residents to the highest degree of surgical craftsmanship. Although they were individualists, each having a particular field of interest, their competence was broad indeed and there were many patients who, following unsuccessful treatment elsewhere, or with major lesions, were referred because of the intricate procedures which their treatment demanded.

The importance which general surgery maintained is indicated by the statistics of 1961: out of 9,500 surgical patients at the hospital, 3,600 were in general surgery while orthopaedics, urology and neurological surgery accounted for from 1,200 to 1,500 patients each; there were also 750 patients treated by the cardiovascular surgeons.

One surgeon of unsurpassed skill and judgment was Dr. Frank Mills, a product of the Gallie course who had completed his postgraduate training at the Leahy Clinic in Boston. During the war he established his reputation during service with the First Field Surgical Unit working with Canadian soldiers in Sicily and Italy. This led to his promotion to Lieutenant-Colonel in charge of surgery at a general hospital. Reference has already been made to his service in general surgery with Dr. F. I. Lewis on Ward A after the death of Roscoe Graham, from which he was appointed to head the service on Ward B in 1957—and the years have proven the value of this quiet unassuming gentleman to the hospital.

Dr. Bruce Tovee was one of the younger surgeons whose training as a resident under Professor Gallie was consolidated during the war by prolonged surgical experience in the front lines. When he returned, Dr. Roscoe Graham arranged an appointment for him with Dr. Lester Dragstedt of the University of Chicago, where he was involved in gastrointestinal surgery and research. He returned to the Graham service with an intimate knowledge of a relatively new procedure for the treatment of gastric ulcer—vagotomy—and also a keen interest in applied basic research. But facilities were lacking, and it was long days spent on the wards and in the operating room which groomed him to become the logical successor of Roscoe Graham and, progressing with experience, to take his place as a leader in the fields of surgery uncovered by borderline specialties.

Apart from his actual practice, one of Tovee's greatest contributions was as Chairman of the Emergency Committee, which faced the problems of maintaining an efficient emergency department. In 1964 it was reported that during the past three years the number of patients had tripled, and it was constantly necessary to keep a considerable number of patients in the beds in the recovery room while waiting for admission to hospital. During 1963, 36,000 patients had been treated in the department, of whom over 11,500 required X-ray examinations. There were 1,350 operations performed, nearly one-third of them in the "dirty" operating room. New problems were throwing an increasing strain on emergency accommodation. These included a growing number of old-age patients, who came with no particular medical condition, and there had also been 125 alcoholics and 55 attempted suicides who had to be kept under close observation and often required urgent treatment.

Dr. Robert Mustard had been a classmate of Bruce Tovee. The war interrupted his postgraduate training, as he spent five years in England and on the Western Front, returning as a lieutenant-colonel with the M.B.E. The completion of his postgraduate training took the form of a travelling fellowship to the United Kingdom and Sweden. During the early years of his appointment to the staff of the General, he was associated with Harold Wookey, and as a result was recognized on Wookey's retirement as the chief proponent of head and neck surgery. Although his skill was recognized in the full field of general surgery, it was in the treatment of oral, laryngeal and oesophageal cancer and extensive dissections, resections and reconstructions in the head and neck that he gained an outstanding reputation at the General Hospital. Mustard's service was of great value to many committees, especially dealing with the constantly thorny problem of maintaining good hospital records, and he undertook, towards the end of Kergin's professorship, the direction of the training program of the department.

Norman Delarue came to his position of leadership in a more roundabout way. During the war he had developed great skill in neurosurgery, but on completing his residency training at the General Hospital after the war went to St. Louis to work under Dr. Evarts Graham, the leading advocate of the surgical treatment of cancer of the lung. Here he began to cultivate his great interest in research as applied to malignant disease. Robert Janes appointed him as Consulting Surgeon to the Department of Surgery in 1948, and he undertook the first long series of adrenalectomies for breast cancer to be done in Toronto. He also became actively involved in thoracic surgery as applied to bronchogenic cancer, and his studies of the importance of sputum cytology in the early diagnosis and the radiological and exploratory assessment of the extent of lung and glandular involvement brought him international recognition. His ceaseless crusade to convince the public and the profession of the dangerous association between cigarette smoking and cancer of the lung convinced all who listened to him or who read what he had written. One of the most important surveys which he undertook was described in his report, in 1965, of the result of the treatment at the General Hospital of 1,200 patients with lung cancer.

The younger surgeons who came to reinforce the general surgical service in the postwar period enjoyed a new atmosphere in which liberal support was available both for research fellowships and for training abroad. J. A. Palmer, who had originally been trained by Dr. Stuart Gordon in plastic surgery, was appointed to the Ward B service in 1957 to work with Mustard in treating the growing volume of cases requiring head and neck surgery. Both Mustard and he were appointed Consulting Surgeons to the Princess Margaret Hospital, which was the source of a large number of surgical problems. But it was Palmer's work in hyperparathyroidism, in association with Dr. E. R. Yendt, which opened a new field in which he became a surgical authority.

F. G. Pearson was one of Kergin's residents, and as a result became particularly interested in thoracic surgery. He went as a McLaughlin Travelling Fellow to various centres in the United Kingdom and Sweden, and spent six months with Belsey in Bristol to familiarize himself with the latter's treatment of oesophageal lesions. Of the young surgeons, Pearson's interest in research was the most intense, resulting in the successful control of post-operative tracheal defects with the use of a Marlex mesh. When Professor Kergin was able to justify establishing a new sub-specialty of thoracic surgery apart from cardiology, Pearson was appointed head of the service in 1967. As a result, mediastinal and oesophageal surgery became drawn into its orbit—a significant encroachment on the work carried out by some of the general surgeons up to this time.

N. T. McPhedran, another of Kergin's residents, returned from a McLaughlin Fellowship to become a full-time member of the surgical staff. Reference has been made to his involvement in the study of pancreatic disease. His work with the medical staff investigators in the clinical investigation unit was conducive to original observations, and his close association with the head of the department was a sound preparation for his appointment as Professor of Surgery to the new Medical School in Calgary, Alberta.

Gastrointestinal surgery remained, as ever, within the practice of the general surgeons. However, there was relatively little liaison with the medical gastroenterologists, and patients were largely direct referrals, the problems technical and treatment often urgent. The radiologists, with ever-increasing efficiency, provided the data to govern the surgeon's activities.

During the time of Duncan Graham, Ernest Cleaver, F. W. Rolph, E. J. Maltby and Robert Dickson constituted a service in the Department of Medicine on Ward H where, on a basis of clinical excellence, they established themselves as authorities in the diagnosis and treatment of gastrointestinal conditions. After Cleaver's death, Maltby and Dickson were joined by one of Graham's senior interns whose work in the problems of deficiency disease was of interest to them. R. M. Taylor left in 1950 to take over his duties with Atomic Energy of Canada, which led to a long and distinguished career with the National Cancer Institute. Almost at the same time, Dickson went to the Wellesley Division and Maltby, despite his unquestionable talents, was absorbed into the all-inclusive specialty of internal medicine. His diagnostic reputation was based on the virtues of the old school, when the intern staff carried out all routine laboratory tests and readily available diagnostic radiology provided evidence beyond that of the palpating hand or a sigmoidoscope.

A series of publications from the General Hospital early in the Farquharson era showed that his staff, as represented by W. R. Campbell, J. A. Dauphinee, R. C. Dickson, E. J. Maltby, Trevor Owen, J. C. Sinclair and K. J. R. Wightman, were at the forefront in studies of jaundice, serum proteins and hepatic disease, acute infections of the liver, diseases of the biliary tract, chronic hepatitis and cirrhosis, and diseases of the pancreas. During the next twelve years improvements in laboratory facilities, both at the hospital and at the Banting Institute, brought about a profound change in the study of gastrointestinal disease. The experience of Dr. J. M. Finlay, as a Fellow in Therapeutics under K. J. R. Wightman, in organizing the first metabolic unit on Ward G, traced the slow step-by-step progress which made possible the biochemical investigation of metabolic disturbances. In 1954, he undertook his first studies of malabsorption, then spent a year at Hammersmith Hospital, London, England, studying calcium metabolism. This gave him a common interest with Dr. E. R. Yendt, who returned from Harvard at this time to be recognized as an international authority in this field of investigation. Finlay's association with gastroenterology had begun during the time of E. J. Maltby and Charles B. Brown, when the first bi-monthly rounds with the general surgeons were organized. Unfortunately, as has been already intimated, very little active cooperation between the physicians and surgeons was achieved. Finlay's own contribution was based on his increasing knowledge of biochemical research, but he sought training and acquired skill in oesophagoscopy and gastroscopy. As a result, he produced the first cine-films of gastroscopy ever done in Canada. When Maltby retired from active service in 1960, Finlay continued to work with Charles Brown. Together they provided a service and knowledge in this particular field, including diseases of the liver, which kept abreast of the investigational demands which had come to apply to all the clinical departments of the hospital.

Under Norman Urquhart's leadership, an efficient and whole-hearted effort from the Board of Trustees was taken for granted. The broadening responsibilities of Dr. John Sharpe resulted in his new designation as Executive Director in 1963, and in preparation for the future Dr. J. D. Wallace became Assistant Director in 1965. At the same time, this administrative staff utilized increasingly efficient organization in facing many questions that had simply dwarfed the problems of the past. W. L. Louth, who succeeded L. V. Campbell as Comptroller in July 1962, became responsible for a budget which in 1965 was in excess of $18,000,000. Professor Kergin and Professor K. J. R. Wightman, during their services as Chairmen of the Medical Advisory Board, made frequent reports to the trustees to keep them aware of the work and opinions of numerous committees in many facets of hospital activity.

Plans developed for the modernization of the medical wards on College Street. With the disappearance of the old long wards and the provision of teaching areas, the bed capacity would decrease by twenty beds on each floor. But it was hoped that greater efficiency, resulting in a shorter average patient's stay and redistribution of departmental accommodation, would to some extent compensate for this. The integration of the hospital into an affiliated group of teaching hospitals was constantly under study, along with the closer association with the Health Science Centre and the growing responsibility of the teaching units of attending staff, resident staff, interns and clinical clerks for the care of all patients admitted to the hospital.

Desirable and inevitable as this might become, integration was only half approved of; to many it would discount the ideals of the medical or the surgical practitioner who had carried in his heart as well as in his mind the problems of those who had come under his personal care in this old hospital. Integration might have to be the answer to the health care of the future, but it would leave with those students and residents of the past a memory of that quality, intangible and undefined, which they had accepted as the character and soul of the good physician—whose contribution could not be entirely submerged in the efficient routine of a clock-ruled institution.

Looking back over the long years from 1965, one might say that this old hospital had never been better served by those in authority. It had gained its pre-eminence in Canadian medicine by the contributions of many who gave unselfishly—but the achievement was corporate as well as individual: as one looked from University Avenue at the great block of buildings it was possible to make a half-turn and see, across Queen's Park, the buildings of the Ontario parliament and of the University of Toronto. Through their close relation with the hospital and understanding of its needs, these institutions too had made their contributions to the health and welfare of the people of Ontario. The city, as well, had both contributed and benefited: the hospital's very name signifies the integral part it has played in the municipality, and the representatives who served as trustees on behalf of its citizens included, from the very beginning, many who have been outstanding in the history of the city of Toronto. Hopefully the partnership will grow in the challenging years to come.

APPENDIX I

In 1888 the staff list for the first time separated physicians and surgeons and some other specialists, including the first designated dentist for the hospital.

CONSULTING PHYSICIANS

Dr. W. T. Aikens
Dr. Norman Bethune
Dr. J. J. Cassidy
Dr. W. B. Geikie
Dr. J. H. Richardson
Dr. J. D. Thorburn
Dr. H. H. Wright

ATTENDING PHYSICIANS

Dr. H. C. Burritt
Dr. J. L. Davidson
Dr. James E. Graham
Dr. A. A. MacDonald
Dr. Alexander McPhedran
Dr. C. Sheard

OCULISTS AND AURISTS

Dr. G. H. Burnham
Dr. R. A. Reeve
Dr. G. Sterling Ryerson

SPECIALIST IN DISEASES OF THE THROAT AND NOSE

Dr. G. McDonagh

PATHOLOGISTS

Dr. W. H. B. Aikens
Dr. G. A. Bingham

ATTENDING SURGEONS

Mr. I. H. Cameron
Dr. F. L. Grasett
Dr. L. MacFarlane
Dr. R. B. Nevitt
Dr. P. W. Strange
Dr. L. Teskey

BURNSIDE LYING-IN DEPARTMENT

Dr. J. H. Burns
Dr. U. Ogden
Dr. J. P. Russell
Dr. J. A. Temple
Dr. Adam H. Wright

EXTERNE STAFF

Dr. Allan M. Baines
Dr. Theodore S. Covington
Dr. George A. Peters
Dr. James F. W. Ross
Dr. Bertram Spencer

DENTIST

Dr. G. S. Caesar

APPENDIX II

The staff list for 1908 was the last to be authorized by the Board of Trustees of the Toronto General Hospital before the establishment of the Joint Hospital Relations Committee linking the hospital and the University of Toronto.

SURGERY

Professor I. H. Cameron (ex officio)

Dr. George A. Bingham

C. B. Shuttleworth—Senior Assistant

T. B. Richardson—Clinical Assistant

A. B. Wright—Clinical Assistant

Dr. Alexander Primrose

F. N. G. Starr—Senior Assistant

E. Stanley Ryerson—Clinical Assistant

Samuel Westman—Clinical Assistant

Dr. H. A. Bruce

W. J. O. Malloch—Senior Assistant

A. A. Beattie—Clinical Assistant

W. W. Jones—Clinical Assistant

John McCollum—Clinical Assistant

MEDICINE

Dr. Alexander McPhedran

Andrew R. Gordon—Senior Assistant

William Goldie—Clinical Assistant

V. E. Henderson—Clinical Assistant

H. C. Parsons—in charge of tuberculosis clinic under Dr. McPhedran's service

Dr. W. P. Caven

J. T. Fotheringham—Senior Assistant

W. B. Thistle—Second Senior Assistant

E. C. Burson—Clinical Assistant

Joseph Graham—Clinical Assistant

Dr. Graham Chambers

R. D. Rudolf—Senior Assistant

G. W. Howland—Clinical Assistant

G. W. Ross—Clinical Assistant

D. K. Smith—Clinical Assistant (dermatology)

GYNAECOLOGY

J. F. W. Ross

F. W. Marlow—Senior Assistant

A. C. Hendrick—Clinical Assistant

W. B. Hendry—Clinical Assistant

Ida E. Lind—Clinical Assistant

Helen McMurchy—Clinical Assistant

OBSTETRICS

K. C. McIlwraith

Frederick Fenton—Senior Assistant

J. A. Kinnear—Clinical Assistant

OPHTHALMOLOGY

Dr. R. A. Reeve

J. M. MacCallum—Assistant

Dr. Maclennan—Assistant

C. Trow—Assistant

Colin Campbell—Clinical Assistant

W. H. Lowry—Clinical Assistant

EAR, NOSE AND THROAT

Dr. George McDonagh

Geoffrey Boyd—Senior Assistant

Perry Goldsmith—Senior Assistant

Dr. D. J. G. Wishart—Senior Assistant
Gilbert Royce—Clinical Assistant
E. M. Stewart—Clinical Assistant

ANAESTHESIA

Dr. Samuel Johnston
Dr. Duncan Anderson—Assistant

ELECTRICAL

C. R. Dickson
Dr. George Balmer—Assistant

Life members of the active staff without service under the provisions of the Burnside Trust Agreement:

F. L. Grasett
Dr. A. G. Temple

CONSULTING STAFF

Medicine

W. H. B. Aikens
A. M. Baines
John Caven
J. L. Davidson
F. F. McMahon

Surgery

R. B. Nevitt
N. A. Powell
Luke Teskey

Obstetrics

Adam H. Wright

Eye and Ear

G. H. Burnham
G. Sterling Ryerson

APPENDIX III

With the appointment in 1921 of C. L. Starr as Surgeon-in-Chief to the Toronto General Hospital and Professor of Surgery at the University of Toronto on a full-time basis, all appointments were his personal responsibility.

FIRST DIVISION—WARD A

G. A. Bingham—Senior Surgeon

C. B. Shuttleworth—Assistant Surgeon

A. B. Wright—Assistant Surgeon

C. B. Parker—Junior Assistant Surgeon

SECOND DIVISION—WARD B

F. N. G. Starr—Senior Surgeon

R. R. Graham—Assistant Surgeon

E. Stanley Ryerson—Assistant Surgeon

H. W. Wookey—Junior Assistant Surgeon

THIRD DIVISION—WARD C

Alexander Primrose—Senior Surgeon

R. A. Gaby—Assistant Surgeon

N. S. Shenstone—Assistant Surgeon

Oliver Mabee—Junior Assistant Surgeon

OUT-PATIENT DEPARTMENT AND EMERGENCY

N. A. Powell—Consulting Physician

George Wilson—Senior Surgeon

R. H. Thomas—Assistant Surgeon

GENITO-URINARY AND VENEREAL SERVICE

W. W. Jones—Surgeon

R. J. A. McComb—Assistant Surgeon

Robin Pearse—Assistant Surgeon

C. H. Hair—Junior Assistant

J. C. McClelland—Junior Assistant

CLINICIANS UNATTACHED

F. A. Cleland

W. A. Costain

G. C. McIntyre

E. E. Shouldice

CONSULTANT IN SURGERY

H. A. Bruce

RESIDENT SURGEON

R. M. Janes

APPENDIX IV

The first postwar staff list (1945) shows the large number of members who were or had been on active service.

DEPARTMENT OF MEDICINE

Physician-in-Chief

Professor Duncan A. L. Graham†

Attending Physicians

Dr. Robert G. Armour—in charge of Neurology Clinic, Out-patient Department

Dr. John Hepburn, Supervisor, Ward 1—in charge of Cardiovascular Clinic, Out-patient Department

Assistant Attending Physicians

Dr. W. Fletcher McPhedran—Medical Clinic, Out-patient Department

Dr. Emerson J. Trow—Dermatology Clinic, Out-patient Department

Dr. Gordon Bates
Dr. Walter R. Campbell
Dr. Ernest E. Cleaver
Dr. R. A. Cleghorn*
Dr. James A. Dauphinee*
Dr. Hammett A. Dixon
Dr. J. Gilbert Falconer
Dr. R. F. Farquharson
Dr. A. Almon Fletcher
Dr. J. Wallace Graham*
Dr. H. Hyland†
Dr. Robert B. Kerr*
Dr. Gladstone W. Lougheed
Dr. R. Ian Macdonald*
Dr. E. J. Maltby
Dr. Trevor Owen
Dr. J. Clifford Richardson*
Dr. H. E. Rykert†
Dr. Wilfred P. Warner*
Dr. Norman Wrong*

Junior Assistant Attending Physicians

Dr. Carl R. Burton
Dr. T. Albert Crowther
Dr. Edward S. Jeffrey
Dr. W. E. Ogden
Dr. Herbert E. Pugsley
Dr. V. F. Stock

Resident Physician

Dr. William F. Greenwood*

Voluntary Assistants in the Medical Out-patient Department

Dr. Allan Burnett
Dr. Harold D. Delamere
Dr. Kenneth E. Ferrie
Dr. Ralph Gerred
Dr. Willson A. McTavish

Tuberculosis Clinic

Dr. E. L. Sexsmith

Assistants in the Venereal (Syphilis) Out-patient Clinic

Dr. Noble Black
Dr. Henry W. Lore
Dr. G. A. McLarty

DEPARTMENT OF THERAPEUTICS AT THE UNIVERSITY OF TORONTO

Dr. C. E. Cooper Cole

DEPARTMENT OF ANAESTHESIA

Dr. H. J. Shields

*On active service
†Returned from active service

Assistant Attending Anaesthetists

Dr. G. R. Balfour
Dr. W. E. Brown
Dr. Stanley M. Campbell†
Dr. John Chassels
Dr. N. S. Clark
Dr. S. J. Evelyn
Dr. A. R. Wilkins

DEPARTMENT OF PHYSICAL THERAPY

Dr. W. J. Gardiner

DEPARTMENT OF SURGERY

Surgeon-in-Chief

Professor W. E. Gallie

Senior Surgeons

Dr. R. R. Graham
Dr. R. I. Harris†
Dr. K. G. McKenzie
Dr. Robin Pearse
Dr. N. S. Shenstone
Dr. H. W. Wookey

Associate Surgeons

Dr. R. M. Janes
Dr. R. J. A. McComb
Dr. C. B. Parker
Dr. R. H. Thomas

Assistant Surgeons

Dr. J. H. Couch
Dr. J. A. MacFarlane*
Dr. J. C. McClelland
Dr. D. W. G. Murray

Junior Surgeons

Dr. Carl Aberhart†
Dr. E. H. Botterell*
Dr. S. D. Gordon*
Dr. F. G. Kergin*
Dr. F. I. Lewis
Dr. J. R. F. Mills*
Dr. D. R. Mitchell*
Dr. W. K. Welsh*

Temporary Junior Surgeons

Dr. M. I. Davis
Dr. Jessie C. Gray
Dr. W. O. Stoddart

Voluntary Assistants in Out-patient Department

Dr. G. W. Carrow
Dr. R. G. McKenzie
Dr. A. N. McKillop
Dr. H. F. Robertson*
Dr. J. V. Tilley*
Dr. J. L. Uren

Resident Surgeon

Dr. D. R. Bohnen

DEPARTMENT OF OBSTETRICS AND GYNAECOLOGY

Chief of Service

Professor W. A. Scott

Senior Obstetricians and Gynaecologists

Dr. W. G. Cosbie
Dr. H. B. Van Wyck

Associate Obstetricians and Gynaecologists

Dr. W. A. Dafoe
Dr. D. M. Low

Senior Assistants

Dr. D. N. Henderson
Dr. H. W. Johnston

Junior Assistants

Dr. J. C. Goodwin
Dr. John C. Mann
Dr. J. R. McArthur*
Dr. M. C. Watson†
Dr. G. L. Watt

Resident

Dr. William D. Flatt

DEPARTMENT OF OPHTHALMOLOGY

Chief of Service

Dr. W. W. Wright

Associate Surgeons

Dr. Clarence E. Hill
Dr. W. R. F. Luke
Dr. A. E. MacDonald

Dr. H. M. Macrae

Assistant Surgeons

Dr. T. H. Hodgson
Dr. J. F. A. Johnson

DEPARTMENT OF RADIOLOGY

Chief of Service

Professor G. E. Richards

Associate

Dr. A. C. Singleton†

Senior Assistants

Dr. Malcolm R. Hall
Dr. Vera Peters

Junior Assistants

Dr. C. L. Ash
Dr. W. A. Hargon

Research Assistant

Dr. H. M. Worth

DEPARTMENT OF OTOLARYNGOLOGY

Chief of Service

Professor Angus Campbell

Associate Surgeon

Dr. C. A. Rae*

Assistant Surgeons

Dr. H. H. Burnham
Dr. H. W. D. McCart†
Dr. G. W. McGregor

Junior Surgeons

Dr. G. A. Fee
Dr. P. E. Ireland*
Dr. Angus M. McLeod*
Dr. G. C. Snell

APPENDIX V

The Board of Trustees appointed in 1947 under N. C. Urquhart included many new members.

BY THE LIEUTENANT-GOVERNOR

Mr. N. C. Urquhart (Chairman)
Mr. J. L. Carson
Mr. J. D. Eaton
Mr. C. S. Hamilton
Mr. B. L. Mitchell
Mr. F. K. Morrow
Mr. James Y. Murdoch
Mr. G. Harrison Smith

BY THE UNIVERSITY OF TORONTO

Mr. Henry Borden
Mr. C. G. McCullagh
Mr. Balmer Neilly (Vice-Chairman)
Lt. Col. W. E. Phillips
Dr. Sidney Smith

BY THE SUBSCRIBERS

Mr. Edgar G. Burton
Mr. W. C. Laidlaw
Mr. H. M. Turner
Mr. E. P. Taylor
Mr. S. M. Wood

BY THE CITY OF TORONTO

Ald. W. H. Butt
Ald. H. F. Fishleigh
Ald. A. A. Lamport
Ald. E. L. Weaver
Ald. M. W. Wilson

EX-OFFICIO

Dr. W. E. Gallie

APPENDIX VI

The staff appointments in 1951 under the new heads of departments ushered in a new era.

DEPARTMENT OF MEDICINE

Chief of Staff

Dr. R. F. Farquharson

Consulting Physicians

Dr. Robert G. Armour
Dr. Gordon Bates
Dr. H. K. Detweiler
Dr. A. Almon Fletcher
Dr. Duncan A. L. Graham
Dr. John Hepburn
Dr. E. S. Jeffrey
Dr. John A. Oille
Dr. F. W. Rolph
Dr. V. F. Stock
Dr. Emerson J. Trow
Dr. G. S. Young

Senior Physicians

Dr. Walter R. Campbell
Dr. Hammett A. Dixon (in charge of Dermatological Clinic, OPD)*
Dr. H. H. Hyland
Dr. E. J. Maltby
Dr. Trevor Owen (in charge of the General Medical Clinic, OPD)
Dr. K. J. R. Wightman

Physicians

Dr. Carl R. Burton
T. Albert Crowther (in charge of Tuberculosis Clinic, OPD)
James A. Dauphinee
Robert C. Dickson (physician in charge of the Medical Service, Wellesley Division)
J. Wallace Graham
Cameron C. Gray
William F. Greenwood
R. Ian Macdonald (General Medical Clinic)
W. A. Oille
Herbert E. Pugsley
J. Clifford Richardson
H. E. Rykert
Arthur H. Squires
A. B. Stokes
J. A. Walters
N. M. Wrong

Assistant Physicians

H. J. M. Barnett
B. Berris
C. B. Brown (Wellesley Division)
W. T. W. Clarke
W. Johnston MacAllister
A. D. McKelvey
D. P. Murnahan (Wellesley Division)
M. A. Ogryzlo
W. A. Rowan (Wellesley Division)
John W. Scott
J. C. Sinclair
G. W. Smith
R. C. Smith
W. B. Spaulding
E. James Trow
O. H. Warwick

Clinical Assistants

Jose Barzelatto
A. Bogoch
R. M. Bremner
K. W. G. Brown
R. M. Clark

*Out-patient Department

J. M. Finlay
Oscar Kofman
R. L. MacMillan
S. Rogers
Irving Rother

Resident Physician

Ramsay W. Gunton

Voluntary Assistants

C. J. Bardawill
H. C. Hare
H. Kalant
Abraham Rapoport

Voluntary Assistants—OPD

W. E. Armour
D. F. Breithaupt
R. F. Gerred
A. F. Graham
Marinus G. Jansen
R. A. MacKay
K. D. McEachern
A. E. Parks
R. H. Penny
E. M. Robinson
Philip A. Ryan
I. H. Schleser
M. P. Schulman
E. L. Sexsmith (Tuberculosis Clinic)
R. C. Sky

Cardiovascular Clinic

M. Stein
N. J. D. Wiggin
C. Wright Young

Assistants—Venereal Clinic—OPD

D. H. Borsook
Henry W. Lore
G. A. McLarty
J. L. Uren

DEPARTMENT OF THERAPEUTICS, UNIVERSITY OF TORONTO

K. J. R. Wightman

Research Fellow in Therapeutics

J. M. Finlay

SERVICE IN ANAESTHESIA

Anaesthetist-in-Chief

H. J. Shields (Associate in Therapeutics in charge of Anaesthesia)

Senior Anaesthetists

G. R. Balfour
G. D. M. Boddington
W. E. Brown
Stanley M. Campbell
John Chassels
N. S. Clark
S. J. Evelyn
R. A. Gordon
A. R. Wilkins

Assistant Anaesthetists

I. M. MacKay
Peter Marchant (Wellesley Division)
George F. Smith (Wellesley Division)

DEPARTMENT OF PHYSICAL THERAPY

Chief of Physical Therapy

W. J. Gardiner

Assistants

A. T. Jousse
Andres Zinovieff

DEPARTMENT OF SURGERY

Surgeon-in-Chief

R. M. Janes

Consultants

W. E. Gallie
R. I. Harris
W. W. Jones
J. C. McClelland
R. J. A. McComb
Robin Pearse
N. S. Shenstone
R. H. Thomas
H. W. Wookey

Senior Surgeons

S. D. Gordon
F. G. Kergin
F. I. Lewis

J. L. McDonald (in charge of Surgical Service, Wellesley Division)
Kenneth G. McKenzie
D. R. Mitchell
D. W. G. Murray

Surgeons

Carl Aberhart
W. G. Bigelow
E. H. Botterell
J. H. Couch
F. P. Dewar
J. R. F. Mills

Assistant Surgeons

N. C. Delarue
I. B. Macdonald
David L. MacIntosh
R. A. Mustard
C. J. Robson
E. B. Tovee

Clinical Assistants

G. W. D. Armstrong (Orthopaedic Service)
W. K. Kerr (Urology)
D. C. Robertson (Ward B)
C. W. Taylor (Neurosurgery)
Donald R. Wilson (Ward C)

Voluntary Assistants in OPD

D. R. Bohnen
A. N. McKillop
H. F. Robertson
A. G. Shaw
W. O. Stoddart

Resident

H. R. Gallie

DEPARTMENT OF OBSTETRICS AND GYNAECOLOGY

Obstetrician and Gynaecologist-in-Chief

D. E. Cannell

Consultants

W. A. Scott
H. B. Van Wyck

Senior Obstetricians and Gynaecologists

W. G. Cosbie
W. A. Dafoe (in charge of Obstetrics and Gynaecology, Wellesley Division)
D. N. Henderson
D. M. Low

Obstetricians and Gynaecologists

J. C. Goodwin
H. W. Johnston
John C. Mann
J. R. McArthur
M. C. Watson
G. L. Watt

Assistant Obstetricians and Gynaecologists

Geraldine Maloney
J. W. Rogers
Crawford Shier
D. J. Van Wyck

Voluntary Assistants

William D. Flatt
L. J. Harris
R. G. Mackenzie
John Oswald
Magnus Spence
Herbert Tait

Residents

W. G. McGarrity (Jan. 1–June 30)
F. Bryans (July 1–Dec. 31)

DEPARTMENT OF OPHTHALMOLOGY

Ophthalmologist-in-Chief

A. J. Elliott

Consultants

Clarence E. Hill
W. W. Wright

Senior Ophthalmologists

W. R. F. Luke
A. E. MacDonald
H. M. Macrae

Ophthalmologists
T. H. Hodgson
J. F. A. Johnston

Assistant Ophthalmologist
J. S. Crawford

DEPARTMENT OF OTOLARYNGOLOGY

Otolaryngologist-in-Chief
P. E. Ireland

Consultants
Angus Campbell
C. A. Rae

Senior Otolaryngologists
H. H. Burnham
H. W. D. McCart

Otolaryngologists
Angus M. McLeod
G. C. Snell

Assistant Otolaryngologist
D. P. Bryce

Clinical Assistant
Hugh Barber

Voluntary Assistant (OPD)
W. E. Goodman

DEPARTMENT OF RADIOLOGY

Acting Radiologist-in-Chief
A. C. Singleton

Senior Radiologists
C. L. Ash
Malcolm R. Hall

Radiologist
Vera Peters

Assistant Radiologists
R. B. Holmes
K. F. MacEwan
O. B. Miller
D. G. Wollin

APPENDIX VII

The continuing growth of the hospital staff is evident from the 1961 appointments.

DEPARTMENT OF MEDICINE

Physician-in-Chief

Dr. K. J. R. Wightman

Consultants

Gordon Bates
Walter R. Campbell
H. K. Detweiler
R. F. Farquharson
A. Almon Fletcher
Duncan A. L. Graham
E. J. Maltby
John A. Oille
Trevor Owen

Senior Physicians

H. H. Hyland
J. C. Laidlaw
R. Ian Macdonald
W. B. Spaulding
J. A. Walters
N. M. Wrong

Physicians

H. J. M. Barnett
B. Berris
K. W. G. Brown
Carl R. Burton
W. T. W. Clarke
T. Albert Crowther
J. A. Dauphinee
J. Wallace Graham
Cameron C. Gray
William F. Greenwood
Ramsay W. Gunton
M. W. Johnston
R. L. MacMillan
A. D. McKelvey
M. A. Ogryzlo
W. A. Oille
J. Clifford Richardson
John W. Scott
J. C. Sinclair
R. C. Smith
A. B. Stokes
E. R. Yendt
D. M. Young

Assistant Physicians

J. H. Crookston
C. Ezrin
J. M. Finlay
E. M. Foreman
J. P. Grant
J. G. Humphrey
E. A. McCullough
P. H. Melville
J. D. Morrow
S. Rogers
B. M. Sanders
H. A. Smythe
D. A. Stinson
G. W. Stock
E. James Trow
E. D. Wigle
C. R. Woolf

Clinical Assistants

H. Aldridge
Robert Anderson
B. Hazlett
Donald Killinger
Sora Lee
D. C. Mortimer
W. C. Nicholas
E. J. Noble
H. H. Rotman
J. L. Ruse
R. Volpe
M. G. Williams

Chief Resident Physician

R. H. Wensel

Resident Physician

D. Cowan

Voluntary Assistants

G. A. Gow
G. W. Smith
Russell Taylor

Voluntary Assistants—OPD

E. A. Allen
S. D. Bain
T. R. H. Box
J. Carson
G. S. Cohen
John E. C. Cole
F. B. Fallis
Erik Foldes
J. L. A. Fowler
J. Garriock
R. F. Gerred
A. F. Graham
Wulf Grobin
Stefan Grzybowski
M. G. Jansen
M. Lenczner
G. J. Mainprize
K. D. McEachern
Robert Moore
A. E. Parks

Voluntary Assistants—Special Clinics

Arthritis Clinic

V. Halmos
J. N. Swanson

Cardiovascular Clinic

J. B. Armstrong
D. B. Campbell
I. H. Shleser
J. Zawadski

Chest Clinic

E. L. Sexsmith

Dermatology Clinic

J. G. Kenny
T. B. Scott

Diabetic Clinic

E. M. Robinson

Endocrine Clinic

M. Cohen
E. G. Cross
N. Green
Joan Vale

Haematology Clinic

Henry Goldenberg
G. Hart
I. Rother
J. S. Senn
H. J. Watt
J. G. Watt

Neurology Clinic

G. W. Fitzgerald
O. Kaufman
L. Mitis
S. Starkman

Venereal Clinic

Dorothy H. Borsook
F. B. Fallis
Oscar Kofman
H. W. Lore

DEPARTMENT OF REHABILITATION AND PHYSICAL MEDICINE

Director

Dr. W. J. Gardiner

Assistants

W. O. Geisler
C. M. Godfrey
A. T. Jousse

DEPARTMENT OF ANAESTHESIA

Anaesthetist-in-Chief

Dr. Stanley M. Campbell

Consultants

John Chassels
N. S. Clark

S. J. Evelyn
H. J. Shields
A. R. Wilkins

Senior Anaesthetists

G. R. Balfour
G. D. M. Boddington
H. B. Fairley
Shirley Fleming
R. A. Gordon
C. W. P. Lunderville
I. M. MacKay
Peter Marchant

Anaesthetists

T. R. Handley
Brian Marshall
Raymond Mathews

Voluntary Assistants

Ann Marie Fehrman
J. E. York

Residents

Marvin Kay
Claude Pouliot

Clinical Assistant

J. H. Kerr

DEPARTMENT OF SURGERY

Surgeon-in-Chief

Dr. F. G. Kergin

Consultants

R. I. Harris
R. M. Janes
F. I. Lewis
J. A. MacFarlane
J. C. McClelland
K. G. McKenzie
D. W. G. Murray
N. S. Shenstone
R. H. Thomas
H. W. Wookey

Senior Surgeons

W. G. Bigelow
E. H. Botterell
F. P. Dewar
S. D. Gordon
J. R. F. Mills
D. R. Mitchell
E. B. Tovee

Surgeons

Carl Aberhart
N. C. Delarue
David L. MacIntosh
R. A. Mustard

Assistant Surgeons

W. R. Harris
R. O. Heimbecker
W. K. Kerr
J. A. Key
W. M. Lougheed
Ian Macnab
N. T. McPhedran
T. P. Morley
J. A. Palmer
F. G. Pearson
D. C. Robertson
C. J. Robson
W. J. Spence

Voluntary Assistants

D. R. Bohnen
L. S. Davies
Phillip Klotz
A. N. McKillop
H. F. Robertson
A. G. Shaw
G. E. P. Wilson

Clinical Assistants

R. J. Baird
Aron M. Rappaport
W. Sapirstein

Chief Resident

R. H. Railton

Residents

P. J. F. Kuypers (Cardiovascular)
B. Langer (General Surgery)
J. K. Murray (Neurosurgery)
J. Sales (Urology)

S. Schatz (Neurosurgery)
E. Silverstein (Orthopaedics)
I. Todd (General Surgery)

DEPARTMENT OF OBSTETRICS AND GYNAECOLOGY

Obstetrician and Gynaecologist-in-Chief

Dr. D. E. Cannell

Consultants

W. G. Cosbie
W. A. Dafoe
D. M. Low

Senior Obstetricians and Gynaecologists

D. N. Henderson
H. W. Johnston
John C. Mann
G. L. Watt

Obstetricians and Gynaecologists

J. R. McArthur
C. B. Shier
M. C. Watson

Assistant Obstetricians and Gynaecologists

William Allemang
J. L. M. Bean
J. L. Harkins
J. A. Low
J. W. Rogers
D. J. Van Wyck

Voluntary Assistants

M. L. Bunker
E. A. Crawford
William D. Flatt
J. D. M. Gillies
W. H. Johnston (Paediatrics)

DEPARTMENT OF OPHTHALMOLOGY

Opthalmologist-in-Chief

A. J. Elliott

Consultants

Clarence E. Hill
A. E. MacDonald
W. W. Wright

Senior Ophthalmologists

W. R. F. Luke
H. M. Macrae

Ophthalmologists

J. S. Crawford
J. C. Hill
G. A. Thompson

Assistant Ophthalmologists

Lois Lloyd
J. S. Speakman

Voluntary Assistants

J. C. C. Alexander
Davidson Black
D. H. Green
D. W. Harper
J. W. Hiltz
G. S. Jakerow
D. E. Sillers

DEPARTMENT OF OTOLARYNGOLOGY

Otolaryngologist-in-Chief

Dr. P. E. Ireland

Consultants

Angus Campbell
C. A. Rae

Senior Otolaryngologists

None

Otolaryngologists

D. P. Bryce
Angus M. McLeod
G. C. Snell

Assistant Otolaryngologists

H. O. Barber
W. S. Goodman
Douglas Snell

Clinical Assistants
None

Voluntary Assistants
W. E. Goodman
M. D. Lunan
J. Stuckler

DEPARTMENT OF DIAGNOSTIC RADIOLOGY

Radiologist-in-Chief
A. C. Singleton

Senior Radiologists
Malcolm R. Hall

Radiologists
R. B. Holmes
R. A. Lobb
D. E. Sanders

Assistant Radiologists
R. M. Parrish
G. Wortzman

Voluntary Assistants
John Gibson

DEPARTMENT OF RADIOTHERAPY

Radiotherapist-in-Chief
C. L. Ash

Radiotherapists
Staff of the Ontario Cancer Institute

DEPARTMENT OF PATHOLOGY

John D. Hamilton—Consultant Pathologist and Acting Head, Division of Pathology, Department of Laboratories

Pathologists
W. Anderson
H. J. Barrie
D. W. Thompson

Assistant Pathologists
None

Assistants in Surgical Pathology
None

Assistants in Autopsy Pathology
A. J. Gelbloom
Peter Lampert
Neill Rewcastle

Neuropathologists
Mary I. Thom

DEPARTMENT OF DENTISTRY

Dental Surgeon-in-Chief
Douglas M. Tanner

Senior Dental Oral Surgeon
Albert Antoni

Dental Surgeons
John Ackerman
E. P. Downton

Voluntary Assistants
B. Crystal
A. Green
R. R. Jones
John Ostler

DEPARTMENT OF LABORATORIES

Consulting Microbiologist
Dr. Philip H. Greey

Index